Prenatal Diagnosis and Prognosis

Prenatal Diagnosis and Prognosis

R. J. Lilford PhD, MRCP, MRCOG
Professor and Head, Department of Obstetrics and Gynaecology,
St James's University Hospital, Leeds, UK

Butterworths
London   Boston   Singapore   Sydney   Toronto   Wellington

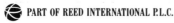
First published 1990

© **Butterworth & Co (Publishers) Ltd, 1990**

British Library Cataloguing in Publication Data

Lilford, Richard J.
  Pre-natal diagnosis.
  1. Antenatal medicine. Diagnosis
  I. Title
  618.22
    ISBN 0–407–01044–0

Library of Congress Cataloging Data applied for

Phototypeset by Scribe Design, Gillingham, Kent
Printed and bound in Great Britain by Courier International Ltd, Tiptree, Essex

Contributors

F. Bryce, MRCOG
Senior Registrar in Obstetrics and Gynaecology, previously Research Fellow at St James's University Hospital, Leeds

H. Cuckle, BA, MSc, DPhil
Senior Lecturer, Department of Environmental and Preventive Medicine, St Bartholomew's Hospital, Charterhouse Square, London

C. Gosden, BSc, PhD, DipRCPath
Professor, MRC Human Genetics Unit, Western General Hospital, Edinburgh; Honorary Professor, Department of Obstetrics and Gynaecology, King's College Hospital, London

H. Irving, MBBS, FRCR
Consultant Radiologist, St James's University Hospital, Leeds

R.J. Lilford, PhD, MRCP, MRCOG
Professor and Head of Department of Obstetrics and Gynaecology, St James's University Hospital, Leeds

R. Mueller, MB, BSc, MRCP
Consultant Clinical Geneticist, Yorkshire Regional Health Authority

C. Rodeck, BSc, FRCOG
Professor in Obstetrics and Gynaecology, Queen Charlotte's Hospital, Royal Postgraduate Medical School, London

M. Super, MD, MSc, FRCP, DCH
Consultant Paediatric Geneticist, Royal Manchester Children's Hospital, Manchester

D. Thomas, FRCS, MRCP
Consultant Paediatric Surgeon, St James's University Hospital, Leeds

J. Thornton, MD, MRCOG
Senior Lecturer in Obstetrics and Gynaecology, St James's University Hospital, Leeds

N. Wald, FFCM, MD
Professor in Department of Environmental and Preventive Medicine, St Bartholomew's Hospital, Charterhouse Square, London

I. Young, MD, FRCP
Senior Lecturer and Consultant in Clinical Genetics, Department of Child Health, University of Leicester, Leicester

Contents

Introduction

R.J. Lilford

Prenatal diagnosis has taken off in the last decade and it is certainly one of the most interesting, controversial and rapidly changing topics in medicine and human affairs generally. The number of articles on this, the cutting edge of genetics, is now enormous and the subject is developing into a speciality in its own right. Books devoted to this subject are starting to appear in libraries, but the vast majority of published material suffers from a fundamental defect – it concentrates on diagnosis not prognosis. This book concentrates on prognosis because it is prognosis, not diagnosis, that is important. Diagnosis in the sense of the absolute immutable truth about the disease afflicting a particular patient, is often an illusion in medicine, and this is particularly true in prenatal diagnosis. When we attach a diagnostic label, we do so mainly to tell us what to do next; when we diagnose appendicitis, what we really mean is that we think the likelihood of appendicitis has crossed the threshold whereby operative treatment has the greatest advantages (greatest expected utility) for the patient. In the case of prenatal diagnosis the most important treatment is termination of pregnancy. Parents do not make this decision on the basis of concrete 'diagnosis', they make the decision on the basis of prognosis.

What is prognosis? – it is the likelihood (or probability) of various outcomes. Parents need to know the probability of a falsely reassuring result on testing for Duchenne dystrophy, the probability of miscarriage with chorionic villus sampling, the probability of neonatal death if the fetus appears to have isolated exomphalos, the probability of mental retardation if the scan has shown apparently isolated ventriculomegaly or the amniocentesis result a 47 XXX karyotype and so on. In each of the above examples the so-called diagnosis is fairly easily made, but in each case the parents will look to the doctor to tell them what it *means*, i.e the prognosis.

This book, therefore, discusses diagnosis, (in-so-far as diagnosis is possible), but gives considerable detail on prognosis so that the clinician has the information that parents need. This detail is required, even when termination is not an option. We, therefore, include information about the paediatric management and surgical complications for many conditions.

Diagnosis has many different levels, differential, clinical, pathological. Until now abnormal ultrasound results have been classified according to the final pathological diagnosis, but this is inadequate because, in clinical practice, we are frequently confronted with a particular ultrasound appearance which is consistent with many different pathologies. Granted, in some cases imaging gives us a high level diagnosis (i.e. a diagnosis which is likely to be pathologically correct, e.g. gastroschisis). Often, however, we get low level diagnosis, e.g. cerebral ventriculomegaly or dilated renal tract. In these cases we do not know the cause of the dilatation. Is it low pressure or high pressure? If the latter, what is the nature of the obstruction? What effect has it had on the brain and kidney respectively?

In this book we have therefore classified disorders detectable by ultrasound according to their prenatal characteristics (Chapters 1, 2 and 3). There are too many articles and books detailing abnormalities which can be picked up on scan while we all know that, in the vast majority of cases, the scan merely picked up a problem whose exact nature, e.g. choledochal cyst, fetus in fetu, etc. was only confirmed after delivery. Thus the first three chapters in this book deal mostly with what is and is not possible in prenatal prognostication and give probabilities linked to the various scan abnormalities as accurately as existing data will allow – often the confidence limits on these probabilities must be very wide because of bias and inadequate follow-up in the literature, so much of which concentrates on the pretty pictures obtained and not the outcome for the child.

Sometimes, in ultrasound diagnosis we are left with almost no idea of what the abnormality was. The posterior cerebral fossa cyst in Figure 1 resolved spontaneously and the neonate is developing well at 2 years of age. We will never know what caused this cyst. The hydrothorax in Figure 2 resolved spontaneously after we had excluded Down's syndrome but without *in-utero* drainage and the neonate was healthy. The mass behind the heart in Figure 3 appeared to be connected to the descending aorta on colour Doppler blood flow mapping and we suspected a sequestered lung lobe or neuroblastoma. In either event, the child was healthy and postnatal X-rays were completely normal, although CT scan was not attempted.

In this book, therefore, we concentrate on the difficulties and uncertainties that confront the prenatal diagnostician in the real world rather than pretending that the issues are resolved and ultrasonic appearances diagnostically specific.

Chapter 4 by Cuckle and Wald deals with one of the most important issues in prenatal diagnosis – biochemical tests for chromosomal abnormalities. The fetus

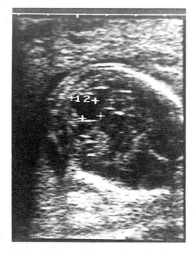
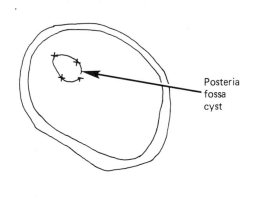

Posteria fossa cyst

Figure 1 A small central cyst in the posterior cerebral fossa which was not associated with any neurological problem in the child

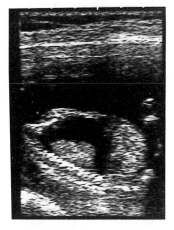
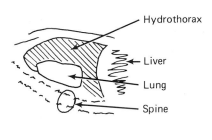

Figure 2 Large hydrothorax (with no hydrops) which resolved spontaneously during pregnancy with good outcome

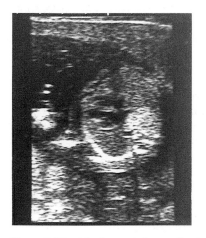
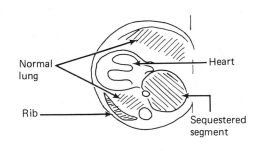

Figure 3 'Mass' in the posterior mediastinum which remains undiagnosed in the healthy baby

with Down's syndrome tends to be biochemically immature for its gestational age and therefore has higher levels of human chorionic gonadotrophin (HCG) and lower levels of oestriol and alpha-fetoprotein. The number of Down's syndrome detectable for a stable number (5%) of amniocenteses increases from 25% to over 65% by triple testing. The chance that a 40-year-old woman will be found by triple testing to have a Down's syndrome risk, under that normally associated with a 35 year old, is 70%. These and many other fascinating details are clearly explained in this chapter. Clinicians will need a good understanding of this information, both in counselling individual patients (the majority of women over 30 years of age at St James's Hospital now opt for triple testing as do many at a younger age) and in deciding on hospital policy.

One of the most vexing problems in medicine concerns counselling for patients where prenatal diagnosis has revealed unexpected abnormalities such as mosaicism, *de-novo* translocation, etc. For example, the majority of mosaics on amniocentesis, even when present in all flasks, are not present in the fetus and are either culture artefacts or, more likely, confined to extra-fetal tissues. The subject of chromosomes is introduced in Chapter 5 and then, in Chapter 6, Christine Gosden looks in detail at the variety of confusing results and pitfalls that beset this subject. Clinicians armed with this knowledge will be better able to walk the tight rope between unnecessary termination and false reassurance and will be able to give the best available information on the likely effects of many of these abnormalities on the child.

Molecular biology has revolutionized the subject of prenatal diagnosis. When I started at St James's Hospital 5 years ago we were still acceding to requests to terminate all males in Duchenne dystrophy carriers – now gene diagnosis is routine for this and many other conditions. In Chapter 7, Maurice Super gently introduces this subject in a delightful chapter, rich in anecdotes from his wide experience. Robert Mueller (Chapter 8) then explains the precise basis of the new genetics in much the clearest chapter on the subject that I have read. The real meat of the subject – precisely how genetic risk is calculated for prenatal diagnosis using linked markers – is then given by Ian Young (Chapter 9). This is essential reading for anyone who wishes to understand and explain, albeit in principle, why there is a finite risk of false reassurance in, for example, the prenatal diagnosis of Huntington's chorea.

Cytogenetics and biochemical diagnosis, however, involve fetal tissue sampling and the risks of these various procedures are discussed in some detail in Chapter 10.

In the last analysis, counselling must be as non-directive as possible, albeit supportive (warm and friendly). Parents must use the information which the doctor has helped them to understand. This information concerns the likelihood (probabilities) of various outcomes. What parents decide will therefore depend on how they value these outcomes. The science of connecting probabilities to values to determine the overall best-bet (the option with the highest expected utility) is called decision theory. It is the key to understanding the logical framework of genetics in general and prenatal diagnosis in particular. This subject also teaches us much about the way that humans use information, the biases or inherent faults in human reasoning and, building on the pioneering work of Pauker and Pauker, Jim Thornton shows us, in Chapter 11, how these 'faulty heuristics' can be addressed in talking to couples. This chapter provides clear logical methods for dealing with complex issues and the methodology described completes the prenatal diagnosis revolution – structural imaging, ultrasound directed invasive procedures, gene probe diagnosis and the means to amalgamate all this complex information with human values – decision theory.

Chapter 1

Antenatal diagnosis of craniospinal defects

F.C. Bryce, R.J. Lilford and C. Rodeck

Introduction

The introduction of routine ultrasound examination of the fetus during the second trimester of pregnancy has led to the detection of a wide range of craniospinal defects (Table 1.1). With the development of high resolution real-time ultrasonography an accurate anatomical diagnosis of many craniospinal abnormalities can be made, but to give a precise prognosis is often more difficult. The presence of some fetal anomalies is known to be associated with chromosomal defects which can be excluded by fetal karyotyping of liquor amni, chorion or fetal blood. Abnormalities such as anencephaly, hydranencephaly or holoprosencephaly are either lethal or associated with such severe mental handicap and high infant mortality that the prognosis may be considered uniformly hopeless.

Improvements in imaging technology have led to the identification of features whose significance is still unclear. While isolated reports of specific anomalies have appeared, very few surveys include patients where the abnormality has been followed up after birth. It is, therefore, very difficult to counsel prospective parents about the probabilities of the various outcomes for their child.

This chapter is based on a review of cases of craniospinal defects reported in the literature and from our own experiences, where the diagnosis has been made early

Table 1.1 Craniospinal defects detectable by ultrasonography

Anencephaly
Spina bifida (open)
Spina bifida (closed)
Encephalocoele
Incencephaly
Isolated hydrocephaly
Holoprosencephaly
Hydranencephaly
Microcephaly
Dandy Walker malformation
Porencephalic cyst
Choroid plexus cysts
Absent corpus callosum
Absent cerebellum
Sacral agenesis

Table 1.2 Prognosis of craniospinal defects

Prognosis	Craniopsinal defect
1. Prognosis uniformly poor	Anencephaly Porencephaly Hydranencephaly Incencephaly Alobar holoprosencephaly Microcephaly
2. Prognosis usually good	Choroid plexus cysts
3. Prognosis usually poor and reasonably well defined	Meningomyelocoele Encephalocoele
4. Prognosis variable/poor	Apparently isolated hydroencephaly Agenesis of corpus callosum Posterior fossa cysts

in the antenatal period. If a craniospinal defect is detected in the developing fetus it must be confirmed by an expert in imaging. Extracranial defects must also be sought (as their presence will usually affect the prognosis adversely). The prognosis may be categorized as uniformly hopeless, usually poor, variable and usually good. The various defects associated with these categories are illustrated in Table 1.2. Counselling of parents concerning possible outcomes for their expected child is relatively straightforward for those pregnancies where the defect falls into group 1 (prognosis uniformly poor) and termination of pregnancy should be offered in these cases. If the defect falls into group 2, the outcome is expected to be good and counselling can reflect this optimistic forecast, although full support should be given to the parents throughout the pregnancy because, despite reassurance, it has been our experience that parents continue to have anxieties about the normality of their child, even after delivery and a normal paediatric assessment. Some consideration may be given as to whether parents should be informed of an abnormality if the prognosis is uniformly good. A small pilot study in antenatal counselling groups has demonstrated that most parents would rather not be told the information if the defect was:

1. minor
2. almost always associated with a good prognosis
3. not likely to influence management.

   Clearly there is a delicate interplay between medical obligations of beneficiance and autonomy in this area.

   It is much more difficult to provide probabilistic information for parents whose child has a defect falling into groups 3 and 4. For group 3 the probabilities of good outcomes are known to be poor and the conditions are lethal in about half of the cases. Termination of pregnancy should be offered before viability. Group 4 presents the most difficult counselling problem. Frequently the information regarding prognosis is not available and much of it is based on neurosurgical series which are potentially biased towards patients with a better prognosis than might be expected for cases diagnosed antenatally. We have collected reports of outcomes for cases diagnosed antenatally and compared these with outcomes of postnatally diagnosed cases. Although the information available is limited it suggests that the antenatal diagnosis of craniospinal defects in this last group has a less favourable outcome than reported in the neurosurgical and paediatric literature. Antenatal diagnosis, however, does enable arrangements to be made for future management of the pregnancy, timing and place of delivery and, if necessary, availability of intensive neurosurgical care.

Group 1: prognosis uniformly poor

This group includes anencephaly, holoprosencephaly, severe porencephaly (cystic cerebral destruction) and microcephaly. Characteristic findings for craniospinal defects occurring within this group have been well documented in the literature (Vintzileos et al., 1987b). The lesions are usually gross and easily detected at 18 weeks' gestation. The prognosis is either lethal or associated with a severe degree of mental handicap whether or not the structural abnormality is associated with chromosomal defects.

Anencephaly and holoprosencephaly are generally easy to detect at 18 weeks' gestation. Holoprosencephaly may be associated with a fluid-filled cranial vault (Figure 1.1) or with a small skull containing no midline echo, disorganized cerebral ventricles and prominent basal nuclei (Figures 1.2, 1.3 and 1.4). Microcephaly is more difficult to detect. Antenatal diagnosis in the second half of pregnancy depends on a demonstration of impaired cranial growth rather than direct visualization of the lesion (Chervenak et al., 1987). The utility of head measurements alone is limited as these can be markedly biased by factors such as incorrect dating or intrauterine growth retardation. Comparison of biometric parameters, e.g. head circumference/abdominal circumference ratio on serial scanning is necessary for this diagnosis (Chervenak et al., 1987). The head size should fall to about three standard deviations below expected values before the diagnosis can be made with confidence. The prognosis for mental function is very poor in microcephaly because impaired head growth is entirely secondary to poor

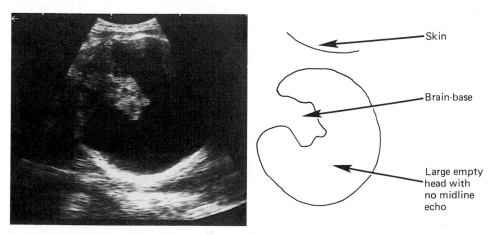

Figure 1.1 Holoprosencephaly with fluid-filled cranium

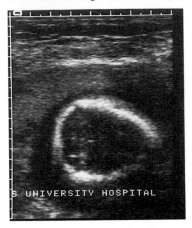

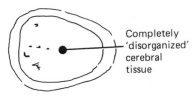

Completely 'disorganized' cerebral tissue

Figure 1.2 Holoprosencephaly without cyst formation at level at which one would normally expect to see the cerebral ventricles and midline structures

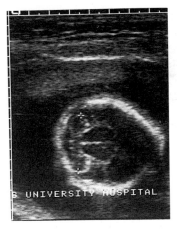

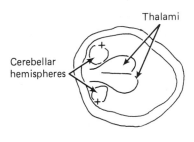

Thalami

Cerebellar hemispheres

Figure 1.3 Cross-section of the cranium in the patient shown in Figure 1.2, but at a lower (inferior) level. Note prominent thalami

brain growth. Some cases of microcephaly are associated with congenital infections (e.g. rubella, toxoplasmosis) but the majority are isolated defects and half of the latter are inherited on an autosomal recessive basis (Warkany, 1971). A recurrence risk of 1 in 8 is often quoted but microcephalic infants with no evidence of viral infection following consanguineous marriage can be regarded as recessive in aetiology.

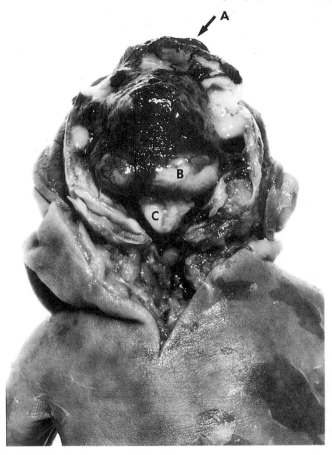

Figure 1.4 Post-mortem examination of patient in Figures 1.2 and 1.3. View from behind. A. Fused frontal folds. B. Cerebellum. C. Medulla oblongata. Thalamus lies between A and B and is partly covered with blood clot

Group 2: prognosis usually good – choroid plexus cysts

The prenatal diagnosis of choroid plexus cysts was first reported by Chaudleigh, Pearce and Campbell (1984) and Ostlere, Irving and Lilford (1987) reported a favourable prognosis. Since then eight further reports have appeared in the literature including a more detailed report by Ostlere, Irving and Lilford (1989) (Table 1.3). If figures from these reports are amalgamated (with the exclusion of Bundy, who reviewed trisomy rather than choroid plexus cysts), 120 antenatally detected choroid plexus cysts have been reported and 10 of these were associated with chromosomal abnormalities (1 trisomy 21 and 7 trisomy 18). In each of seven cases with trisomy 18 where a follow-up scan is reported, the cyst was noted to persist beyond 23 weeks' gestational age. Amalgamation of these series almost certainly overestimates risk due to publication and selection bias. Choroid plexus

Table 1.3 Summary of world literature reports of outcome for choroid plexus cysts diagnosed antenatally

Author	Number	Trisomy	Outcome
Friday, Schwartz and Tuffli (1985)	1	0	Normal infant
Nicolaides, Rodeck and Gosden (1986)	4	3(18)	All trisomy pregnancies terminated. Cysts persistent up to termination at 24 weeks. One normal outcome, cyst had resolved by 23 weeks
Ostlere, Irving and Lilford (1989)	42	3	Two trisomy 18 and one trisomy 21
Bundy et al. (1986)	1	1	Reviewed 12 cases of trisomy 18. One had a choroid plexus cyst
Benacerraf (1987)	2	0	Normal outcome
Furness (1987)	30	3	Not given. (2 trisomy 18 and 1 other trisomy unspecified)
Chitkara et al. (1988)	41	1	39 normal outcome. Hydrocephaly – 1 Fetus papyraceus – 1

cysts are usually small (1 cm or less) and may be unilateral or bilateral; single or multiple. They have no significant long-term effects if chromosomes are normal. Six of the eight well-documented cases associated with trisomy were over 12 mm in diameter. If a cyst is over 12 mm in diameter or if it persists beyond 23 weeks' gestation, then chromosomal analysis (fetal blood or chorion) should be considered, or at least a very detailed scan carried out to search for features of trisomy 18, such as cardiac defect, overlapping fingers, cleft lip, abnormal feet and diaphragmatic hernia (Figure 1.5). Other cases should undergo a cardiac scan (since an abnormality will suggest trisomy) and if this is normal the prognosis is excellent (see Figure 1.6).

Group 3: prognosis usually poor and reasonably well defined

Spina bifida

The major craniospinal abnormality falling into this group is spina bifida (Figures 1.7, 1.8, 1.9, 1.10, 1.11 and 1.12). Lorber and Salfield (1981) found that of 42 *selected* neonatal cases (with small lesions and other favourable features), six died despite surgery and of the remaining 36, half survived with no or minimal handicap; all 71 unoperated cases died. This is the best reported series and in our opinion gives an optimistically misleading prognosis. Overall, at least half of the cases die if neonatal surgery is restricted to infants with a reasonably good prognosis and less than 10% of cases detected antenatally will survive without paralysis. Eighty per cent will develop hydrocephalus and require shunting, although this seldom results in mental retardation. (The neonatal outcome is reviewed in greater detail by Tyrrell et al., 1988.) Real time ultrasound scanning provides a specific diagnosis and can therefore define the position and extent of the lesion. This information should be included in any assessment of long-term prognosis. Debate over the

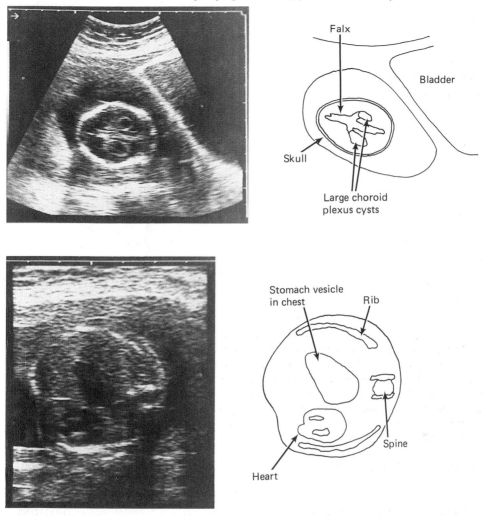

Falx

Bladder

Skull

Large choroid
plexus cysts

Stomach vesicle
in chest   Rib

Spine

Heart

Figure 1.5 Large bilateral choroid plexus cysts. These cysts were associated with a diaphragmatic hernia. Fetal blood confirmed trisomy 18 and labour was induced at 20 weeks' gestational age. The placenta was analysed by direct analysis and this showed the trisomy. Trisomy 18 is, however, sometimes associated with false-negative direct (or short-term) analysis of chorion because of mosaicism of the trophoblast. Thus, fetal blood sampling or placental culture are needed before the parents can be given a high level of reassurance regarding chromosomes. This particular patient only wanted to end the pregnancy in the face of a hopeless prognosis

relative merits of ultrasound versus maternal serum alpha-fetoprotein (MSAFP) for screening for neural tube defects has come down in favour of ultrasound because:

1. reported pick-up rates (sensitivity) are similar (between 60 and 90%)
2. specificity is much higher
3. ultrasound has many other advantages (confirmation of gestational age, diagnosis of multiple gestation, detection of other anomalies).

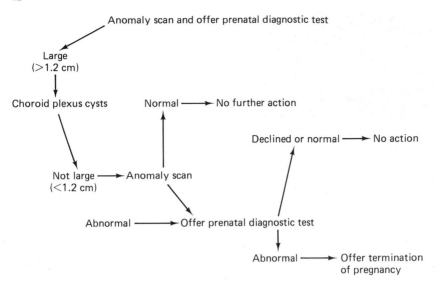

Anomaly scan and offer prenatal diagnostic test

Large
(>1.2 cm)

Choroid plexus cysts

Normal ——→ No further action

Declined or normal ——→ No action

Not large ——→ Anomaly scan
(<1.2 cm)

Abnormal ——→ Offer prenatal diagnostic test

Abnormal ——→ Offer termination
of pregnancy

Figure 1.6 Suggested scheme in the management of fetal choroid plexus cysts (from Ostlere, Irving and Lilford, 1989)

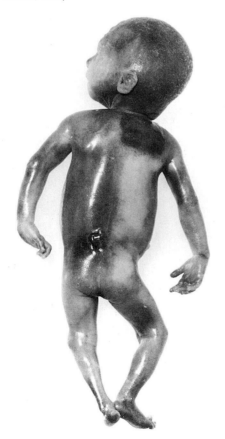

Figure 1.7 Small neural tube defect

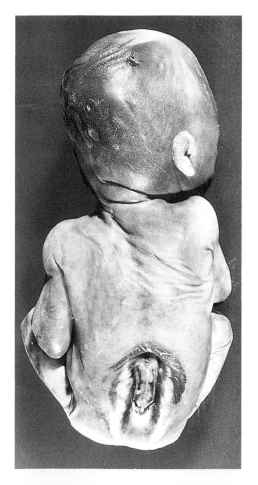

Figure 1.8 Large neural tube defect

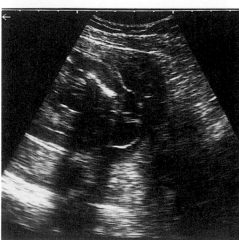

Figure 1.9 Meningocoele and spina bifida

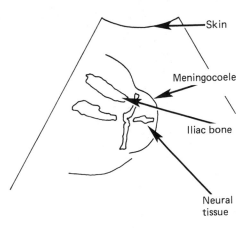

Skin

Meningocoele

Iliac bone

Neural
tissue

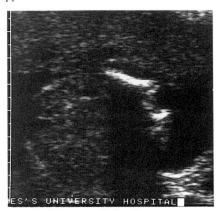 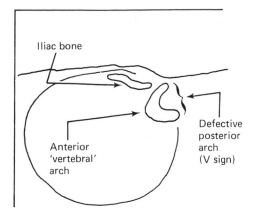

Figure 1.10 Transverse scan of defective neural arch. Spinous processes and posterior position of arch are absent causing the V sign

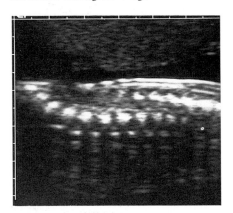 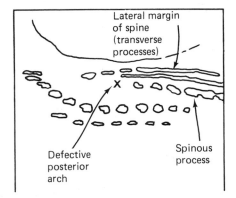

Figure 1.11 Same patient as in Figure 1.10; longitudinal (sagittal) scan showing spinal defect

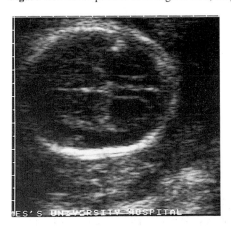 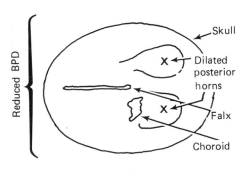

Figure 1.12 Dilated posterior horns of lateral ventricles in patient demonstrated in Figures 1.10 and 1.11 – an early sign of hydrocephalus due to Arnold-Chiari malformation. The posterior fossa is usually abnormal in such cases (banana cerebellum), the biparietal diameter (BPD) is smaller (on average) and the anterior cranial vault flattened (causing the 'lemon' sign)

Strategy 1: ultrasound only

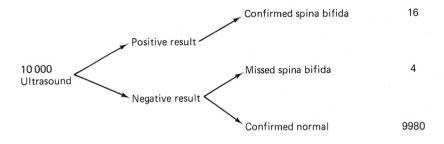

	Confirmed spina bifida	16
Positive result		
10 000 Ultrasound	Missed spina bifida	4
Negative result		
	Confirmed normal	9980

Strategy 2: ultrasound, MSAFP test and amniocentesis

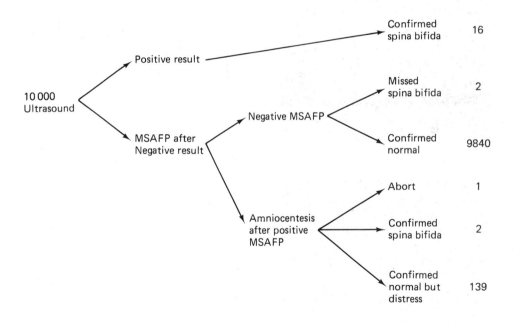

Figure 1.13 Two schemes aimed at offering a prenatal diagnosis service for neural tube defects. The trade-off is between a slightly higher detection rate with MSAFP and scan versus less anxiety (and unnecessary amniocentesis) among those offered a scan only. This argument will probably become obsolete with the introduction of the triple test for Down's syndrome. However, some authorities may favour screening for aneuploidy by oestriol and HCG only, since these offer the greatest discrimination in detection of Down's syndrome and will eliminate the anxiety from frequent false-positive diagnoses with MSAFP

The question of whether MSAFP should be carried out in addition to ultrasound hinges on the extra cases detected and the number of false positives. Since these two tests are unlikely to be independent (large lesions on scan are more likely to cause abnormal MSAFP levels) the extra pick-up rate in high prevelance areas is about 2:10 000 women screened (Figure 1.13) falling to 1:10 000 where prevalence is low at the cost of about 400 false-positive, anxiety provoking, results (Tyrrell *et al.*, 1988). However, it is impossible to ignore a high level when MSAFP is used primarily for Down's syndrome screening.

Encephalocoele

An encephalocoele is a defect in the cranial vault (usually occipital but occasionally frontal, basal or parietal). Defects may range from a small bony defect without brain tissue in herniated meninges to a major vault defect with large quantities of brain tissue in the herniated sac. Like other craniospinal defects it may occur as an isolated lesion or as part of an autosomal syndrome (e.g. autosomal recessive Meckel syndrome, where the condition is associated with cystic kidneys and polydactyly). Encephalocoele may also occur as part of Robert's, Chemke, Knoblock and cryptophthalmos syndromes and in dyssegmental dwarfism, which are all autosomal recessive. Ultrasound diagnosis is made by observing the presence of a cystic lesion outside the skull and a bony defect in the skull. If large amounts of brain tissue have herniated through the defect then this is usually easily seen. Smaller defects may be much more difficult to diagnose. Associated abnormalities are frequently observed, commonly as a second neural tube defect or hydrocephalus.

The prognosis for a fetus with encephalocoele depends largely on the quantity of brain tissue which protrudes into the herniated sac. Several studies have looked at the outcome for children born with encephalocoele (McLauren, 1964; Lipshitz, Beck and Froman, 1969; Mealey, Ozenitis and Hockey, 1970; Lorber and Schofield, 1979). Children with pure meningocoele generally have normal development after surgery. Herniation of brain tissue through the defect is associated with an extremely poor prognosis. There is little information on the significance of a small amount of brain herniation. Chervenak *et al.* (1984) reported the outcome of two such children who are currently alive with moderate developmental delay. Hydrocephalus, if present, in the absence of brain tissue herniation and other associated anomalies has a relatively favourable prognosis providing postnatal shunting is carried out. Parents who have an antenatal diagnosis of a child with an encephalocoele should be counselled to consider termination of pregnancy if brain tissue has herniated, particularly if microencephaly is present, as the prognosis is poor. If no brain tissue has herniated the outlook is much more favourable but surgery will be necessary to repair the defect after delivery.

Group 4: prognosis variable – poorly defined

The craniospinal defects falling into this group cause the obstetrician the most difficulty when counselling prospective parents about outcome. As mentioned previously, caution must be used in extrapolating the prognosis from neurosurgical cases to those detected antenatally.

Apparently isolated ventriculomegaly

Most cases of fetal ventriculomegaly are associated with spina bifida, congenital infection, chromosomal abnormalities or other structural anomalies. The most difficult counselling situation arises when none of these features is detected and the diagnosis of apparently isolated ventriculomegaly is made. This diagnosis depends on a good understanding of the normal cross-sectional anatomy of the cerebral hemispheres (Figure 1.14). Even then, the label hydrocephalus (which some

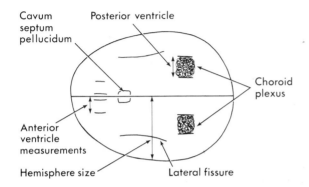

Figure 1.14 Normal cross-sectional anatomy of the fetal head. In the second trimester, hydrocephalus manifests as ventricular dilatation only and the skull, if anything, tends to be small

restrict to cases of high-pressure dilatation) or ventriculomegaly represents a very low-level diagnosis. The causes (high level diagnoses) which underlie ventriculo-megaly are shown in Figure 1.15. Note that in many instances, high-level diagnosis is not very high level since many cases are idiopathic. The diagnosis of ventriculomegaly is often clear-cut (Figure 1.16), but border-line cases occur and should be managed conservatively unless associated with other abnormalities or until unequivocal ventricular dilatation occurs.

A review of the literature (Figure 1.17) suggests that the outcome of antenatally detected ventriculomegaly is worse than that reported in the neurosurgical literature. (See: Laurence and Coates, 1962; Lorber, 1962; Overton and Snodgram, 1965; Lorber and Zachary, 1968; Mealey, Gilmor and Bubb, 1973; Glick *et al.*, 1984; Harrod *et al.*, 1984; Williamson *et al.*, 1984; Clewell *et al.*, 1985; Oberbaur, 1985; Pober, Greener and Holmes, 1986; Serlo *et al.*, 1986; Ricketts, Lowe and Patel, 1987; Vintzileos *et al.*, 1987a; .) Approximately one-quarter of fetuses with apparently isolated ventriculomegaly will survive with normal intelligence. Survival rates are artificially low because head decompression at delivery is frequently fatal. Mental impairment, when present, is severe in about 50% of cases. These figures might still underestimate the severity of prognosis for cases ascertained in time for termination of pregnancy, as they are based almost exclusively on cases ascertained in the third trimester. The prognosis may well be worse for those that are obvious in the middle trimester. The extent of the ventricular dilatation has very little prognostic value and fetal surgery (Manning, 1985) would appear to offer no benefit (Table 1.4). Since carrying out this review another important series of 47 cases has been published by Hodgins *et al.* (1988) with slightly more optimistic prognostic figures. Twenty-five had other severe anomalies on sonogram and 19 of these cases had termination of pregnancy while

Aetiology of Ventriculomegaly

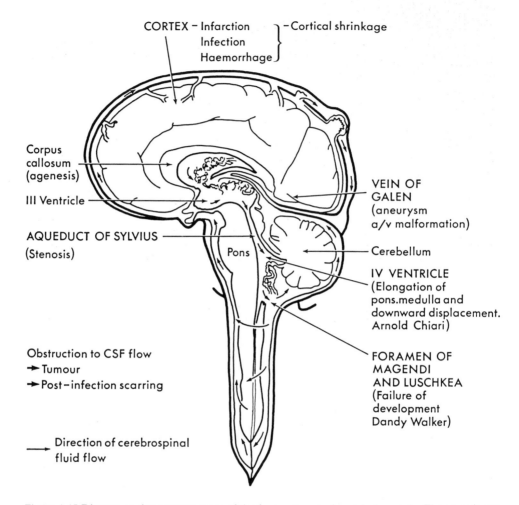

Figure 1.15 Diagram to demonstrate some of the *known* causes of ventriculomegaly. The cause is not always obvious even at post-mortem

the remaining six died after birth. Twenty-two cases of apparently isolated ventriculomegaly were reported. Seven of these were found to have other anomalies at birth; three died, three survived with severe handicap and one is intellectually normal. Fifteen of 22 cases were confirmed to have isolated ventriculomegaly. All survived, 12 normally, one with severe and two with moderate mental handicap. Thus, of 22 cases of apparently isolated ventriculomegaly detected *in-utero*, three died, four had severe mental handicap, two moderate handicap and 13 normal intellectual development. The gestational age at time of diagnosis is not given. All data confirm that the outcome for fetal

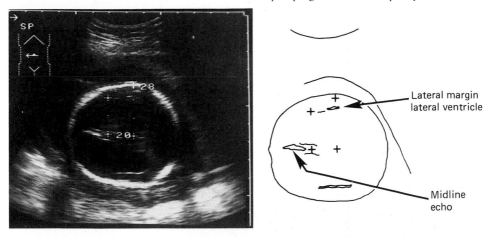

Figure 1.16 Typical case of ventriculomegaly. Normally the ventricle to hemisphere (VH) ratio is less than 0.6 at 16 weeks' gestational age and less than 0.5 by 20 weeks. Sometimes the VH ratio becomes abnormal only in late pregnancy, or it may start off abnormal and then become normal. We have seen cases start off as abnormal, become normal and then again abnormal as pregnancy advances. In general, a firm diagnosis with the offer of termination of pregnancy should only be made in cases of apparently isolated ventriculomegaly when the diagnosis is confirmed beyond all reasonable doubt

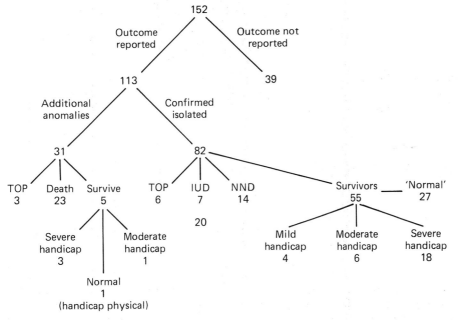

Figure 1.17 Literature review of 152 cases of antenatally diagnosed fetal ventriculomegaly. Even when no other lesions are detected, they are still often present. Of 113 cases of apparently isolated ventriculomegaly, nine had termination of pregnancy (TOP) (most were identified in the third trimester). Of the remaining 104, 60 survived. Of these survivors, 28 had severe or moderate handicap and 32 had mild handicap. There would be more survivors if Caesarean section was carried out more often than head decompression and vaginal delivery. Impaired mental development is usually a parent's greatest fear and yet this is uncertain in isolated ventriculomegaly. This is one of the most difficult situations in prenatal diagnosis. IUD, intrauterine death; NND: neonatal death

Table 1.4 Outcome of fetal ventriculomegaly according to treatment

	In-utero *treatment*	Ex-utero *treatment*
Normal	11	13
Mild delay	3	4
Moderate delay	0	3
Severe delay	18	0

ventriculomegaly is much worse when other congenital abnormalities are present and around 33% of cases of apparently isolated ventriculomegaly will subsequently be found to have other anomalies after delivery.

By comparison, amalgamated reports in the neurosurgical literature for outcome in cases diagnosed following delivery show that 58.5% survived and 41% had an IQ of more than 70.

At present there does not appear to be any other method by which the prognosis of apparently isolated ventriculomegaly can be determined more accurately. Authors have related prognosis to brain mass-cortical thickness and while some find a correlation (Jansen *et al.*, 1982; McCullough and Balzer-Martin, 1982; Amacher and Wellington, 1984), others find no relationship (Foltz and Shurtleff, 1963; Shurtleff, Kronmal and Foltz, 1975). The reason for this relates to the cause of the ventriculomegaly, and the time of onset. Moderate ventriculomegaly, for example, may be the result of brain shrinkage due to infarction with a very poor prognosis, while a more severe degree of ventricular dilatation may be due to obstruction of cerebrospinal fluid (CSF) (e.g. Arnold-Chiari malformation) with a relatively good prognosis, because the brain is intrinsically normal in these cases. Aqueductal stenosis, however, has a poor prognosis, perhaps because of increased pressure at an earlier and more critical stage of development. For these reasons it is unlikely that the size of the third ventricle or measurement of CSF pressure will provide good prognostic discrimination, although there is a possibility that nuclear magnetic resonance spectroscopy may be helpful along with electrophysiological measurement of brain function.

We have recently encountered two cases of brain shrinkage and ventricular dilatation at St James's Hospital which were due to ischaemic necrosis secondary to carotid occlusion and cases of this sort might in the future be identifiable on the basis of Doppler assessment of cerebral blood flow resistance. For the management of the fetus diagnosed antenatally to have apparently isolated ventriculomegaly, we would suggest the plan in Figure 1.18. Sensitive counselling must be given and the

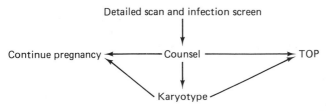

Figure 1.18 Suggested management scheme for ventriculomegaly. TOP: termination of pregnancy

option to terminate the pregnancy discussed. Despite its wide advocacy in the literature urgent fetal karyotyping is only necessary for the minority of parents whose decision to request termination of pregnancy hinges on this result, although it should also be offered antenatally if termination of pregnancy is preceded by urea instillation since this prevents tissue culture from the stillborn infant. In other cases antenatal karyotyping may be useful in planning delivery since Caesarean section may be selected in preference to rapid head decompression and vaginal delivery in cases with gross head enlargement. The latter is almost invariably fatal to the fetus.

Agenesis of corpus callosum

This is an infrequent craniospinal abnormality with a reported prevalence of 1 – 3/1000 population, however, it is found much more commonly among developmentally disabled persons. Nevertheless, many cases are asymptomatic and the actual

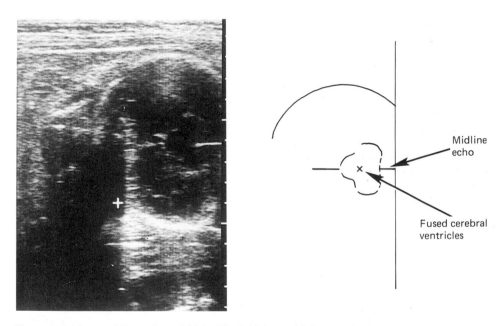

Figure 1.19 Absent midline echo and 'high-riding' third ventricle is agenesis of the corpus callosum. This diagnosis was confirmed by postnatal CT scan, and the baby is developing normally at 2 years of life

frequency in the population remains unknown. Sonographic features have been described in detail in the neonate and more recently there have been six reports of detection in the fetus. The ultrasonic features (Figure 1.19) are:

1. dilatation of third ventricle
2. high position of third ventricle
3. dilatation of occipital horns
4. increased separation of frontal horns and bodies of lateral ventricles

Table 1.5 Large collected reports of anomalies associated with agenesis of corpus callosum (postnatal)

Author	Number	Associated anomalies
Larsen and Osborn (1982)	44	13 interhemisphere cysts – hydrocephalus 5 Dandy Walker cysts 3 Arnold-Chiari malformation
Babcock (1984)	5	
Parrish, Rooessman and Levinsohn (1979)	47	85% – CNS anomalies 62% – anomalies outside CNS 62% – 1 or more organ systems involved 38% – 3 or more organ systems involved 13% – no other lesions
Jeret *et al.* (1987)	705	85% – mental retardation 42% – ocular abnormalities 32% – gyral abnormalities 23% – hydrocephalus 29% – other CNS lesions 24% – corticovertebral lesions

5. concave medial wall of frontal horns of lateral ventricle
6. absence of cavum septum pellucidum of corpus callosum.

The significance of agenesis of the corpus callosum lies in the high incidence of associated malformations (Table 1.5). Thirteen out of 44 patients reported by Larsen and Osborn (1982) had interhemispheric cysts and hydrocephalus, five had Dandy Walker cysts and three had the Arnold-Chiari malformation. Babcock (1984) reported additional abnormalities in four of five cases. Although most cases are sporadic and of unknown cause, agenesis of corpus callosum is a frequent finding in trisomy 8, 13, 18 and is a feature of four well-defined syndromes: the Aicardi syndrome (which is sex-linked); Anderman's syndrome and the Acrocallosal syndrome – all associated with severe mental retardation, and the Shapiro syndrome, characterized by defective temperature control leading to recurrent spontaneous hypothermia. Several other syndromes have also been associated with agenesis of corpus callosum in frequencies greater than in the normal population (Jeret *et al.*, 1987). These include fetal alcohol syndrome, Arnold-Chiari II, West syndrome, and the oral facial digital syndrome.

In the largest review of cases of agenesis of corpus callosum (705 cases confirmed by neurological techniques and collected from literature reports), Jeret *et al.* (1987) reported a selection of clinicopathological findings frequently associated with agenesis of the corpus callosum. Common abnormalities included mental retardation 85%, seizures 42%, ocular anomalies 42%, gyral anomalies 32%, hydrocephalus 23% and other CNS lesions 29%. Developmental abnormalities are not attributed to the absence of the corpus callosum *per se* but are due to the other CNS malformations or dysfunction which may be genetic or non-genetic.

It is important to realize that the above cases were ascertained postnatally and therefore represent a biased selection where associated anomalies and their features brought the abnormality to medical attention. Agenesis of the corpus is an

Table 1.6 Outcome of antenatally diagnosed agenesis of corpus callosum

Author	Number	Gestation at diagnosis (weeks)	Outcome
Verco and LeQuesne (1987)	1.	36	Diagnosis confirmed post-delivery. Also absent cavum septum pellucidum. Eventual outcome not reported
	2.	24	Diagnosis confirmed postnatally. Also absent cavum septum pellucidum, dilatation of atria, associated deformity of lateral ventricles. No report of eventual outcome
	3.	20	Diagnosis at 20 weeks plus congenital diaphragmatic hernia. Pregnancy terminated. Diagnosis confirmed at post-mortem
	4.	23	Preterm delivery at 34 weeks. Absent corpus callosum, cavum septum pellucidum. Mild dilatation of atria, posterior and temporal horns of lateral ventricles. No report of outcome
Comstock *et al.* (1985)	1.	16 confirmed at 33 weeks	Prominent occipital horns of lateral ventricles from 16 weeks. Midline cystic structure at 33 weeks. Delivered at 36 weeks – lower segment caesarean section (LSCS). Absent corpus callosum confirmed. No report of outcome
	2.	30	Posterior fossa cyst 30 weeks. Enlarged third ventricle. Preterm labour at 34 weeks – LSCS. Neonatal ultrasound scanning – absence of corpus callosum. Dandy Walker cysts, small encephalocoele. Outcome not reported
Bryce and Lilford (1989)	1	31	Cystic area anterior cerebral hemisphere. Apparently continuous with lateral ventricles. Diagnosis of absent corpus callosum. Confirmed post-delivery. Normal development at 24 months

incidental finding at adult post-mortem and often exists with no symptoms. It is sometimes said that Leonardo da Vinci had simple agenesis of the corpus callosum with no apparent ill effect!

Antenatal diagnosis of the abnormality has been reported in six cases (Table 1.6). The eventual outcome and developmental progress has not been reported in any of these series. We can report one case diagnosed antenatally and confirmed by postnatal ultrasonography. This baby is developing normally at 2 years of age (Bryce and Lilford, 1989). What is the obstetrician to tell the parents when an antenatal diagnosis of agenesis of the corpus callosum has been made? First, in view of the very high chance of associated cerebral anomalies a detailed ultrasound scan of the cranial and extra-cranial systems should be carried out. If any other anomaly is detected, then the prognosis is essentially that of the other condition and this is usually very poor. If no other anomaly is detected but the parents would request termination of a fetus which was certain to die or be mentally retarded, then karyotyping should be offered. If the pregnancy continues then careful postnatal scans and follow-up are required so that superimposed hydrocephalus can be detected early and treated by shunting.

Intracranial cerebrospinal fluid cysts

Intracranial cerebrospinal fluid (CSF)-containing cysts are usually congenital but frequently remain asymptomatic during infancy. Only rarely do they remain symptom-free until adulthood (Smith and Smith, 1976). The cyst may communicate with the ventricular system as does the Dandy Walker cyst or they may lack this communication as in the case of arachnoid cysts.

The Dandy Walker malformation

The Dandy Walker malformation is the most important of the cysts to be found in the posterior cerebral fossa. It was originally described as a malformation caused by atresia of the foramen of Magendie and Luschka. However, this has been disputed since atresia of both foramina would cause severe non-communicating hydrocephalus and Hirsch *et al.* (1984) demonstrated a communication between the fourth ventricle and subarachnoid space in more than 80% of cases. Hydrocephalus may develop antenatally or more commonly postnatally and may in some cases be due to intraventricular bleeding at the time of delivery.

The antenatal detection of the Dandy Walker malformation has been described in eight cases in the literature (Table 1.7). Features on an ultrasound examination which would suggest the Dandy Walker malformation are:

1. large posterior fossa cyst
2. hypoplastic cerebellar vermis – displaced anteriolaterally
3. dilatation of third ventricle.

In reports of antenatal diagnosis by ultrasonography the most consistent finding has been a defect in the vicinity of cerebellar vermis. We do not believe it is possible to differentiate this from complete absence of the cerebellar vermis (Joubert's syndrome) which has a universally bad prognosis.

In the event of a Dandy Walker malformation being diagnosed during the antenatal period, a careful search for associated anomalies must be made as they occur frequently (Hart, Malamud and Ellis, 1972; Brown, 1977; Hirsch *et al.*, 1984). Among the central nervous system malformations we have already said that agenesis of the corpus callosum is particularly relevant and this is present in 7 – 17% of cases (Sawaya and McLaurin, 1981; Hirsch *et al.*, 1984). This combination of birth defects is believed to carry a poor prognosis for intellectual development.

Associated systemic anomalies occur to a lesser degree than cerebral malformations and very often are not serious (facial dysmorphism, polydactyly, syndactyly) (Hart, Malamud and Ellis, 1972; Brown, 1977). Congenital heart defects (mainly ventriculoseptal defects) have also been described and if these are suspected then fetal echocardiography should be performed.

Table 1.7 Outcome of cases of Dandy Walker malformation diagnosed antenatally

Author	Number	Gestation of USS	USS findings	Outcome
Pilau (1986)	5	30	Retrocerebellar cyst. Defect in vermis. Enlarged lateral and third ventricles. Macrocrania	Induced vaginal delivery at 37 weeks. Dandy Walker malformation confirmed. Ventriculo-peritoneal shunting. Survival (? quality)
		32	Retrocerebellar cyst. Defect in vermis. Normal lateral and third ventricles. Macrocrania	Caesarean section 37 weeks (abruption). Dandy Walker malformation confirmed. Agenesis of corpus callosum, cyst, peritoneal shunting. Survival (? quality)
		24	Retrocerebellar cyst. Defect in vermis. Enlarged lateral and third ventricles	Termination of pregnancy. Hypoplasia of vermis. Agenesis of corpus callosum
		24	Retrocerebellar cyst. Defect in vermis. Enlarged lateral ventricles. Macrocrania	Termination of pregnancy. Dandy Walker malformation
		18	Occipital meningocoele. Defect in vermis. Normal lateral and third ventricles	Termination of pregnancy. Occipital meningocoele. Dandy Walker malformation
Serlo, Kirkinen and Jouppila (1985)	3	24	Occipital triangular defect. Lateral ventricles slightly dilated	Elective Caesarean section 39 weeks. Dandy Walker malformation confirmed. Ventriculo-cystoperimeostomy. 5-years developmentally normal
		28	Occipital triangular defect. III ventricles dilated	Spontaneous vaginal at 39 weeks. Dandy Walker cysts. Ventriculo-cystoperimeostomy. 5-years developmentally normal
		22	Occipital triangular defect. Lateral ventricles slightly dilated	Elective LSCS at 37 weeks. Dandy Walker cyst. Ventriculo-cystostomy. 4–5 years normal development

USS: ultrasound scanning

The prognosis for the Dandy Walker malformation is difficult to determine due to ascertainment bias of the various postnastal surveys. Some prenatal surveys consist mainly of cases where termination of pregnancy was carried out, e.g. Pilau *et al.* (1986). Others are postnatal neurosurgical series in which children have presented with hydrocephalus which may have worsened the prognosis. Fischer (1973), in the first large postnatal series of published results of treatment of the anomaly, reported a mortality rate of 50%; of the survivors, half were reported as severely intellectually impaired. Two more recent studies (Sawaya and McLaurin,

Table 1.8 Cases of Dandy Walker malformation ascertained on the basis of symptoms after delivery with follow-up of mental development

Author	Total cases	Cases with IQ > 80	
		No	%
Udvarhelyi and Epstein (1975)	12	8	67
Hirsch *et al.* (1984)	27	16	59
Fischer (1973)	14	8	57
Carmel, Antunes and Hilal (1977)	13	6	46
Tal *et al.* (1980)	8	3	37
Carteri, Gerosa and Gaini (1979)	8	3	37
James *et al.* (1979)	6	2	33
Sawaya and McLaurin (1981)	14	4	29
Total	102	50	49

1981; Hirsch *et al.*, 1984) reported survival rates following treatment of 77% and 88% respectively, but of the survivors only 30 – 40% had an IQ greater than 80. Details of associated anomalies, onset of hydrocephalus and relationship to subsequent IQ are not given. One series of prenatal diagnosis also gives full postnatal follow-up. Serlo, Kirkinen and Jouppila (1985) reported a series of three cases of antenatal diagnosis of isolated Dandy Walker cysts made at 22 – 28 weeks' gestation by ultrasound examination (Table 1.8). All cases were monitored for the development of hydrocephalus during pregnancy. However, biparietal growth and severity of the anomaly remained constant and allowed delivery to occur at term. Postnatally the diagnosis was confirmed, early neonatal shunting procedures were performed and subsequent follow-up for up to 2 years has shown normal mental and physical development. In Pilau's series of five cases diagnosed antenatally, two pregnancies continued to term and required shunting, survival is reported but details of neurological and developmental progress are not given. We can add a further case of apparent Dandy Walker malformation, plus ventriculomegaly, diagnosed at 28 weeks who developed normally to one year of age but who has since died. In contrast to most conditions, the prognosis for *in-utero* diagnosis of isolated Dandy Walker malformation appears better than for cases reported postnatally. This may be because of a reversal of the usual selection bias. A proportion of other cases never come to surgery because of fetal or neonatal death, while in the case of Dandy Walker malformation some cases would never cause symptoms. Early presymptomatic treatment of hydrocephalus may help prognosis in other cases. Already Tal *et al.* (1980) have reported an improvement in outcome for infants treated aggressively following early postnatal diagnosis of the Dandy Walker syndrome.

Obstetric management should, therefore, aim to exclude associated anomalies. Regular ultrasonography should be carried out to detect hydrocephaly. Even if this occurs, the chance of normal intellectual development is at least 50% and cephalocentesis at delivery has somewhat less justification than in other cases of hydrocephalus. The possibility of mild cerebral trauma at delivery precipitating hydrocephaly in the neonate must also be considered. In the cases reported antenatally, two out of five were delivered vaginally and both developed normally although they have required shunting following delivery. As with isolated hydrocephalus, the parents of a child diagnosed to have Dandy Walker malformation antenatally must be counselled that if they choose to continue the pregnancy, then there is a large probability that the child will require surgery.

Arachnoid cysts

Arachnoid cysts occurring in the posterior cranial fossa may be exceedingly difficult to distinguish from the Dandy Walker malformation. Criteria for diagnosis include visualization of a fourth ventricle with a normal configuration and no apparent communication between the cyst and the ventricular system. However, the outcome for arachnoid cysts is generally favourable although this depends on the situation of the cyst. Arachnoid cysts are rarely multiple and associated anomalies are rare. Even large cysts may be asymptomatic when situated in the cerebellar hemisphere, but if in the vicinity of the third ventricle, even small cysts may cause ataxia, head bobbing or endocrinological disturbances such as precocious puberty. Galassi et al. (1985) reported a series of 10 cases of arachnoid cysts of the posterior fossa – age range 17 months–58 years. A high rate of birth-related trauma was reported (50%). Following craniotomy and excision of the cyst, one patient died the day following surgery, one patient had recurrence of the cyst, one remained unchanged and the remaining seven cases all improved after treatment. Serlo et al. (1985) reported 12 cases of arachnoid cyst at ages ranging from one month to 12 years treated by shunting. Follow-up showed two with ataxia, two with hemiplegia and slight intellectual retardation and eight were developing normally although one has had a cyst recurrence. It may be seen from these two reports that the prognosis for arachnoid cysts may also be considered to be optimistic provided the cyst is not in the area of the quadrigeminal plate (i.e. near the third ventricle).

References

Amacher, A. L. and Wellington, J. (1984) Infantile hydrocephalus: long term results of surgical therapy. *Child's Brain*, **11**, 217–229

Babcock, D.S. (1984) The normal absent and abnormal corpus callosum sonographic findings. *Radiology*, **151**, 449

Benacerraf, B.R. (1987) Asymptomatic cysts of fetal choroid plexus in the second trimester. *Journal of Ultrasound Medicine*, **6**, 475

Brown, J.E. (1977) The Dandy-Walker syndrome. In *Handbook of Clinical Neurology*, Vol 30, (edited by P.J. Vinken and G.W. Bruyn). Amsterdam: Elsevier, pp. 623–646

Bryce, F.C. and Lilford, R.J. (1989) Antenatal diagnosis of agenesis of the corpus callosum. Case report and literature review..(Submitted for publication)

Bundy, A.L., Saltzman, D.H., Pober, B., Fine, C., Emerson, D. and Doubilet, P.M. (1986) Antenatal sonographic findings in trisomy 18. *Journal of Ultrasound Medicine*, **5**, 361–364

Carmel, P.W., Antunes, J.L. and Hilal, S.K. (1977) Dandy-Walker syndrome: clinico-pathological features and re-evaluation of modes of treatment. *Surgical Neurology*, **8**, 132–138

Carteri, A., Gerosa, M. and Gaini, S.M. (1979) The dysraphic state of the posterior fossa. Clinical review of the Dandy-Walker syndrome and the so-called arachnoid cysts. *Journal of Neurosurgical Science*, **23**, 53–59

Chaudleigh, P., Pearce, M. and Campbell, S. (1984) The prenatal diagnosis of transient cysts of the fetal choroid plexus. *Prenatal Diagnosis*, **4**, 135

Chervenak, F.A., Isaacson, G., Mahoney, M.J., Berkowitz, R.L., Tortora, M. and Hobbins, J.C. (1984) Diagnosis and management of fetal cephalocele. *Obstetrics and Gynecology*, **64**, 86–90

Chervenak, F.A., Rosenberg, J., Brightman, R.C., Chitkara, U. and Jeanty, P. (1987) A prospective study of the accuracy of ultrasound in predicting fetal microcephaly. *Obstetrics and Gynecology*, **69**, 908

Chitkara, U., Cogswell, C., Norton, K., Wilkins, I.A., Mehalek, K. and Berkowitz, R.L. (1988) Choroid plexus cysts in the fetus: a benign anatomic variant or pathologic entity. Report of 41 cases and review of the literature. *Obstetrics and Gynecology*, **72**, 185–189

Clewell, W.U., Meier, D.R., Mancuester, D.R., Manco-Johnson, M.L., Pretorias, D.K. and Nendee, R.W. (1985) Ventriculomegaly: evaluation and management. *Seminars in Perinatology*, **9**

Cochrane, D.D. and Myles, T. (1982) Management of extra-uterine hydrocephalus. *Journal of Neurosurgery*, **57**, 590–596

Comstock, C.H., Culp, D., Gonzalez, J. and Boal, D.B. (1985) Agenesis of the corpus callosum in the fetus. Its evaluation and significance. *Journal of Ultrasound Medicine*, **4**, 613–616

Fischer, E.G. (1973) Dandy-Walker syndrome: an evaluation of surgical treatment. *Journal of Neurosurgery*, **34**, 615–621

Foltz, E.L. and Shurtleff, D.B. (1963) Five year comparative study of hydrocephalus in children with or without operation (113 cases). *Journal of Neurosurgery*, **20**, 1064–1078

Friday, R.O., Schwartz, D.B. and Tuffli, G.A. (1985) Spontaneous intrauterine resolution of intraventricular cystic masses. *Journal of Ultrasound Medicine*, **4**, 385

Furness, M.E. (1987) Choroid plexus cysts and trisomy 18. *Lancet*, ii, 693

Galassi, E., Tognetic, F., Franco, F., Fagioli, L., Nasi, M.T. and Gaist, G. (1985) Intratentorial arachnoid cysts. *Journal of Neurosurgery*, **63**, 210–217

Glick, P.L., Harrison, M.R., Nakayoma, D.K. *et al.* (1984) Management of ventriculomegaly in the fetus. *Journal of Pediatrics*, **105**, 97

Harrod, M.J.E., Friedman, J.M., Santos-Ramos, R., Rutledge, J. and Weinberg, A. (1984) Etiologic heterogeneity of fetal hydrocephalus diagnosed by ultrasound. *American Journal of Obstetrics and Gynecology*, **150**, 38

Hart, M.N., Malamud, N. and Ellis, W.G. (1972) The Dandy-Walker syndrome. A clinicopathological study based on 28 cases. *Neurology*, **27**, 771–780

Hirsch, J.F., Pierre-Khan, A., Renier, D., Sainte-Rose, C. and Hoppe-Hirsch, E. (1984) The Dandy-Walker malformation. A review of 40 cases. *Journal of Neurosurgery*, **61**, 515–522

Hodgins, R.J., Edwards, M.S.B., Goldstein, R. *et al.* (1988) Natural history of fetal ventriculomegaly. *Paediatrics*, **82**, 642–697

James, H.E., Kaiser, G., Schut, L. and Bruce, D.A. (1979) Problems of diagnosis and treatment of the Dandy-Walker syndrome. *Child's Brain*, **5**, 24–30

Jansen, J., Gloerfelt-tarp, B., Pederson, H. and Zastorff, K. (1982) Prognosis in infantile hydrocephalus: follow-up in adult patients born 1946–1955. *Acta Neurologica Scandinavica*, **65**, 81–93

Jeret, J.S., Serur, D., Wisniewski, K.E. and Lubin, R.A. (1987) Clinicopathological findings associated with agenesis of the corpus callosum. *Brain Development*, **9**, 255–264

Larsen, P. and Osborn, A. (1982) Computed tomographic evaluation of corpus callosum agenesis and associated malformations. *Journal of Computer Assisted Tomography*, **6**, 225

Laurence, K.M. and Coates, S. (1962) The natural history of hydrocephalus. Detailed analysis of 182 unoperated cases. *Archives of Disease in Childhood*, **43**, 516–527

Lipshitz, R., Beck, J.M. and Froman, C. (1969) An assessment of the treatment of encephalo-meningoceles. *South African Medical Journal*, **43**, 609

Lorber, J. (1962) The results of early treatment of extreme hydrocephalus. *Developmental Medicine and Child Neurology*, (suppl. 16), 21–29

Lorber, J. and Salfield, S.A.W. (1981) Results of selective treatment of spina bifida cystica. *Archives of Disease in Childhood*, **56**, 822–830

Lorber, J. and Schofield, J.K. (1979) The prognosis of occipital encephalocele. *Zeitschrift fuer Kinderchirurgie*, Z **28**, 347

Lorber, J. and Zachary, R.B. (1968) Primary congenital hydrocephalus. Longterm results of controlled therapeutic trial. *Archives of Disease in Childhood*, **43**, 518

Manning, F.A. (1985) International Fetal Surgery Registry. *Clinical Obstetrics and Gynaecology*, **29**, 551–557

McCullough, D.C. and Balzer-Martin, L.A. (1982) Current prognosis in overt neo-natal hydrocephalus. *Journal of Neurosurgery*, **57**, 387

McLaurin, R.L. (1964) Parietal cephaloceles. *Neurology*, **14**, 764

Mealey, J., Gilmor, R.L. and Bubb, M.P. (1973) The prognosis of hydrocephalus overt at birth. *Journal of Neurosurgery*, **39**, 348–355

Mealey, J., Ozenitis, A.J. and Hockey, A.A. (1970) The prognosis of encephaloceles. *Journal of Neurosurgery*, **32**, 209

Nicolaides, K.H., Rodeck, C.H. and Gosden, C.M. (1986) Rapid karyotyping in non-lethal fetal malformations. *Lancet*, **i**, 286

Oberbaur, R.W. (1985) The significance of morphological details for developmental outcome in infantile hydrocephalus. *Child's Nervous System*, **1**, 329–336

Ostlere, S.J., Irving, H.C. and Lilford, R.J. (1987) Choroid plexus cysts in the fetus. *Lancet*, **i**, 1491

Ostlere, S.J., Irving, H.C. and Lilford, R.J. (1989) A prospective study of the incidence and significance of fetal choroid plexus cysts. *Prenatal Diagnosis*, **9**, 205–211

Overton, M.C. and Snodgram, S.R. (1965) Ventriculovenous shunts for infantile hydrocephalus. A review of 5 years experience with this method. *Journal of Neurosurgery*, **23**, 517–521

Parrish, M., Rooessman, U. and Levinsohn, M. (1979) Agenesis of the corpus callosum: a study of the frequency of associated malformations. *Annals of Neurology*, **6**,

Pilau, G., Romero, R., De Palma, L. *et al.* (1986) Antenatal diagnosis and obstetric management of Dandy-Walker syndrome. *Journal of Reproductive Medicine*, **31**, 1017–1022

Pober, B.R., Greene, M.F. and Holmes, L.B. (1986) Complexities of intraventricular abnormalities. *Journal of Pediatrics*, **108**, 545–551

Ricketts, N.E.M., Lowe, E.M. and Patel, N.B. (1987) Prenatal diagnosis of choroid plexus cysts. *Lancet*, **i**, 213

Sawaya, R. and McLaurin, R.L. (1981) Dandy-Walker syndrome. Clinical analysis of 23 cases. *Journal of Neurosurgery*, **55**, 89–98

Serlo, W., Kirkinen, P. and Jouppila, P. (1985) Ante and postnatal evaluation of the Dandy-Walker syndrome. *Child's Nervous System*, **1**, 148–151

Serlo, W., Wendt, L., Heikkinen, E. and Saukkonen, A.L. (1985) Shunting procedures in the management of intra-cranial cerebrospinal fluid cysts in infancy and childhood. *Acta Neurochirurgica*, **76**, 111–116

Serlo, W., Kirkinen, P., Jouppila, P. and Herva, R. (1986) Prognostic signs in fetal hydrocephalus. *Child's Nervous System*, **2**, 93–97

Shurtleff, D.B., Kronmal, R. and Foltz, E.L. (1975) Follow up comparison of hydrocephalus with and without myelomeningocele. *Journal of Neurosurgery*, **42**, 61–68

Smith, R.A. and Smith, W.A. (1976) Arachnoidal cysts of the middle cranial fossa. *Surgical Neurology*, **5**, 246–252

Tal, Y., Freigang, B., Dunne, H.G., Durity, F.A. and Moyes, P.D. (1980) Dandy-Walker syndrome: analysis of 21 cases. *Developmental Medicine and Child Neurology*, **22**, 189–201

Tyrrell, S., Howel, D., Bark, M., Allibone, E. and Lilford, R.J. (1988) Should maternal alphafetoprotein estimation be carried out in centers where ultrasound screening is routine? A sensitivity analysis approach. *American Journal of Obstetrics and Gynecology*, **158**, 1092

Udvarhelyi, G.B. and Epstein, M.H. (1975) The so-called Dandy-Walker syndrome. Analysis of 12 operated cases. *Child's Brain*, **1**, 158

Verco, P.W. and LeQuesne, G.W. (1987) Agenesis of the corpus callosum in fetus, neonate and infant. *Australas Radiology*, **31**, 129–135

Vintzileos, A.M., Cambell, W.A., Weinbaum, P.J. and Nochimson, D.J. (1987a) Perinatal management and outcome of fetal ventriculomegaly. *Obstetrics and Gynecology*, **69**, 5–11

Vintzileos, A.M., Cambell, W.A., Weinbaum, P.J. and Nochimson, D.J. (1987b) Antenatal evaluation and management of ultrasonically detected fetal anomalies. *Obstetrics and Gynecology*, **69**, 640

Warkany, J. (1971) Microcephaly congenital malformations. *Chicago Year Book*. Medical publishers 237–244

Williamson, R.A., Schauberger, C.W., Varner, M.W. and Ascuenbrener, C.A. (1984) Heterogeneity of pre-natal onset hydrocephalus: management and counselling implications. *American Journal of Medical Genetics*, **17**, 497–508

Chapter 2

Extra-craniospinal anomalies (excluding renal system)

F.C. Bryce, R.J. Lilford and C. Rodeck

Introduction

Most significant extra-craniospinal morphological abnormalities can now be diagnosed by ultrasonography during the antenatal period. Some can only occasionally be diagnosed by ultrasound, while others may only be easily detectable in the third trimester. For example, current real-time ultrasound equipment does not permit an accurate diagnosis of most cardiac anomalies until the middle of pregnancy and other anomalies, e.g. duodenal atresia may not manifest themselves until later still, (although the stomach vesicle can be viewed as early as 16 weeks' gestational age, the quantity of amniotic fluid swallowed at this gestation is only 2–7 ml/day). In general, anomalies which are viewed directly (e.g. exomphalos) are diagnosable earlier than those where diagnosis relies on secondary effects (e.g. obstruction to flow in duodenal atresia) or differential growth ratios (achondroplasia, microcephaly). Nevertheless, there are exceptions to this rule, especially in the renal tract where dilatation of the bladder or ureters with oligohydramnios may be apparent well before the middle of pregnancy (*see* Chapter 3). Similarly the lethal limb reductive deformities (e.g. type 2 osteogenesis imperfecta and thanatophoric dwarfism) can be detected at approximately 16 weeks' gestational age.

Once the best possible diagnosis of an anatomical anomaly has been made, the therapeutic options will depend on parental wishes. These in turn depend on the possible prognosis, and it is prognosis rather than diagnosis which is required by the prenatal diagnostician who must be able to provide the patient with the information about the short- and long-term outlook and the surgical treatments which may be available. We present a collection of commonly diagnosed extra-cranial anomalies and review the expected prognosis for these conditions when diagnosed antenatally. As is the case with central nervous system abnormalities, karyotyping may enable an improved prognosis to be given. For example isolated hydro- or (chylo-) thorax has a good prognosis, i.e. it may disappear spontaneously or may require *in-utero* drainage if severe. Nevertheless, this appearance is associated with Down's syndrome and parents will often wish to exclude this diagnosis before deciding on further options.

Congenital gastrointestinal anomalies

The gastrointestinal tract is a common site for congenital defects, in many cases ultrasonic demonstration of these anomalies is possible and surgical correction after birth is often successful. The anomalies which most commonly present are:

oesophageal atresia   1:1500 – 2500 births
exomphalos and gastroschisis   1:2500 – 10000 births
congenital duodenal atresia   1:2700 – 10000 births.

A number of rarer anomalies such as diaphragmatic hernia and distal atresia of the intestine may be diagnosed antenatally. Fetal ascites is a more common finding which we discuss later.

Proximal intestinal obstruction

Duodenal atresia

This is the most common of the fetal small bowel atresias. It is associated with preterm delivery in 54% of cases and hydramnios in 45%. Like many other congenital abnormalities, the prognosis is strongly influenced by the presence of associated anomalies which are present in 48% of affected infants (Loveday, Barr and Aitken, 1975). The most common of these are trisomy 21 (30%), malrotation of gut (22%) and congenital heart disease (20%). Prenatal diagnosis of duodenal atresia is feasible and was first reported by Loveday, Barr and Aitken (1975) who noticed the 'double vesicle' sign (Figure 2.1). False negative diagnosis is possible

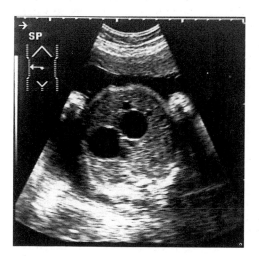 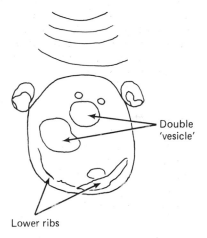

Figure 2.1 The 'double vesicle' in duodenal atresia

and Nelson *et al.* (1982) reported two cases where serial ultrasound scans had been entirely normal throughout the second trimester. Most cases are diagnosed after 24 weeks' gestation, but Baker, Grant and Bieber (1984) reported one case diagnosed at 22 weeks' gestational age and Miro and Baird (1988) reported a further case which was suspected at 20 weeks' but not confirmed until 35 weeks' gestation.

Prenatal diagnosis is generally made too late for termination of pregnancy, but the parents may be prepared for the possibility of associated multiple malformations or chromosomal abnormalities. Parents should decide whether to have prenatal diagnosis to exclude Down's syndrome but the point should be made that it is not clear how prenatal detection of Down's syndrome in late pregnancy should influence obstetric management. It does not follow, for example, that this knowledge should affect intrapartum care in the case of fetal distress. Failure to intervene in such cases will not necessarily result in fetal death, but may compound the disability of Down's syndrome with superadded hypoxic cerebral damage. Thus, the most cogent basis for the offer of an invasive prenatal diagnostic test to exclude Down's syndrome is to give parents an opportunity to prepare themselves for this possible diagnosis. We are persuaded by the argument that the moment of birth is often best separated from the moment of diagnosis. Amniocentesis may also help in the diagnosis, since bile acids and optical denisty are increased in this abnormality (Deleze, Sideropoulos and Paumgartner, 1977).

Prognosis

Early surgical correction of duodenal atresia has a survival rate of 90% and results are even better in the absence of associated defects.

Two recent reports from Miro and Baird (1988) and Romero *et al.* (1988), suggest that prenatal diagnosis of duodenal atresia may contribute to improving the outlook of affected infants (Table 2.1) by reducing the incidence of pneumonia,

Table 2.1 Outcome of antenatal diagnosis versus postnatal diagnosis in duodenal atresia

Author	Number of cases	Associated anomalies	Comments
Miro and Baird (1988)	26 12 (prenatal diagnosis)	38.5% 6 – trisomy 21 3 – cardiac malformation 1 – tracheo-oesophageal fistula	Showed definite benefit of prenatal diagnosis with less metabolic disturbances and less delay before surgery
Romero *et al.* (1988)	18 11 (prenatal diagnosis)	6 – trisomy 21 1 – cardiac anomaly 1 – neural tube defect 1 – diaphragmatic hernia	All infants diagnosed in prenatal period treated immediately. No preoperative or postoperative complications. 5 of 7 cases diagnosed neonatally developed metabolic complications attributable to duodenal atresia

hypovolaemia and hypokalaemic alkalosis. The risk of recurrence in subsequent pregnancies is less than 1:100 and the risk for the offspring of an affected parent is of a similar magnitude. The fetus with congenital obstruction of the gut at a high level may also be at risk of intrauterine growth retardation (Cozzi and Wilkinson, 1969; Pierro *et al.*, 1987). Various theories have been advanced, such as reduced capacity of intestinal absorption of amniotic fluid or reduced nutrition of the fetus via the alimentary tract, although this explanation sounds facile to us.

Oesophageal atresia

Hobbins *et al.* (1979) suggested that the inability to detect fetal stomach or loops of intestine ultrasonically, along with hydramnios, should alert the obstetrician to the possibility of oesophageal atresia. However, cases of oesophageal atresia often have a fistula between respiratory tract and gastrointestinal tract, distal to the oesophageal obstruction and this will permit a variable amount of amniotic fluid to enter the fetal stomach. Isolated reports of *in-utero* diagnosis appear in the literature, but along with these are cases where antenatal detection was not feasible. Like other obstructions of the upper gastrointestinal tract, *in-utero* diagnosis is probably beneficial to the neonate as it enables immediate suction of the upper pouch to be carried out after delivery and feeding to be withheld, so that aspiration pneumonia can be prevented.

Prognosis

In a large series reported by Spitz, Kiely and Brereton (1987), the outcome for 148 infants with oesophageal atresia (none diagnosed antenatally) has been reviewed – 47% of these patients had associated abnormalities; 21.6% cardiovascular, 12.2% gastrointestinal, 16.8% anorectal, 12.2% genitourinary, and 3% chromosomal. Mortality in the group studied was directly related to the severity of associated anomalies, especially those of the heart. Survival rates depended on the type of lesion; 100% survival was reported for proximal oesophageal atresia with distal oesophageal fistula; 86% for proximal oesophageal fistula; 23% for cases with both distal and proximal fistulae. The overall survival rate was 85.1%. It should be noted that in 90% of cases of oesophageal atresia, only one major operation is required, but 10% have an atretic segment and these are managed by a two-stage procedure. The initial operation enables direct intragastric feeding and a pharyngeal stoma is created so that sham feeding can be practised in order that the skill of swallowing is still retained. Definitive surgery is then carried out at about 1 year of age. Even in cases where primary anastomosis is possible, there is a significant incidence of stricture which may require dilatation during childhood.

Distal intestinal obstruction

Obstruction distal to the ligament of Treitz is more difficult to diagnose during the antenatal period, but this is sometimes possible when multiple echo-free areas are observed in the abdomen. They can be distinguished from renal cysts by their position and the presence of peristalsis. In contrast to duodenal atresia, intestinal atresia is infrequently associated with other anomalies; 2% are found to have trisomy 21 and 2% cardiovascular abnormalities.

Following diagnosis of a lower gastrointestinal tract obstruction, careful monitoring of the pregnancy must be considered as there is a possibility of perforation and meconium peritonitis, which may manifest with the sudden onset of fetal ascites. Meconium begins to accumulate in the fetal bowel from the fourth month of gestation and if perforation occurs, large amounts of meconium may escape into the peritoneal cavity and form a meconium pseudocyst. This is demonstrated ultrasonically as an echo-free mass with irregular walls formed by matted coils of intestine. In general, obstruction of the distal gastrointestinal tract will not influence timing or mode of delivery.

Prognosis

Providing no other congenital anomalies are detected the parents can be given a good prognosis with surgery.

Congenital diaphragmatic hernia

Three features on the ultrasound examination may indicate the presence of a congenital diaphragmatic hernia (CDH):

1. polyhydramnios
2. shift of the mediastinum
3. absence of an intra-abdominal stomach, with demonstration of abdominal organs in the thorax usually on the left side (Figure 2.2).

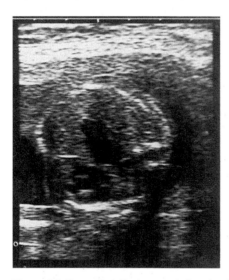
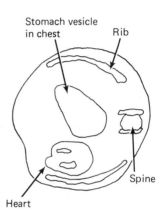

Figure 2.2 Congenital diaphragmatic hernia with stomach displaced into chest, alongside the heart

Routine ultrasound examination at 18 weeks' gestation is nevertheless an insensitive diagnostic method for diaphragmatic hernia. Harrison *et al.* (1986), reported normal ultrasound examination in three affected fetuses scanned serially at 20, 26 and 38 weeks' gestation. It is noteworthy that in contrast to the general poor prognosis, all three of these infants survived and it has been suggested that such cases missed by ultrasound are more likely to have either late gestational herniation of viscera or smaller diaphragmatic defects with relatively little thoracic displacement. The latter explanation is more plausible in terms of embryology. False-positive diagnosis is uncommon. We have encountered this in one case (ascertained in the third trimester) which turned out to have congenital eventration of the diaphragm.

Prognosis
Overall mortality for antenatally diagnosed cases is 80%. Prognosis is influenced by three sonographic features:

1. the presence of polyhydramnios
2. the size of the defect (i.e. the amount of abdominal content in the chest)
3. displacement of the heart (also a reflection on the amount of herniated viscera)
4. alteration in the relative sizes of right and left ventricles.

The aetiology of polyhydramnios is unclear, but it is postulated that it is caused by impaired fetal swallowing of amniotic fluid due to the compression or twisting of the oesophagus by herniated abdominal organs. Adzick *et al.* (1985) reported 82 cases of antenatally diagnosed congenital diaphragmatic hernia, 62 cases were diagnosed to have polyhydramnios and only 11% of these survived; 55% of the 20 remaining cases survived. Polyhydramnios may not develop until the third trimester and the absence of this feature should not give too much encouragement in early pregnancy. The presence of a large defect with a large quantity of fetal gut displaced into the thorax is also associated with a poor prognosis as this is strongly associated with pulmonary hypoplasia, the main cause of death in infants with CDH. Neonates with severe pulmonary hypoplasia will not survive, even with prompt surgical correction and optimal neonatal care. The pathogenesis of pulmonary hypoplasia is most probably the result of compression of the developing lung by fetal gut.

Iritani (1984) and more recently Bohn *et al.* (1987) and Sakai *et al.* (1987) have proposed that the primary pathological mechanism for development of congenital diaphragmatic hernia is inhibition of growth of the embryonic lung and that the diaphragmatic defect is a secondary phenomenon. We disagree with this

Table 2.2 Diaphragmatic hernia. Outcome following antenatal diagnosis

Author	Number of cases	Mortality (%)	Findings	Outcome
Sarda *et al.* (1983)	2	100	Both diagnosed antenatally at 17 and 21 weeks	Both died following surgery
Jouppila and Kirkinen (1984)	7	85	Diagnosed antenatally	2 – associated anomalies, died 2 – still born 3 – surgical treatment in first 24 h, only 1 survived
Adzick *et al.* (1985)	94	80	88 – prenatal diagnosis	North American survey on CDH 19 – survived (20%) 27 – prenatal or preoperative death (50% congenital abnormality) 46 – postoperative death 2 – interoperative death 89% of those with polyhydramnios died
Barss, Benacerraf and Frigoletto (1985)	1	100	Diagnosed at 29 weeks	Died of pulmonary hypoplasia
Grisoni *et al.* (1986)	6	66	All diagnosed antenatally	2 – with associated omphalocoele – died 2 – with large defects and pulmonary hypoplasia died 2 – survived surgery
Nakayoma *et al.* (1985)	20	75	9 – cases antenatal detection 11 – not detected	15 – died All 9 cases diagnosed antenatally died 11 false negative. No false positive on antenatal diagnosis

Table 2.3 Diaphragmatic hernia. Outcome following postnatal diagnosis

Author	Number of cases	Mortality (%)	Comments
Dibbins and Wiener (1974)	20	60	All diagnosed before 24 h of age. 6 of the 8 survivors had minimal pulmonary hypoplasia
Harrison *et al.* (1978)	70	66	37 died. Of those that died 34 presented before 24 h of age and had no treatment. 33 had treatment, 10 of whom died
Shochat *et al.* (1979)	18	38	All infants operated on in first 24 h of life
Sumner and Frank (1981)	4	0	All presented cyanosed at birth. Immediate repair of defect undertaken
Marshall and Sumner (1982)	62	33	All cases had primary repair. Of those presenting after 6 h of age 22 (100%) survived
Puri and Gorman (1984)	36	97	11 still births diagnosed at autopsy. 25 live births 15 died prior to transfer 10 had surgery and 9 died All still births had associated lethal pulmonary abnormality
Hamson *et al.* (1984)	75	43	Outcome is that reported following corrective surgery in first 24 h of life

hypothesis, since maldevelopment of one lung is not fatal and the poor prognosis of CDH is most plausibly related to compression of both lungs. Nevertheless, *in-utero* surgery to correct CDH, technical problems aside, will not necessarily correct the lung defect which may be irreversible before such surgery can be contemplated. Harrison, Ross and de Lorimier (1981) reported successful experimental outcomes of fetal surgery in the lamb, but simulated CDH was induced relatively late in pregnancy, by which time the lung buds would already be almost developed. At least three attempts at correction surgery have been made on the human fetus but none of the patients has survived the neonatal period. Other congenital defects are associated with CDH although reported incidence varies considerably. About 5% will have trisomy 18 or partial tetrasomy of the short arm of chromosome 12 (Pallister Killian syndrome, *see* Chapter 6).

In summary the mortality rate for antenatally diagnosed CDH is 80% even in the best centres. It is possible to individualize. We offer a probability of survival of about 50% if there is no polyhydramnios and a small amount of bowel in the chest, and a prognosis of about 10% survival if many adverse factors are present. Invasive karyotyping may be offered, but again we think that this is most appropriate for those people who:

1. do not wish termination of pregnancy anyway
2. who would wish termination, but only if they could be certain that the prognosis was hopeless. We discuss the appropriate action for rapid karyotyping (*see* Chapter 6).

The management of pregnancy will depend on the severity of the lesion, the stage of gestation when the diagnosis is made and the presence of associated anomalies, in particular polyhydramnios. If the parents decide to continue the pregnancy, then there is no advantage for abdominal or elective premature delivery. We favour *in-utero* transfer to a unit specializing in neonatal surgery.

Tables 2.2 and 2.3 show that antenatal diagnosis has contributed little to improving outcome with that reported in the standard surgical literature and that our probabilistic mortality estimates are realistic.

Abdominal wall defects

Gastroschisis and omphalocoele (exomphalos)

Omphalocoele and gastroschisis are congenital ventral wall defects with herniation of the abdominal viscera. However, they have very different prognostic implications. The birth prevalence reported by Baird and MacDonald (1981) in a review of over 500 000 live births was 0.08/1000 for gastroschisis and 0.21/1000 for omphalocoele. Hauge *et al.* (1983) documented a prevalence among still births and live births combined of 0.19/1000 and 0.14/1000 for omphalocoele and gastroschisis respectively.

Embryologically, the congenital defect of omphalocoele arises from a primary failure of the lateral cephalic and caudal folds to form the umbilical ring. If the cephalic fold fails to progress, the defect is associated with abnormalities in the diaphragm and ectopia cordis. If the caudal folds fail to progress, the omphalocoele may be associated with imperforated anus or extrophy of the bladder. The most common defect arises from failure of fusion of the lateral folds resulting in a large central omphalocoele – the eviscerated organs are usually small intestine and liver covered by a sac of peritoneum and amnion.

Gastroschisis arises from a defect between two normal rectus muscles. The primary body folds develop normally, forming the umbilical ring at 21 days. At 35 – 50 days the intestine normally elongates and enters the umbilical cord. In gastroschisis the intestine ruptures out of the base of the cord, possibly because of a failure of formation of the umbilical coelom. The rupture is usually on the right (as the right umbilical vein has become absorbed leaving a slight defect on the right of the umbilical cord). Unlike omphalocoele, only intestine is extruded and this lies free in the amniotic cavity. This may lead to inflammation of the intestinal walls which become matted together. Incomplete strangulation is also said to lead to exudation and matting.

Antenatal diagnosis of a ventral wall defect is possible as early as 12 – 13 weeks of gestation. By 18 weeks' gestation it should be possible to demonstrate whether the herniated viscera are surrounded by an amnioperitoneal membrane (omphalocoele) or floating freely (gastroschisis) (Figure 2.3). If omphalocoele is suspected, examination of the transverse sagittal and coronal views will help in defining the integrity of the ventral diaphragm, sternum, heart, bladder and site of lesion with respect to the umbilical ring. Omphalocoele, especially if large, is often associated with kinking of the spine, and this appearance does not necessarily imply spina bifida. Occasionally omphalocoele may herniate through the covering membrane, but it remains a central defect rather than herniation alongside the cord, as in gastroschisis.

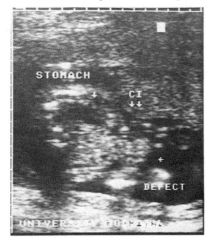
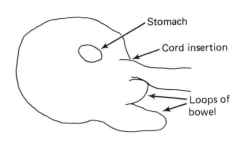

Figure 2.3 Gastroschisis showing free loops of bowel

Associated anomalies are common in the case of omphalocoele but not gastroschisis. This was confirmed in a review by Moore and Nar (1986) which consisted of 490 cases of gastroschisis (203) and omphalocoele (287). None of the cases of gastroschisis had associated extra-abdominal malformations, while these were present in over half the cases of omphalocoele: 74% of these were multiple and 14% were part of a named syndrome, 4% of all cases of omphalocoele had chromosomal trisomies and 16% had cardiac malformations which were usually severe and multiple. The largest number of malformations involved the musculoskeletal and central nervous systems. A more recent report of 35 prenatally diagnosed cases of omphalocoele (Gilbert and Nicolaides, 1987) showed 54% to have chromosomal abnormalities (17 trisomy 18, 1 triploidy, 1 Klinefelter's syndrome). It is common for the incidence of chromosomal abnormalities to be higher in a series diagnosed antenatally by ultrasound than in the paediatric surgical literature, because many cases with aneuploidy may be still born or die before referral in the early hours of life, while yet others are not referred because of the recognized poor prognosis. Structural anomalies were found in a total of 74% of fetuses, the most frequent (47%) being cardiac. Other studies, e.g. Carpenter *et al.* (1984), confirm the high rate of anomalies with omphalocoele in contrast to gastroschisis (Tables 2.4 and 2.5).

The frequent association of chromosomal abnormalities with omphalocoele, along with the relatively good prognosis if other anomalies are not present, suggests that patients should consider prenatal chromosome analysis. Gastroschisis is not a strong reason for termination of pregnancy, but omphalocoele, if very large (involving liver or bladder) or if associated with other anomalies, is good reason to offer termination of pregnancy.

Preterm labour is more common in these conditions, particularly in association with gastroschisis. The timing of delivery may be an important consideration. Tibboel *et al.* (1986) have suggested that bowel damage in cases of gastroschisis accelerates after 30 weeks' gestation due to changes in amniotic fluid osmolality and sodium, creatinine and urea concentrations. In addition, the abdominal wall defect becomes relatively smaller with advancing gestational age and this may lead

Table 2.4 Outcome following postnatal diagnosis of omphalocoele

Author	Number of cases	Anomalies	Outcome
Colombani and Cunningham (1977)	17	12 associated (71%). 59 concomitant 3 trisomies	Overall mortality 47%. In absence of associated or concomitant anomalies 20%. Reported increased risk with maternal age and increasing birth order
Stringel and Filler (1979)	74	38% associated anomalies 8 trisomies	Overall mortality 43% 66% – major anomalies 12% – minor or no associated anomaly
Mayer et al. (1980)	28	66% associated anomalies 40% trisomies	Mortality 34%
Grosfield, Daues and Weber (1981)	47	66% associated anomalies 6 trisomies	Overall mortality 27.6%
Baird and Macdonald (1981)	126	58% associated anomalies 8 trisomies 50% additional unrelated defects	Overall mortality not given
Klein, Kosloske and Hertzler (1981)	6	66% associated anomalies	50% mortality
Wladimiroff et al. (1984a)	46	78% associated defects	63% mortality
Kirk and Wah (1983)	38	42% major 13% minor	29% mortality
Carpenter et al. (1984)	25	64% (16) 3 trisomies	40% mortality
Moore and Nar (1986)	287	14% (syndrome associated) 74% overall associated anomalies 12% trisomy (4%)	International survey of 16 paediatric surgery centres. Overall mortality not given

to compression of mesenteric vessels. For these reasons, elective preterm delivery has been suggested and Caesarean section has been advocated to allow precise timing of delivery and avoid further compression of fetal abdomen and bowel (Fitzsimmons et al., 1988). Davidson et al. (1984) and Kirk and Wah (1983) have questioned the benefit of elective Caesarean section on the basis of their review. The current literature would suggest that if a central wall defect is associated with another major anomaly or is present in a very low birthweight fetus, then the outcome is poor regardless of route of delivery and Caesarean section is not justified. However, if no other anomaly is present and the infant weighed over 1500 g, the baby should be delivered in a hospital in a neonatal unit and surgical correction should follow in 12 h. We are inclined to the view that:

1. delivery should not be brought forward before 37 weeks because any improvement in the condition of the intestine is more than offset by the disadvantage of prematurity

Table 2.5 Outcome following postnatal diagnosis of gastroschisis

Author	Numbers studied	Associated anomalies	Outcome
Colombani and Cunningham (1977)	20	20%	Overall mortality 40%. In absence of associated anomalies 31%. High incidence of growth retardation
Stringel and Filler (1979)	44	5%	High incidence of growth retardation. Overall mortality 27%
Mayer et al. (1980)	47	23% (main anomalies, bowel 15% and cardiac 8.5%)	High incidence of prematurity, 12.7%
King, Savrin and Bales (1980)	64	37% additional anomalies but only 9% of major significance	6% postoperative mortality
Baird and Macdonald (1981)	29	48%	Overall mortality not given
Klein, Kosloske and Hertzler (1981)	18	36% Defects all related to gastroschisis except 1 case with ventricular septal defect	Mortality 18%
Kirk and Wah (1983)	74	6.8% major additional anomalies	Mortality 13.5%
Carpenter et al. (1984)	13	1 case had additional defect	1 case died 10 cases had associated growth retardation
Moore and Nar (1986)	203	16% (6% non-digestive)	International survey of 16 paediatric surgical centres. Overall mortality not given
DiLorenzo, Yasbeck and Darharme (1987)	54	27% (10% non-digestive)	Overall mortality 13.6%

2. the vaginal route of delivery should be used unless there are separate indications for Caesarean section, such as breech presentation.

Prognosis

The outcome for gastroschisis is good. Kirk and Wah (1983) reported a mortality rate of 13.5% for infants with gastroschisis. The mortality for omphalocoele was 29% with a much smaller percentage undergoing surgery (*see below*). Carpenter *et al.* (1984) reported a mortality of 7.7% for gastroschisis. For infants with omphalocoele the mortality rate for cases with lateral or caudal fold defects was 18.8% compared with 78% for those with a cephalic fold defect. Thus, large defects containing a large portion of liver, have a much worse surgical prognosis. These patients may require multistage operations if the abdomen is unable to accommodate all of the herniated viscera in the first instance. The lungs may be

Table 2.6 Gastroschisis-omphalocoele (exomphalos): outcome following prenatal diagnosis

Author	Number	Associated anomalies	Outcome

Mann and Ferguson Smith (1984)	88
	16 gastroschisis
	72 omphalocoele
		37.5% gastroschisis
		No trisomies
		
		62% omphalocoele
		11% trisomy
			39 TOP
			20 spontaneous stillbirths
			29 live births:
			  5 gastroschisis – 1 died
			  24 omphalocoele – 10 died

Nakayama et al. (1984)	13
	  2 gastroschisis
	11 omphalocoele
		82% (9) of omphalocoele	Both gastroschisis survived
			82% mortality with
			  omphalocoele

Redford, McNay and Whittle (1985)	6 gastroschisis		All cases treated surgically following delivery. 50% mortality (3) 2 died from sepsis, 1 from respiratory distress syndrome

Jouppila and Kirkinen (1984)	5 omphalocoele
	
	5 gastroschisis
		80% had multiple associated anomalies All had trisomy 18
		All 5 cases had associated multiple anomalies (heart, CNS, lower limbs)
			4 died in utero
			1 born alive but died at 3 h
			
			All 5 died
			  4 in utero
			  1 survived 24 h

Barss, Benacerraf and Frigoletto (1985)	1 gastroschisis 3 omphalocoele	Detected at 20 weeks 1 – additional anomaly 1 – ascites 1 – omphalocoelectomy	Surgery at birth – survived 2 died 1 with no associated anomaly survived following surgery
Hasan and Hermonsan (1986)	47 9 detected antenatally: 5 omphalocoele 4 gastroschisis	65% omphalocoele 10% gastroschisis	Mortality 65% omphalocoele 13% gastroschisis
Grisoni et al. (1986)	2 gastroschisis 9 omphalocoele	No associated anomalies 8 had multiple associated anomalies	Both survived 6 died 3 survived surgery
Sermer et al. (1987)	25 17 omphalocoele 8 gastroschisis	71% omphalocoele 50% gastroschisis	Mortality 59% omphalocoele 38% gastroschisis
Gilbert and Nicolaides (1987)	35 omphalocoele	73% additional anomalies 47% congenital heart disease 17 trisomy 18 1 triploidy 1 Klinefelter's syndrome	63% elective TOP 11.4% died 25% survived
Fitzsimmons et al. (1988)	16 gastroschisis	1 had additional anomalies	1 antepartum death

TOP: termination of pregnancy

hypoplastic in the most severe cases. Togama (1972) found a similar poor survival rate in cases of cephalic fold defects. More recently DiLorenzo, Yazbeck and Darharme (1987) reported an overall mortality rate of 13.6% for gastroschisis and Fitzsimmons et al. (1988) reported 100% survival in 14 neonates with an antenatal diagnosis of gastroschisis. (See Tables 2.4, 2.5 and 2.6.)

In the cases of gastroschisis the intestinal damage might delay the onset of enteral feeding and parents should be warned that prolonged convalescence with intravenous feeding is sometimes required. They should also be warned that two-stage surgery may be necessary if the abdominal cavity cannot accommodate all the herniated viscera. DiLorenzo, Yazbeck and Darharme (1987) reported a 15-year experience of 59 cases of gastroschisis and these figures showed an increasing trend to attempt primary closure (32% primary closure attempted before 1978, 82.5% after 1978). The complication rate for primary closure was reported as 25.6% with a 12.8% mortality rate – interestingly in the higher birthweight group. In contrast the silicon pouch had a 75% complication rate with a 15% mortality and a considerably longer stay in hospital.

Other ventral defects

Body stalk anomaly results in direct fusion of the abdominal contents with the placenta and spinal skeletal deformities are due to the abnormal posture. The prognosis for this disorder, where the incidence is 1:15 000, is hopeless.

Bladder extrophy may occur in association with exomphalos or as an isolated defect. The latter, with an incidence of 1:30 000, is seldom diagnosed antenatally but repeated failure to identify a bladder is the cardinal ultrasound feature. Postnatal treatment is by urinary division or bladder repair but continence is seldom reported. The mortality rate is low for the isolated defects but very high for full cloacal extrophy.

Miscellaneous fetal intra-abdominal anomalies by ultrasound

Cystic fibrosis

Meconium ileus may be an important manifestation of cystic fibrosis in the fetus. Ultrasonically this may appear as enlarged bowel loops seen in the third trimester of pregnancy and a highly echogenic mass seen in the second and to a less extent in the third trimester. Several authors, Denholme et al. (1984), Muller et al. (1986), Papp et al. (1985), Boue et al. (1986), have described these echogenic intra-abdominal areas with subsequent confirmation of cystic fibrosis. The appearance is an almost certain sign of the disease if the parents are carriers but a highly echogenic mass seen in a fetal abdomen between 16 – 20 weeks' of gestation, in non-carrier parents may be associated with completely normal outcome. This appearance is therefore very difficult to interpret in the fetus of Caucasian parents with no history of cystic fibrosis. In the future the prior risk status of such parents may be determined by testing parents for high risk DNA markers which are in linkage disequilibrium with the abnormal gene or by testing for a deletion. In the meantime, our association with a handful of parents and informal consultations with colleagues inclines us against intervention on the basis of this ultrasound appearance when the parents are not known carriers.

Ovarian cysts

Fetal ovarian cysts are probably related to the FSH peak between 20 – 30 weeks' gestation. They are almost always benign (serous follicular cysts). In reported cases (Wilson, 1982; Babut *et al.*, 1983; Bourgeot and Cockenpot, 1985) the gestational age at the time of detection has been greater than 28 weeks' gestation. The typical appearance is a homogeneous echo-free mass in the hypochondrium and this is usually mobile during sonographic examination. *In-utero* torsion may occur (Bourgeot and Cockenpot, 1985; Gaudin *et al.*, 1988), with the appearance of intracystic flocculation followed by sedimentation and the appearance of a liquid interface. Smaller cysts (less than 50 mm) frequently resolve spontaneously. The differential diagnosis is of other intra-abdominal cysts such as those of the bile duct, pancreas, kidney or gut duplications or volvulus. Neonatal ovarian cysts are rarely associated with life-threatening complications and the method and timing of delivery should not be influenced by the ultrasound diagnosis. Treatment should be decided neonatally, cysts over 50 mm may be removed surgically or the cyst may be aspirated under ultrasonic control. Long-term morbidity and mortality are negligible.

Sacrococcygeal teratoma

Teratomas are the most commonly presenting tumours of newborns. Sacrococcygeal teratomas occur in approximately 1:40 000 live births (and nasopharyngeal lesions are rarer still). The lesions may be totally cystic (15%) but are more likely to be solid or mixed. Malignant change is possible and risk of this is quoted at 10% but rises to 65 – 90% if diagnosis and surgical excision are delayed beyond 4 months of age; 75 – 80% of tumours occur in females.

Antenatal diagnosis of this tumour using ultrasonography has been reported on a number of occasions. Ultrasound findings describe a hyperechoic solid or mixed solid cystic tumour mass of variable shape with occasional bizarre internal echoes. The lesion may extend into the abdomen around the lower end of the spine. A similar lesion seen on the back and loin consisting of multiple loculated cysts is the lumbosacral cystic hygroma. Spina bifida is associated with a vertebral lesion and is in the midline.

Those cases not diagnosed by routine ultrasound scan (USS) at 16 – 18 weeks generally present at 22 – 34 weeks' gestation with polyhydramnios. The literature suggests that cases detected after 30 weeks' gestation have a better prognosis than those that present symptomatically prior to 30 weeks. It has also been noted that the presence of placental enlargement and/or hydrops in association with fetal sacrococcygeal teratomas is highly predictive of fetal death. Associated congenital anomalies or chromosomal anomalies are rare.

Fetal death in cases of sacrococcygeal teratomas appear to result from the secondary effects of the tumour. Tumour mass and polyhydramnios give an increased risk of preterm labour and delivery. Massive haemorrhage into the tumour with secondary fetal exsanguination may occur spontaneously *in utero* or be precipitated by labour and delivery. Dystocia secondary to tumour bulk or tumour rupture may occur during either vaginal delivery or Caesarean section. Finally, placental hypertrophy and hydrops may be associated with high output cardiac

Table 2.7 Summary of findings and outcome in reported cases of sacrococcygeal teratoma

Author	Gestation at diagnosis (weeks)	Hydramnios	Placenta hypertrophy	Hydrops	Clinical course	Outcome
Santos Ramos and Duenhoeffer (1975)	Unknown	Unknown	Unknown	Unknown	Eclampsia Ruptured tumour	Died at birth
Sand and Brock (1976)	26	Yes	Yes	Yes	Terminated	Still born
	25	Yes	Yes	Yes	Induced abortion after intrauterine death	
Horger and McCarter (1979)	31	Yes	Unknown	No	Preterm labour 32 weeks – LSCS	Alive
Vermer et al. (1979)	24	Yes	Unknown	Unknown	Preterm labour LSCS	Still born
Cousins et al. (1980)	25	Yes	Yes	Yes	Eclampsia	Still born
Bendel and Alexander (1980)	30	Unknown	Unknown	No	Preterm labour 32 weeks – LSCS	Alive
Dabe et al. (1980)	30	Yes	Unknown	Unknown	Eclampsia LSCS	Alive
Gergley et al. (1980)	24	Yes	Yes	Yes	Preterm labour	Still born
Kohgac, Nambu and Tanaka (1980)	28	Yes	Yes	Yes	Induced abortion after intrauterine death	Died
	28	Yes	Yes	Yes	Induced abortion after intrauterine death	Died
Lees, Williamson and Brenbridge (1980)	31	Yes	No	No	Preterm labour Vaginal delivery	Died at birth
Seeds et al. (1982)	16	Unknown	No	No	Termination	
Feige et al. (1982)	25	Yes	Yes	Yes	Termination	

Zaleski, Cooperberg and Kliman (1982)	28	Unknown	Unknown	Unknown	Preterm labour / Vaginal delivery	Died at birth
Rayburn and Barr (1982)	34	Yes	Unknown	No	Elective LSCS 34 weeks	Alive
Hecht and Kaiser-Hecht (1982)	24	Yes	Unknown	Unknown	Preterm labour	Died *in utero*
Moerman *et al.* (1982)	28	Yes	Yes	Yes	LSCS	Died at birth
Mintz, Mennuti and Fishman (1983)	34	No	No	No	Aspiration LSCS	Alive
Brock, Richmond and Liston (1983)	19	Unknown	Unknown	Yes	Induced abortion after intrauterine death at 24 weeks	Died
Holzgreve, Mahoney and Guck, (1985)	19	Yes	No	No	Termination	
	22	Yes	No	No	Termination	
	20	Yes	No	No	Preterm labour 33 weeks – LSCS	Lumbosacral plexopathy
	24	Yes	Unknown	No	Preterm labour after intrauterine death	
	31	Yes	Yes	No	Elective LSCS at 32 weeks	Died after birth
	33	Yes	No	No	Pre-eclampsia 34 weeks – LSCS	Alive
Flake *et al.* (1986)	22	Yes	No	No	Preterm labour 28 weeks – LSCS	Died at birth
Grisoni *et al.* (1988)	30	Yes	Unknown	No	LSCS term	Survived
	24	Yes	Unknown	No	Vaginal delivery at 36 weeks	Survived
	35	No	Unknown	No	Vaginal delivery at 37 weeks	Survived
	26	No	Unknown	Yes	32 weeks – LSCS	Died at 2 h
	21	No	Unknown	Yes	28 weeks – LSCS	Died at 15 h
	26	No	Unknown	No	Vaginal delivery at 31 weeks	Died *in utero*
	32	No	Unknown	No	Vaginal delivery at 33 weeks	Survived

LSCS: Lower segment Caesarean section

failure. Mechanisms causing this may be anaemia from tumour haemorrhage, or the high blood flow requirement of the tumour with arteriovenous fistulization.

Grisoni *et al.* (1988) suggested that the ratio of body size to tumour size may have prognostic value. Overall mortality is about 45% (Table 2.7). We suggest that delivery should be carried out by Caesarean section as soon as lung maturity is adequate. Operative delivery may reduce the chances of dystocia or fetal exsanguination. The development of hydrops or placental hypertrophy would appear immediately to precede fetal death. *In-utero* surgery to debulk the tumour or to ligate an arteriovenous fistula is a possible development in the future as a treatment of high output cardiac failure.

Abnormalities of the musculoskeletal system

The most common anomalies of the musculoskeletal system may be logically divided into disorders of muscle and bone. Bone anomalies may be further analysed into disorders of number, size or mineralization. However, in many instances it is impossible to distinguish between the primary defect and the sequelae.

There are at least 21 types of skeletal dysplasia which are identifiable at birth and the majority can be detected *in utero*, although precise diagnosis is seldom possible (Hobbins *et al.*, 1979). It is, however, possible to separate the lethal from non-lethal deformities. For example when we encountered the severely shortened and bent long bones shown in Figure 2.4, we knew that we were dealing with a lethal condition. The differential diagnosis was between osteogenesis imperfecta type 2 (our first diagnosis), congenital hypophosphatasia and one of the severe dwarfing conditions, particularly camptomelic dwarfism which causes bowing of bones. We thought one of the first two diagnoses was most likely because of the

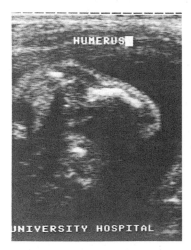
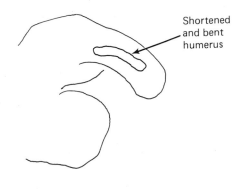

Figure 2.4 Severe shortening and bowing of long bone. Asymmetry and evidence of poor calcification of skull suggested osteogenesis imperfecta type II or hypophosphatasia, rather than a dwarfing condition with bowing, e.g. camptomelia. Either way, we were 99% certain the condition was lethal. Antenatal X-ray is not usually helpful until the third trimester

beaded ribs and decalcified skull, but this was academic since we were 99% certain that the condition was lethal. In this particular case the diagnosis was congenital hypophosphatasia.

In this section we deal mainly with the more dramatic conditions which may be discovered antenatally, often by chance, and which present difficulty in counselling. A large number of more subtle defects have been described in the literature but they are seldom chance findings. Like many abnormalities of the face, they are features for which a search should be made to exclude specific autosomal syndromes when relevant, e.g. thrombocytopenia with absent radius or the Jarcho-Levis syndrome (fused vertebrae and splayed ribs). In addition, polydactyly is an important feature of autosomal genetic disorders (e.g. Meckel syndrome, short rib-polydactyly syndrome) and trisomies 13, 4p and 10q.

Bone disorders

Disorders of the long bones

As a general rule the majority of the congenital syndromes that affect limb growth involve multiple segments, although some may have a predilection for certain bones, e.g. absence of radius in radial dysplasia and thrombocytopenia syndrome or short unequal femora and talipes in the femoral hypoplasia atypical facies syndrome. Most of the congenital syndromes have a defined inheritance (Table 2.8), either autosomal recessive or dominant. The latter may be regarded as new mutations if a parent is not affected and thanatophoric dwarfism is a good example. Anomalies may also be present in addition to shortening of the long bones, e.g. hydrocephalus, abnormal ribs, cleft lip or palate. In the absence of these specific features which might suggest a syndrome, it is seldom possible to diagnose the precise form of the condition *in utero*. This is not a great practical problem, as it is usually possible to distinguish the dwarfing conditions which are likely to be lethal, although two very rare examples (diastrophic dysplasia and chondroectodermal dysplasia) are not incompatible with survival. The main features demonstrated by ultrasonography of the fetal skeletal dysplasias are examined in Table 2.8. Inspection of the table will show that many of the dysplasias have similar features. The ultrasound examination should also include a careful search for defects in other systems and the presence of oligo- or polyhydramnios. In general, the more severe the anomaly the worse the prognosis and many may abort or die *in utero*. Those that survive until delivery may die due to respiratory insufficiency as a result of small thorax and pulmonary hypoplasia. A small number of patients with trisomy 13 or 18 may have skeletal dysplasias. Post-mortem examination (including X-ray) is the most important method for establishing a precise classification and therefore prediction of recurrence risks.

Details of skeletal dysplasias

Thanatophoric dysplasia
This is one of the commonest dysplasias with an incidence of approximately 1:6400. Unlike other dysplasias it is not inherited from affected parents nor in an autosomal recessive fashion. It is always lethal. *In-utero* diagnosis during the third trimester and more recently during the second trimester has been reported by Cremin and Shaff (1977), Camera, Dodero and DePascale (1984) and Elejalde and deElejalde

Table 2.8 Commonly described anomalies detected by skeletal dysplasias

Skeletal dysplasia	Inheritance	Limb lengths	Bone density	Shape	Associated findings	Outcome
Achondrogenesis	AR	Very short	Decreased		Hydrops	Lethal
Thanatophoric dysplasia	? (AD)	>2 s.d. at 20 weeks (below mean)	Decreased spine ossification	Bowed telephone receiver femora	Hydramnios Excess skin Hydrops Small thorax – very short ribs	Lethal Death due to pulmonary hypoplasia
Short rib polydactyly Type I	AR	Very short	Slightly decreased		Polydactyly Occasional transposition of great vessels Polycystic kidneys Occasional hydrops	Lethal
Type II	AR	>2 s.d. at 16 weeks (below mean)	Normal	Bowed long bones	Polydactyly Occasional transposition	Lethal
Camptomelic dysplasia	AR	> s.d. at 16 weeks (below mean)	Decreased	Bowed long bones	50% of chromosomal males demonstrate female external genitalia Small scapulae Ventriculomegaly Cleft palate	Neonatal death Respiratory insufficiency
Achondroplasia heterozygous	AD 85% new mutations	Femur 50% at 18 weeks 30% at 20 weeks <1% at 22 weeks Upper limbs – mild shortening only	Normal		Megalocephaly Ventriculomegaly	Survive Rhizomelic dwarf

Achondroplasia (homozygous)	AR	Femur <1% at 18 weeks Humerus very short. Other limbs shortened Earlier shortening than heterozygote		Megacephaly Ventriculomegaly Very small thorax	Early death due to respiratory insufficiency
Diastrophic dysplasia	AR	>3 s.d. at 16 weeks (below mean)	Bowed long bones	Cleft lip Micrognathia Scoliosis Talipes 'hitchhiker thumbs'	25% mortality in early infancy
Chondroectodermal dysplasia		Femur >2 s.d. at 17 weeks (below mean)	Normal	Polydactyly Short ribs, small thorax 50% atrioseptal defect	50% lethal pulmonary hypoplasia
Osteogenesis imperfecta I	AD	Femur >1.4 s.d. (below mean) Other limbs short	Decreased	Bowed femora at 24 weeks	10% intrauterine fractures	Survive
II	AR 20% 80% new mutation	Limbs >2 s.d. at 16 weeks	Markedly decreased	Severe bowing	Multiple fractures Thin indentable skull Beaded ribs Raised pyrophosphate	Lethal
III	AR	Femur normal at 15 weeks. >2 s.d. at 19 weeks (below mean)	Decreased	Severe bowing	Intrauterine fractures	Most die in childhood with cardiorespiratory defects
IV	AD		Decreased	Marked bowing	Fractures potentially increased with age	Survive

AR: autosomal recessive
AD: autosomal dominant

(1985). Characteristically the ribs and long bones are extremely short. The vertebral bodies are also reduced in height. Thanatophoric dysplasia is associated with clover-leaf skull, which consists of hydrocephalus and congenital synostosis. The limbs may be so severely shortened that it is difficult to identify the individual bones. The chest is small with consequent pulmonary hypoplasia and polyhydramnios is common.

Camptomelic dysplasia

This is a lethal autosomal recessive skeletal dysplasia characterized by severe bowing (camptomelia) of the tibulae and mild bowing of femora, hypoplastic or absent fibulae and shortening of all long bones. Talipes equinovarus, hypoplastic scapulae and small thorax are also prominent features. Male infants may be feminized. The great majority of these infants die as neonates from cardiorespiratory failure.

Achondroplasia

Achondroplasia may be hetero- or homozygous. Heterozygous achrondroplasia is an autosomal dominant condition distinguished by shortening of the proximal long bones (rhizomelia), lumbar lordosis and mega-encephaly; the typical 'circus dwarf'. Hydrocephaly may be present in some cases – 65 – 85% of cases are new mutations. Leonard, Sanders and Lau (1979) and Filley et al. (1981), plotted femur length against biparietal diameter in three affected fetuses and observed the slope of the growth curve to be normal until 20 weeks of gestation with a dramatic fall to less than the first percentile by 24 weeks. Likewise, Kurtz and Wapner (1983) noted mean femur lengths at the 50th percentile at 17 weeks, 30th percentile at 20 weeks and the first percentile at 24 weeks, suggesting the prenatal diagnosis is best achieved by documenting sequential fetal limb measurements during the second trimester of pregnancy. The main importance of prenatal diagnosis is to separate this heterozygous condition from the homozygous form when both parents are carriers.

Homozygous achondroplasia results in early death from respiratory insufficiency, secondary to an extremely small thorax. Hydrocephaly may be more pronounced. Bowie (1982) observed a decreased femur length to biparietal diameter (BPD) ratio at the earlier gestational age of 18 weeks. It appears that this condition can be distinguished reliably from the heterozygous form and this is very important when both parents are carriers.

Diastrophic dysplasia

This is another autosomal recessive disorder characterized by short tubular bones (especially the first metacarpal), talipes equinovarus, severely abducted (hitchhiker) thumbs, hypertrophied auricular cartilage and progressive scoliosis. The mortality rate in infancy is 25%. O'Brien, Rodeck and Queenon (1980) made the first antenatal diagnosis by detecting short femurs at 14 weeks' gestation and subsequently demonstrated micrognathia and cleft lip and palate by fetoscopy. Mantagos et al. (1981) noted severe rhizomelic and acromelic limb shortening with femur length over four standard deviations below the mean at 20 weeks. Wladimiroff et al. (1984b) diagnosed the disorder following the appearance of severe shortening and bowing of all long bones with femur, humerus, tibia and fibula, radius and ulna all more than three standard deviations below the mean.

Chondro-ectodermal dysplasia

Another autosomal recessive condition characterized by short-limbed dysplasia (especially in the distal portions of the extremities), polydactyly, hypoplastic nails and dental anomalies. The condition is lethal in 50% of cases due to pulmonary hypoplasia and cardiac anomalies. Mahoney and Hobbins (1977) diagnosed the condition at 17 weeks' gestation, in a fetus with humerus and femur lengths more than two standard deviations below the mean.

Asphyxiating thoracic dystrophy (Jeune syndrome)

Yet another autosomal recessive condition characterized by a small thorax, short extremities (especially metacarpals, ulnae and fibulae). Pulmonary hypoplasia and renal dysplasia are common. Pulmonary hypoplasia leads to death in over 70% of cases. Lipson et al. (1984) reported femur lengths over two standard deviations below the mean at 16, 18 and 23 weeks. Mild bowing of the femora has also been observed. Elejalde, deElejalde and Pansch (1985) reported all limb lengths between the fifth and 25th percentile at 14 weeks and, at 18 weeks, measurements of the ulna, radius, tibia and fibula were all less than the third centile. Humerus and femur lengths, however, were at the fifth and 25th centiles respectively. Bowing was apparent in all long bones by 18 weeks.

Disorders of long bone growth and mineralization

Achondrogenesis

Achondrogenesis is another severe autosomal recessive lethal defect involving the limbs. Its presentation is essentially the same as thanatophoric dysplasia but it is much less common. Unlike the skeletal dysplasias described above, achondrogenesis involves not only shortening of the long bones but also deficient ossification, most notably in the vertebrae, bones of pelvic girdle and the ribs. Smith, Breitweiser and Dinno (1981) reported the first case detected sonographically and demonstrated short extremities and cranial achondrogenesis. Clearly these features are similar not only to thanatophoric and camptomelic dwarfism (which are also lethal) but also to type 2 (lethal) osteogenesis imperfecta. The genetics of these conditions are different and they must therefore be distinguished at post-mortem X-ray and examination.

Disorders of mineralization

Hypophosphatasia

This is another autosomal recessive condition with a varying outcome ranging from intrauterine death to a small degree of handicap in adulthood. The disorder is characterized by varying degrees of deficient bone mineralization. The bones may appear bowed with multiple fractures but severe shortening of the bone is not a typical finding; only the neonatal lethal form is important to the obstetrician and this can be diagnosed reliably as a lethal bone abnormality by ultrasound in utero and this is important to confirm apparently normal enzyme activities in first trimester chorion samples (Blau et al., 1985).

Osteogenesis imperfecta

Four types of osteogenesis imperfecta have been defined (Sillence, Senn and Danks, 1979).

Type I   The commonest type is Type I or osteogenesis imperfecta tarda levis. This is inherited as an autosomal dominant disease, characterized by osteoporosis, excessive bone fragility and blue sclerae. Antenatal ultrasound findings have been reported – Hobbins, Bracken and Mahoney (1982) documented femur lengths of 1.4 standard deviations below the mean at 19 weeks and visualized a femoral fracture (up to 10% of affected neonates may have fractures at delivery). Chervenak *et al.* (1982) noted femur lengths at 20 weeks to be 1.5 standard deviations below the mean, the femurs were noted to be bowed at 24 weeks and demineralized at 32 weeks.

Type II   This invariably lethal condition is autosomal recessive (Type IIb) in about 20% of cases and dominant (Type IIa) in the remainder. The latter are obviously new mutations and gonadal mosaicism (rather than 20% recessive inheritance) may explain the overall 5% recurrence rate. Characteristic findings are severe osteopenia and bone fragility, causing the long bones to appear crumpled and shortened, with the thighs fixed at right angles to the trunk. The skull is soft and easily deformable, the ribs appear beaded secondary to the callus to multiple healed fractures. This condition can be reliably diagnosed at least as a lethal bone disorder in the first half of pregnancy with no complete false-negative diagnosis reported.

Type III   This is autosomal recessive and characterized by extreme bone fragility. Most cases succumb during childhood due to cardiorespiratory complications. The reliability of antenatal diagnosis is not known. Aylsworth *et al.* (1984) reported normal findings at 10.5 weeks and 16 weeks, while at 19 weeks both femurs appeared bowed with shortened tibiae, fibulae, humeri, radii and ulnae.

Type IV   Type IV is an autosomal dominant condition notable for mild bone fragility and normal sclera. Significant limb bowing at birth may present as the only manifestation of the syndrome. At present there are no reports of antenatal diagnosis of the syndrome.

Disorders of the muscular system

The most frequent muscular disorders are Duchenne muscular dystrophy, facio-scapulo-humeral dystrophy, limb girdle musculodystrophy, distal and ocular myopathy and the oculopharyngeal muscular dystrophy. Antenatal diagnosis of these conditions by ultrasonography is not possible and diagnosis will depend on biochemical or chromosomal analysis, although this is limited to a very small number of conditions.

One exception is arthrogryposis multiplex congenita, which results from abnormal development of muscles and produces a characteristic stiffness of joints. Ultrasonically, abnormal positioning of the joints is observed, including internal rotation of the femur with hyperflexion or contraction of knee and elbow joints.

Cardiac abnormalities

Cardiac anomalies can be divided into those of structure and those of rhythm, although the latter are often caused by structural defects. Eighty-five per cent of

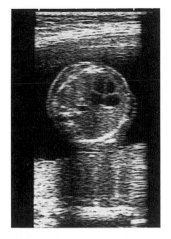
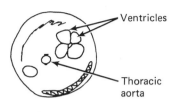

Figure 2.5 Four chamber, transverse view of heart obtained in routine screening. Longitudinal views to check connections to the great arteries are more difficult to obtain, especially in a highly mobile fetus at 18 weeks' gestational age. Sixty per cent of serious anomalies can be excluded by a four-chamber view. One half to 1% of babies are born with congenital heart disease and this rises to about 2% if a first line relative is affected and 10% if two first degree relatives are affected. If more than two first degree relatives have a defect then the condition can be regarded as autosomal dominant. Recurrences occur in the same form in half of the cases. Some anomalies (ventricular septal defect (VSD), atrial septal defect (ASD), Fallot's tetrology) appear to have a higher recurrence risk (3%) than others (coarctation and transposition – 2%; Ebstein's anomaly and tricuspid atresia – 1%). Colour Doppler is helpful in diagnosis of heart abnormalities in high risk patients

abnormalities occur without any obvious predisposing factors and routine screening consists essentially of examination of the standard four-chamber view (Figure 2.5). High risk groups include those with a family history (*see* Figure 2.5), diabetes, hydrops, arrhythmia, lithium (Ebstein's anomaly), alcohol and phenytoin (VSD), coxsackie B virus and rubella infection and associated abnormalities, e.g. omphalocoele, spina bifida.

Structural heart defects

Some major structural abnormalities are diagnosed reliably. These include single atrium or large atrial septal defects, muscular ventricular septal defects, hypoplasia or single ventricles, Ebstein's anomaly, ectopia cordis and tumours. Other anomalies are difficult to detect or classify including tetralogy of Fallot, anomalous venous return, aortic and pulmonary stenosis, transposition of vessels and small septal defects. From the practical point of view anomalies may be divided into four prognostic groups assuming that expert cardiac surgery is available. Those where prognosis is:

1. almost hopeless with less than 10% survival to adolescence (ectopia cordis, severe aortic stenosis, hypoplastic left ventricle)
2. bad with 10–50% survival (hypoplastic right ventricle)

3. reasonable with 50–90% survival (atrioventricular septal defects, single ventricle, Ebstein's anomaly, tetralogy of Fallot, transposition of vessels)
4. good with over 90% survival (most septal defects).

Where reliable detection is possible a fairly accurate prognosis can be given, e.g. hypoplastic ventricle. Very often, however, ultrasound will reveal an anomaly but the haemodynamic severity and presence of other features will be difficult or impossible to determine. For example, with care and skill it is possible to trace the ventriculo-arterial connections, especially if the fetus is in a suitable position, and make a diagnosis of transposition of the great arteries. The prognosis, however, depends on other features which are seldom detectable ultrasonically, e.g. pulmonary stenosis, aortic coarctation or transposed connection of the atria and ventricles (so-called corrected transposition). In this example we would give a prognosis of 50–90% to cover the more benign and serious forms of the disease. Routine scanning will often miss cardiac lesions, especially those which do not disrupt the cuspid valves or intraventricular septa. These structures are seen on the standard four-chamber (cross-sectional) view. Expert cardiac scanning should be carried out when:

1. congenital heart disease has occurred in a first degree relative
2. a suspicious cardiac scan was noted
3. the heart is enlarged or there is an arrhythmia or non-immune hydrops
4. other defects known to be associated with cardiac anomalies are discovered (e.g. omphalocoele, tracheo-oesophageal syndrome, Dandy Walker malformation).

Disturbance of heart rhythm

Disturbance of the heart's rhythm is diagnosed by means of an M-mode echocardiogram since both atrial and ventricular movement can be studied by this technique and the direction of the beam can be selected by simultaneous real-time image. Apart from occasional ventricular or atrial ectopic beats (which are benign), the important arrhythmias are supraventricular tachyarrhythmia and heart block. Supraventricular tachycardia (and other supraventricular tachyarrhythmias such as atrial flutter) results in cardiac failure (non-immune hydrops) if ventricular filling is inadequate and 5% have structural abnormalities, especially atrial–septal defects. The mortality, even with treatment, is about 10% and respiratory distress syndrome is more severe than normal with premature delivery. If the fetus is premature and evidence of hydrops is present, then pharmacological cardioversion is necessary. Prolonged arrhythmia should probably also be treated prophylactically even if there is no heart failure. Digoxin is widely used, 2.5 mg as a loading dose and then 0.5–1 mg/day to achieve a natural level of 2 µg/ml, although this is frequently unsuccessful. Verapamil may be added in a dose of 80 mg 8-hourly if this is unsuccessful but it may be necessary to reduce the digoxin dose since exertion is impaired by verapamil. Congenital atrioventricular block occurs once in 20 000 births and half the cases are associated with a wide range of structural anomalies while many of the remainder are associated with anti-ribonucleoprotein antibodies or full blown systemic lupus erythematosus. Heart failure is usually a sign of structural disease and has a very poor prognosis.

References

Adzick, N.S., Harrison, M.R., Glick, P.L., Nakayama, D.K., Manning, F.A. and de Lorimer, A.A. (1985) Diaphragmatic hernia in the fetus. Prenatal diagnosis and outcome in 94 cases. *Journal of Paediatric Surgery*, **20**, 357–361

Aylsworth, A.S., Seeds, J.W., Guilford, W.A. *et al.* (1984) Prenatal diagnosis of a severe deforming type of osteogenesis imperfecta. *American Journal of Medical Genetics*, **14**, 202

Babut, J.M., Boog, G., Dellenbach, P., Gillet, J.Y., Harrison, R. and Vallette, C. (1983) *Diagnostic antenatal des malformations foetalis par l'echographic.* Edition vigot, Paris, pp. 136–143

Baird, P.A. and MacDonald, E.C. (1981) An epidemiologic study of congenital malformations of the anterior abdominal wall in more than half a million consecutive live births. *American Journal of Human Genetics*, **33**, 470–478

Baker, F., Grant, D.C. and Bieber, F.A. (1984) Antenatal detection of Down's syndrome by sonography. *American Journal of Roentgenology*, **143**, 29

Barss, V., Benacerraf, B.R. and Frigoletto, F.D. (1985) Antenatal sonographic diagnosis of fetal gastro-intestinal malformations. *Pediatrics*, **76**, 445–449

Bendel, R.P. and Alexander, G.L. (1980) Prenatal diagnosis of sacrococcygeal teratoma by ultrasound. *Minnesotta Medicine*, **62**, 623–624

Blau, K., Maxwell, J.D., Johnson, R.D. and Lilford, R.J. (1985) Activities of alkaline phosphatase in first trimester chorion biopsy tissue. *Prenatal Diagnosis*, **5**, 283–286

Brock, D.J.U., Richmond, D.U. and Liston, W.A. (1983) Normal second trimester amniotic fluid alphafetoprotein and acetylcholinesterase associated with fetal sacrococcygeal teratoma. *Prenatal Diagnosis*, **3**, 343–345

Bohn, D., Tamara, M., Perrin, D., Barker, G. and Rabinoveich, M. (1987) Ventilatory predictors of pulmonary hypoplasia in congenital diaphragmatic hernia confirmed by morphologic assessment. *Journal of Pediatrics*, **111**, 423–431

Boue, A., Muller, F., Nazdof, C. and Boue, J. (1984) Prenatal diagnosis in 200 pregnancies with a 1:4 risk of cystic fibrosis. *Human Genetics*, **74**, 288–297

Bourgeot, P. and Cockenpot, P. (1985) Les kystes de l'ovaire dui nouveau-ne. Aspects echographiques. Pre et post-nataux. A propos de 9 observations. *JEMU*, **6**, 285–292

Bowie, J. (1982) (Cited in Filly, R.A. and Golbus, M.S.) Ultrasonography of the normal and pathologic fetal skeleton. *Radiology Clinics*, **20**, 311

Camera, G., Dodero, D. and DePascale, S. (1984) Prenatal diagnosis of thanatophoric dysplasia at 24 weeks. *American Journal of Medical Genetics*, **18**, 39

Carpenter, M.W., Carci, M.R., Dibbins, A.W. and Haddow, J.E. (1984) Perinatal management of ventral wall defects. *Obstetrics and Gynecology*, **64**, 646

Chervenak, F.A., Romero, R., Berkolvitz, R.L. *et al.* (1982) Antenatal sonographic findings of osteogenesis imperfecta. *American Journal of Obstetrics and Gynecology*, **143**, 228

Colombani, P.M. and Cunningham, D.M. (1977) Perinatal aspects of omphalocele and gastroschisis. *American Journal of Disease of Children*, **131**, 1386–1388

Cousins, L., Benirschke, K., Porreco, R. *et al.* (1980) Placentomegaly due to fetal congestive failure in a pregnancy with a sacrococcygeal teratoma. *Journal of Reproductive Medicine*, **25**, 142–144

Cozzi, F. and Wilkinson, A.W. (1969) Intra-uterine growth rate in relation to anorectal and oesophageal anomalies. *Archives of Disease in Childhood*, **44**, 59–62

Cremin, B.J. and Shaff, M.I. (1977) Ultrasonic diagnosis of thanatophoric dwarfism *in-utero*. *Radiology*, **124**, 479

Dabe, S., Legros, G., Rosenfield, R. *et al.* (1980) Sacrococcygeal tumour in infancy. *Canadian Journal of Surgery*, **23**, 363–364

Davidson, J.M., Johnson, R.B., Rigdon, D.T. *et al.* (1984) Gastroschisis and omphalocele: prenatal diagnosis and perinatal management. *Prenatal Diagnosis*, **4**, 355–363

Deleze, G., Sideropoulos, D. and Paumgartner, G. (1977) Determination of bile acid concentration in human amniotic fluid for prenatal diagnosis of intestinal obstruction. *Pediatrics*, **59**, 657

Denholme, T.A., Crow, H.C., Edwards, W.H., Simmons, G.M., Marin Padella, M. and Bartrum, R.J. (1984) Prenatal sonographic appearance of meconium ileus in twins. *American Journal of Radiology*, **143**, 371–372

Dibbins, A.W. and Wiener, E.S. (1974) Mortality from neonatal diaphragmatic hernia. *Journal of Pediatric Surgery*, **9**, 653–662

DiLorenzo, M., Yazbeck, S. and Darharme, J.C. (1987) Gastroschisis a fifteen year experience. *Journal of Pediatric Surgery*, **22**, 710–712

Elejalde, B.R. and deElejalde, M.M. (1985) Thanatophoric dysplasia fetal manifestations and prenatal diagnosis. *American Journal of Medical Genetics*, **22**, 669

Elejalde, B.R., deElejalde, M.M. and Pansch, D. (1985) Prenatal diagnosis of Jeune syndrome. *American Journal of Medical Genetics*, **21**, 433

Feige, A., Gille, J., Von Maillot, K. and Malz, N. (1982) Praenatale diagnostik lines Stenbeinteratomas mit hypertrophic der plazenta. *Geburtshilfe and Frauenheilkunde*, **42**, 20–24

Filly, R.A., Golbus, M.S., Convey, J.C. and Hall, J.G. (1981) Short limbed dwarfism: ultrasonographic diagnosis by mensuration of fetal femoral length. *Radiology*, **138**, 653

Fitzsimmons, J., Nyberg, D.A., Cyr, D.R. and Hatch, E. (1988) Perinatal management of gastroschisis. *Obstetrics and Gynecology*, **71**, 910

Flake, A.W., Harrison, M.R., Adzick, M.S., Laberge, J.M. and Wursof, S.L. (1986) Fetal sacrococcygeal teratoma. *Journal of Pediatric Surgery*, **21**, 563–566

Gaudin, J., le Treguilly, C., Parent, P., Le Guern, H., Boog, G. and Jehannan, B. (1988) Neonatal ovarian cysts. Twelve cysts with antenatal diagnosis. *Pediatric Surgery*, **3**, 158–164

Gergley, R.Z., Eden, R., Schifrin, B.S. *et al.* (1980) Antenatal diagnosis of congenital sacral teratoma. *Journal of Reproductive Medicine*, **24**, 229

Gilbert, W.M. and Nicolaides, K.H. (1987) Fetal omphalocele associated malformations and chromosomal defects. *Obstetrics and Gynecology*, **70**, 633

Grisoni, E.R., Gauderer, M.W.L., Wolfson, R.M. and Izant, R.J. (1986) Antenatal ultrasonography. The experience of a high risk perinatal centre. *Journal of Pediatric Surgery*, **21**, 356–361

Grisoni, E.R., Gauderer, M.W.L., Wolfson, R.M., Jassoni, M.N. and Olsen, M.M. (1988) Antenatal diagnosis of sacrococcygeal teratomas: prognostic features. *Pediatric Surgery International*, **3**, 173–175

Grosfield, J.L., Daues, L. and Weber, T.R. (1981) Congenital abdominal wall defects. Current management and survival. *Surgical Clinics of North America*, **61**, 1037–1048

Hamson, J., James, S., Barrington, J. and Whitfield, J. (1984) The decreasing incidence of pneumothorax and improving survival of infants with congenital diaphragmatic hernia. *Journal of Pediatric Surgery*, **19**, 385–388

Harrison, M.R., Ross, N.A. and de Lorimier, A.A. (1981) Correction of congenital diaphragmatic hernia *in-utero* III. Development of a successful surgical technique using abdominoplasty to avoid compromise of umbilical blood flow. *Journal of Pediatric Surgery*, **16**, 934–941

Harrison, M.R., Adzick, S., Nakayama, D.K. and de Lorimier, A.A. (1986) Fetal diaphragmatic hernia: pathophysiology, natural history and outcome. *Clinical Obstetrics and Gynaecology*, **29**, 490–501

Harrison, M.R., Bjordal, R.I., Langmark, F. and Knatrid, O. (1978) Congenital diaphragmatic hernia: the hidden mortality. *Journal of Pediatric Surgery*, **13**, 3

Hasan, S. and Hermonsan, M.C. (1986) The prenatal diagnosis of ventral wall defects. *American Journal of Obstetrics and Gynecology*, **155**, 842–845

Hauge, M., Bagge, M., Nielson, J. *et al.* (1983) Early prenatal diagnosis of omphalocoele constitutes indications for amniocentesis. *Lancet*, **ii**, 507

Hecht, F. and Kaiser-Hecht, B. (1982) Sacrococcygeal teratoma. Prenatal diagnosis with elevated alphafetoprotein and acetylcholinesterase in amniotic fluid. *Prenatal Diagnosis*, **2**, 229–231

Hobbins, J.C., Bracken, M.B. and Mahoney, M.J. (1982) Diagnosis of fetal skeletal dysplasias with ultrasound. *American Journal of Obstetrics and Gynecology*, **142**, 306

Hobbins, J.C., Grannum, P.A.T., Berkowitz, R.I. *et al.* (1979) Ultrasound in the diagnosis of congenital anomalies. *American Journal of Obstetrics and Gynecology*, **134**, 331

Holzgreve, W., Mahoney, B.S. and Guck, P.S. (1985) Fetal sacrococcygeal teratoma. *Prenatal Diagnosis*, **5**, 245–252

Horger, E.O. and McCarter, L.M. (1979) Prenatal diagnosis of sacrococcygeal teratoma. *American Journal of Obstetrics and Gynecology*, **53**, 660–663

Iritani, I. (1984) Experimental study on embryogenesis of congenital diaphragmatic hernia. *Anat Embryol*, **169**, 13–19

Jouppila, P. and Kirkinen, P. (1984) Ultrasonic and clinical aspects in the diagnosis and prognosis of congenital gastro-intestinal anomalies. *Ultrasound in Medicine and Biology*, **10**, 465–472

King, D.R., Savrin, R. and Bales, E.T. (1980) Gastroschisis update. *Journal of Pediatric Surgery*, **15**, 953–957

Kirk, P.E. and Wah, R. (1983) Obstetric management of the fetus with omphalocele or gastroschisis. A review of 112 cases. *American Journal of Obstetrics and Gynecology*, **146**, 512

Klein, M.D., Kosloske, A.M. and Hertzler, J.U. (1981) Congenital defects of the abdominal wall. *Journal of the American Medical Association*, **245**, 1643–1646

Kohgac, S., Nambu, T. and Tanaka, K. (1980) Hypertrophy of the placenta and sacrococcygeal teratoma. A report of two cases. *Virchows Archives [A]*, **386**, 223–229

Kurtz, A.B. and Wapner, R.J. (1983) Ultrasonic diagnosis of second trimester skeletal dysplasias: a prospective analysis in a high risk population. *Journal of Ultrasound Medicine*, **2**, 99

Lees, R.F., Williamson, B.R. and Brenbridge, M.A. (1980) Sonography of benign sacrococcygeal teratoma *in utero*. *Radiology*, **134**, 717–718

Leonard, C.O., Sanders, R.C. and Lau, U.L. (1979) Prenatal diagnosis óf Turner's syndrome, a familial chromosomal rearrangement and achondroplasia by amniocentesis and ultrasonography. *Johns Hopkins Medical Journal*, **145**, 25

Lipson, M., Waskey, J., Rice, J. *et al.* (1984) Prenatal diagnosis of asphyxiating thoracic dysplasia. *American Journal of Medical Genetics*, **18**, 273

Loveday, B.J., Barr, J.A. and Aitken, J. (1975) The intrauterine demonstration of duodenal atresia by ultrasound. *British Journal of Radiology*, **48**, 1031

Mahoney, M.J. and Hobbins, J.C. (1977) Prenatal diagnosis of chondroectodermal dysplasia. (Ellis-Van Creveld syndrome) with fetoscopy and ultrasound. *New England Journal of Medicine*, **297**, 258

Mann, L. and Ferguson Smith, M.A. (1984) Prenatal assessment of anterior abdominal wall defects and their prognosis. *Prenatal Diagnosis*, **4**, 427–435

Mantagos, S., Weiss, R.R., Mahoney, M. and Hobbins, J.L. (1981) Prenatal diagnosis of diastrophic dwarfism. *American Journal of Obstetrics and Gynecology*, **139**, 111

Marshall, A. and Sumner, E. (1982) Improved prognosis in congenital diaphragmatic hernia. Experience of 22 cases over a two year period. *Journal of the Royal Society of Medicine*, **75**, 607–612

Mayer, T., Black, R., Matlak, M.E. and Johnson, D. (1980) Gastroschisis and omphalocele an 8 year review. *Annals of Surgery*, **192**, 787–788

Mintz, M.C., Mennuti, M. and Fishman, M. (1983) Prenatal aspiration of sacrococcygeal teratoma. *American Journal of Radiology*, **141**, 367–368

Miro, J. and Baird, M. (1988) Congenital atresia and stenosis of the duodenum. The impact of a prenatal diagnosis. *American Journal of Obstetrics and Gynecology*, **158**, 551–559

Moerman, P., Fryns, J.P., Goddeeris, P. *et al.* (1982) Non-immunologic hydrops fetalis. *Archives of Pathology and Laboratory Medicine*, **106**, 635–640

Moore, T.C. and Nar, K. (1986) An international survey of gastroschisis and omphalocele 490 cases. *Pediatric Surgery International*, **1**, 46–50

Muller, F., Frot, J.C., Aubrey, M.C., Bowe, J. and Brie, A. (1986) Meconium ileus in cystic fibrosis. *Lancet*, **ii**, 223

Nakayama, D.K., Harrison, M.R., Chinn, D.U. *et al.* (1985) Prenatal diagnosis and natural history of the fetus with a congenital disphragmatic hernia. Initial clinical experience. *Journal of Pediatric Surgery*, **20**, 118–125

Nakayama, D.K., Harrison, M.R., Gross, B.N. *et al.* (1984) Management of the fetus with an abdominal wall defect. *Journal of Pediatric Surgery*, **19**, 408–413

Nelson, L.N., Clark, E., Fishborne, J.I., Urban, R.B. and Penry, M.F. (1982) Value of serial sonography in the *in utero* detection of duodenal atresia. *Obstetrics and Gynecology*, **59**, 657

O'Brien, G.D., Rodeck, C. and Queenon, J.T. (1980) Early prenatal diagnosis of diastrophic dwarfism by ultrasound. *British Medical Journal*, **280**, 1300

Papp, Z., Toth, Z., Szabo, M. and Szeifert, C.T. (1985) Early prenatal diagnosis of cystic fibrosis by ultrasound. *Clinical Genetics*, **28**, 356–358

Pierro, A., Cozzi, F., Colarossi, C., Irving, I.M., Pierce, A.M. and Lister, J. (1987) Does fetal gut obstruction cause hydramnios and growth retardation? *Journal of Pediatric Surgery*, **22**, 454–457

Puri, P. and Gorman, F. (1984) Lethal non-pulmonary anomalies associated with congenital diaphragmatic hernia. Implications for early intrauterine surgery. *Journal of Pediatric Surgery*, **19**, 29–32

Rayburn, W.F. and Barr, M. (1982) Teratomas: concordance in mother and fetus. *American Journal of Obstetrics and Gynecology*, **144**, 110–112

Redford, D.N.A., McNay, M.B. and Whittle, M.J. (1985) Gastroschisis and exomphalos. Precise diagnosis by mid pregnancy ultrasound. *British Journal of Obstetrics and Gynaecology*, **92**, 54

Romero, R., Ghindini, A., Costigan, K., Touloukian, R. and Hobbins, J.C. (1988) Prenatal diagnosis of duodenal atresia: does it make any difference? *Obstetrics and Gynecology*, **71**, 739

Sakai, N., Tamura, M., Hosokawa, Y., Bryan, A.C., Barker, C.A. and Bohn, D.J. (1987) Effect of surgical repair on respiratory mechanics in congenital diaphragmatic hernia. *Journal of Pediatrics*, **111**, 432–438

Sand, H. and Brock, J.E. (1976) Prenatal diagnosis of soft tissue malformations by ultrasound and X-ray. *Acta Obstetrica et Gynaecologica Scandinavica*, **55**, 191

Santos Ramos, R.S. and Duenhoeffer, J.F. (1975) Diagnosis of congenital fetal abnormalities by sonography. *Obstetrics and Gynecology*, **45**, 276

Sarda, P., Bard, H., Teasdale, F. and Grignon, A. (1983) The importance of antenatal ultrasonography diagnosis of correctable fetal malformation. *American Journal of Obstetrics and Gynecology*, **147**, 443–445

Seeds, J.W., Mittelstaedt, C.A., Cefalo, R.C. and Parker, T.F. (1982) Prenatal diagnosis of sacrococcygeal teratoma: an anechoic caudal mass. *Journal of Clinical Ultrasound*, **10**, 193–195

Sermer, M., Benzce, R.J., Pulson, L. *et al.* (1987) Prenatal diagnosis and management of congenital defects of the anterior abdominal wall. *American Journal of Obstetrics and Gynecology*, **156**, 308

Shochat, S.J., Naeye, R.L., Ford, W.D.A., Whitman, V. and Maisels, M.J. (1979) Congenital diaphragmatic hernia – a new concept in management. *Annals of Surgery*, **190**, 332–339

Sillence, D.O., Senn, A. and Danks, D.M. (1979) Genetic heterogeneity in osteogenesis imperfecta. *Journal of Medical Genetics*, **16**, 101

Smith, W.L., Breitweiser, T.D. and Dinno, N. (1981) *In utero* diagnosis of achondrogenesis type I. *Clinical Genetics*, **19**, 51

Spitz, L., Kiely, E. and Brereton, R.J. (1987) Esophageal atresia: five year experience with 148 cases. *Journal of Pediatric Surgery*, **22**, 103–108

Stringel, G. and Filler, R.M. (1979) Prognostic features in omphalocele and gastroschisis. *Journal of Pediatric Surgery*, **14**, 515–519

Sumner, E. and Frank, D.J. (1981) Tolazoline in the treatment of congenital diaphragmatic hernia. *Archives of Disease in Childhood*, **56**, 350–353

Tibboel, D., Vermey-Keen, C., Kluck, P. *et al.* (1986) The natural history of gastroschisis during fetal life. Development of the fibrous coating on the bowel loops. *Teratology*, **33**, 267

Togama, W.M. (1972) Combined congenital defects of the anterior abdominal wall, sternum, diaphragm, pericardium and heart. A case report and review of the syndrome. *Pediatrics*, **50**, 778

Vermer, U., Weiss, R.R., Almonte, R. *et al.* (1979) Early prenatal diagnosis of soft tissue malformation. *Obstetrics and Gynecology*, **53**, 660–663

Wilson, A. (1982) Ultrasound screening for abdominal masses in the neonatal period. *American Journal of Diseases of Children*, **136**, 147–151

Wladimiroff, J.W., Molenaar, J.C., Niermeijer, M.F. *et al.* (1984a) Prenatal diagnosis and management of omphalocele. *European Journal of Obstetrics, Gynecology and Reproductive Biology*, **16**, 19

Wladimiroff, J.W., Niermeifer, M.F., Laar, J. *et al.* (1984b) Prenatal diagnosis of skeletal dysplasia by real time ultrasound. *Obstetrics and Gynecology*, **63**, 360

Zaleski, A.M., Cooperberg, P.L. and Kliman, M.R. (1982) Ultrasonic diagnosis of extrafetal masses. *Journal of the Canadian Association of Radiology*, **30**, 55–56

Chapter 3

Renal tract anomalies

R.J. Lilford, H. Irving and D. Thomas

Introduction

There are many accounts of the ultrasound features of renal disease classified by diagnosis. Here we produce a more useful classification by ultrasound features. While accurate and specific diagnosis is possible in some cases (e.g. bilateral renal agenesis), this is impossible in others (dilatation of bladder and ureters). Almost 1% of babies have a congenital uropathy of some kind (Grieg *et al.*, 1989). In many cases, however, appropriate follow-up may prevent long-term renal damage (Smith, Egginton and Brookfield, 1987; Arthur *et al.*, 1989; Greig *et al.*, 1989; White, 1989). Thus, ultrasound can identify fetuses requiring detailed investigation in postnatal life.

Approximately 80% of prenatally diagnosed uropathies are asymptomatic in the neonatal period. This group of infants includes some with deteriorating renal function (Thomas, Irving and Arthur, 1985). At least half of all cases of renal failure in infancy and childhood are secondary to congenital disease and it appears that fetal screening will reduce this morbidity by enabling prophylactic surgery and medical treatment to be carried out before irreversible damage has occurred. However, maximal sensitivity will probably come from combined second and third trimester screening.

The obstetrician requires a basic knowledge of paediatric nephrology in order to counsel parents appropriately. Unfortunately, all existing literature is based on final diagnosis and in this chapter, therefore, we classify patients according to the ultrasound features available to the doctor when counselling patients with an abnormal scan result.

Absent kidneys (bilateral renal agenesis)

The hallmark of this lethal condition is profound oligohydramnios and the differential diagnosis is that of severe idiopathic oligohydramnios, often in association with raised maternal serum alpha-fetoprotein. The latter also has a very bad prognosis because the cause of the oligohydramnios is likely to be a serious fetal disease (Richards *et al.*, 1988) and because profound oligohydramnios, of any cause, usually results in severe pulmonary hypoplasia. Lack of filling of the fetal bladder is another sign of renal agenesis, along with failure to visualize the kidneys themselves. Diagnosis was highly accurate, even with earlier ultrasound equipment

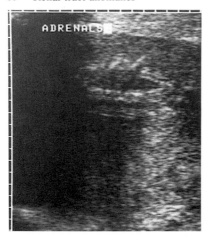
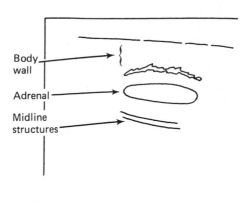

Figure 3.1 Fetal adrenal gland in patient with renal agenesis

and should have improved considerably in recent years (Romero *et al.*, 1985). With the best high resolution equipment it is possible to differentiate kidney (which has a characteristic shape and a demonstrable calyceal system) from the adrenal gland (Figure 3.1). We are not impressed with the frusemide test of fetal renal function, whereby maternal administration of this drug is said to produce fetal bladder filling if the kidneys are present.

Cystic kidney disease

Four conditions are possible when renal cysts are found: infantile (Potter's type 1) and adult polycystic diseases (Potter's type 3); multicystic dysplastic kidney disease (Potter's type 2); and isolated renal cysts. The polycystic kidney diseases are the result of dilatation of the collecting tubules (the distal portions of the ureteric buds). Multicystic kidney is usually associated with atresia of the upper ureter and/or renal pelvis although a 'hydronephrotic' form has been demonstrated in which ureteric patency is maintained. Infantile polycystic disease often causes *in-utero* renal failure (oligohydramnios/absent bladder filling) and is characterized by an enlarged and bright kidney. The increased echogenicity is due to multiple small cysts. False-positive diagnosis is rare if parents are known carriers, but normal findings do not exclude this autosomal recessive disease which will have normal ultrasound features prior to viability in 10% of cases. We have encountered apparent false-positive diagnosis where bright kidneys have been seen in fetuses of parents not known to be carriers.

The adult form of polycystic kidney disease may occasionally produce renal cysts *in utero*. Discrete cysts and enlarged kidneys may be seen. Although the disease is always bilateral the ultrasound appearance *in utero* may be unilateral and this appearance is similar to unilateral multicystic kidney. Parental renal ultrasound is, therefore, useful in cases of renal cystic disease of unknown cause, since if either parent has cystic renal disease, then the adult form of polycystic kidney may be inferred.

Multicystic kidney disease is associated with larger cysts and in almost all cases total absence of function in the affected kidney. It may, however, be unilateral

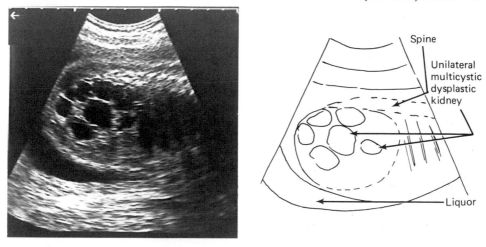

Figure 3.2 Unilateral multicystic kidney in longitudinal 'section'. Note normal liquor volume. The contralateral kidney had normal features

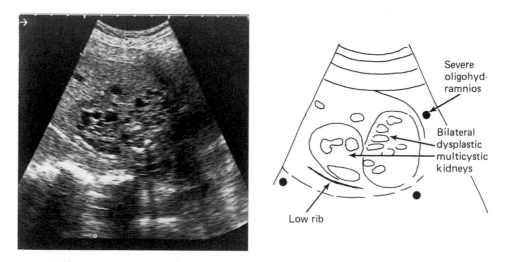

Figure 3.3 Bilateral multicystic dysplastic kidneys in transverse 'section'. Note absence of liquor. The bladder was not seen

(90% of cases are unilateral, Figure 3.2). Bilateral cases are invariably fatal and this outcome can be inferred if oligohydramnios is present and the bladder does not fill (Figure 3.3). Occasionally only one cyst will be seen and the condition must then be distinguished from unilateral pelviureteric junction obstruction. The latter is associated with a greater amount of normal parenchyma and an intact but dilated calyceal system which can be recognized on scan. Unilateral multicystic kidney disease has a good prognosis. Previously, surgeons removed the abnormal kidney to prevent hypertension but this is almost certainly unnecessary (Gordon *et al.*, 1988). The majority of paediatric urologists believe that the risk of late

complications (hypertension, pain, malignant change) is so small as not to justify
the routine 'prophylactic' removal of these lesions.

Dilatation of the renal tract

Apparent pelviureteric junction obstruction

It is difficult to make a precise anatomical diagnosis in most cases of renal
dilatation, but one of the most characteristic appearances is that of ureteropelvic
junction obstruction (PUJ obstruction). This is a partial obstruction, perhaps
caused by tortuosity of the pelviureteric junction or 'fetal folds'. It is unilateral in
two-thirds of cases, but may be associated with other renal anomalies (especially
reflux) and PUJ obstruction on one side with a multicystic (and therefore
non-functioning) kidney on the other is a well recognized finding.

Ultrasonically PUJ obstruction is associated with dilatation of the renal pelvis to
over 10 mm in anteroposterior diameter and distension of the calyces (Figure 3.4).

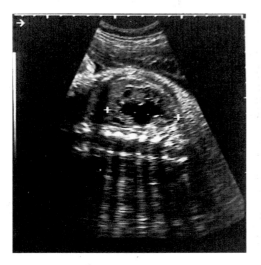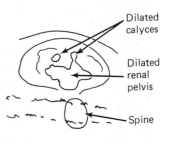

Figure 3.4 Dilated pelvis and calyces in patient with unilateral pelviureteric junction obstruction. There
were no further cystic dilatations in the ureteric area and the bladder was normal

Many cases of mild dilatation resolve before delivery. When dilated renal collecting
systems are seen bilaterally, follow-up scans should be performed 4 or 8-weekly to
ensure that oligohydramnios does not develop. However, we have never seen this
feature of *in-utero* renal failure in bilateral apparent PUJ obstruction. The
prognosis is excellent, even in cases of bilateral apparent PUJ obstruction and
intervention before delivery is seldom, if ever, required.

The postnatal management of PUJ obstruction is controversial. The majority of
obstructed kidneys (60%) retain normal levels of renal function. Some prenatally
diagnosed obstructions resolve spontaneously. Therefore, if renal function is well
preserved, there is little evidence to support the concept of neonatal pyeloplasty
and serial ultrasound will be carried out at 6 months and one year. But evidence of
impaired function, measured by isotope scanning, is a reasonable indication for

early surgical intervention. In very poorly functioning kidneys there may be benefit in a period of percutaneous nephrostomy drainage to assess recoverability of function prior to surgery.

Mega-ureter and normal bladder

This appearance is different to PUJ obstruction and can be caused by:

1. infravesical obstruction (e.g. posterior urethral valves). In theory, this should cause a large bladder but occasionally only the ureters are dilated
2. ureterovesical junction obstruction
3. vesico-ureteric reflux
4. non-obstructive dilatation ('burnt out obstruction'). Again, the bladder is usually dilated in these cases. (*See below.*)

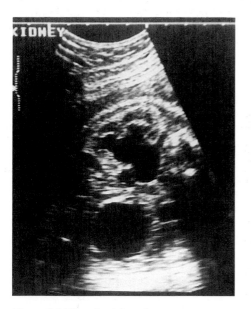 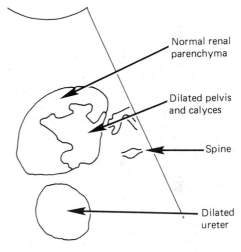

Figure 3.5 Dilated pelvis and ureter

A series of echo-free vesicles are seen along the expected course of the ureter with variable dilatation of the renal pelvis (Figure 3.5). We do not think that it is possible to differentiate the possible causes listed above. Reflux is probably the commonest cause of ureteric dilatation but normal bladder and it is for this reason that, as with PUJ obstruction, all infants should be followed up. In addition, some cases with bilateral mega-ureter but normal sized bladders will turn out to have mild urethral obstruction. Thus, if postnatal scans confirm a dilated urinary tract then a micturating cystogram should be performed. Bladder outlet obstruction (e.g. valves) should be treated by endoscopic surgery. If reflux is found to be the cause, then serial checks for urinary infection, renal ultrasound and selected isotope assessments should be made. Most cases of vesico-ureteric reflux can be managed conservatively (continuous antibiotic prophylaxis) provided that the urine can be maintained free of infection. Ureteric re-implantation may be required if this approach fails. Reflux identified at follow-up of abnormal intrauterine scan differs from reflux presenting initially in postnatal life in, the high proportion of males (80% in our series), the higher grade of reflux, and the higher incidence of associated anomalies in the prenatal cases. Nevertheless, renal function is generally well preserved if the kidneys have been exposed only to sterile, low pressure reflux. Renal damage results from both renal tract infection or (less frequently) as a consequence of an early defect of nephrogenesis – renal dysplasia.

Mega-ureter and megacystis

The most likely diagnosis when this picture is seen is urethral obstruction. This will be due to atresia or posterior urethral valves. Sometimes a short segment of dilated upper urethra will be seen. In some cases profound oligohydramnios will already be present and fetal bladder aspiration almost always shows high urinary sodium levels (over 100 μmol/l after 20 weeks) and other biochemical changes (such as beta-microglobulin) indicative of renal failure in these cases. This renal failure is the result of severe and early back pressure which causes renal dysplasia. Frequently there is no oligohydramnios and these cases hardly ever develop renal failure, although exceptions are reported (Vintzileos et al., 1985). Overall, the prenatal assessment of renal function is accurate (Arthur et al., 1989). This appearance (dilated renal tract and normal liquor volume) usually results from valves and a dilated upper urethra may be seen on scan. Dilated bladder and ureters but normal liquor may also be caused by:

1. severe bilateral vesico-ureteric reflux (the reason for bladder enlargement is presumably a neuropathic problem connected with the cause of the reflux)
2. low pressure dilatation of the renal tract (prune belly syndrome). Some prune belly syndrome patients appear to be the result of a very early urethral obstruction which has resolved, while others may be the result of a primary maldevelopment of the abdominal and urinary tract muscle. The prognosis is good but limb defects sometimes occur and chromosomal abnormalities may be present
3. the megacystis microcolon intestinal hypoperistalsis syndrome. This lethal autosomal recessive condition (Lilford and Penman, 1989) should be suspected if upper intestinal tract dilatation accompanies the dilated renal tract.

Posterior urethral valves (PUV) without renal failure may be associated with chromosomal abnormalities (±20% of prenatal series), especially trisomies 18 and 13, which should be excluded before a good prognosis is given. PUV do not occur in the female infant and sex determination is, therefore, an important part of antenatal assessment. Rarely a urethrocoele may cause bladder outlet obstruction in a female, but this is vanishingly rare. Ascites (due to urine leak) is seen in some cases.

If renal failure or a lethal chromosome abnormality is present, then there is little point in continuing the pregnancy. In other cases the prognosis is good. There are, therefore, few patients who stand to benefit from in-utero surgery. The prognosis for cases without adverse features is at least 95% healthy survival, although surgery is often required after birth. This will usually consist of transurethral valve resection and survival is virtually guaranteed provided that pulmonary function is adequate. In the past, posterior urethral valve obstruction presented typically with severe urinary sepsis in the first few months of life. Up to one-third of affected boys were ultimately destined for chronic renal failure. It is likely that the major benefits of prenatal diagnosis may lie in the prevention of severe urinary infection and renal scarring in early childhood.

Treatment generally consists of endoscopic resection of valve tissue in the neonatal period. Further surgery may be required at a later date in some cases (e.g. unilateral nephro-ureteronephrectomy to remove grossly refluxing non-functional systems). It is possible that intrauterine drainage might ultimately prove to be of value in a small percentage of boys with urethral valves – but many years follow-up would be required to confirm this.

Since less than 5% of cases with good prognostic signs (normal sodium, normal liquor, normal renal parenchyma) will develop renal failure, and since *in-utero* surgery will cause fetal loss more often than this (Elder, Duckett and Synder, 1987) and may fail, we can find little place for attempts to drain the bladder permanently *in utero*. The only exceptions are cases where:

1. urinary sodium is normal but oligohydramnios is already present (fetal surgery will not necessarily prevent pulmonary hypoplasia in such cases)
2. good prognostic criteria are present at presentation but oligohydramnios then develops before fetal viability.

In our experience of over 80 cases, none have fulfilled these criteria and we regard most attempts at fetal bladder drainage as unnecessary; Lilford's maxim of fetal surgery usually applies; either the damage is so severe and so early that any surgery is too late or the prognosis is so good that no intervention is required. The San-Francisco group have experience with 200 cases. Only five required *in-utero*

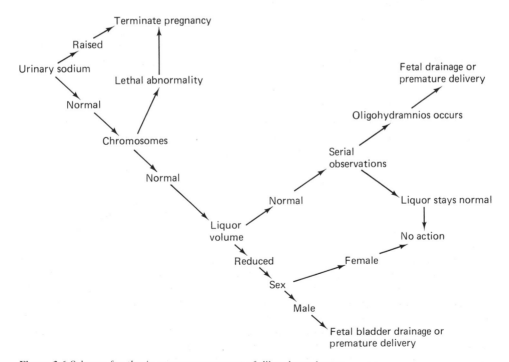

Figure 3.6 Scheme for the *in-utero* management of dilated renal tract

drainage (oligohydramnios but normal fetal urine sodium) and three of these survived (Longaher, Adzick and Harrison, 1989). It should be recognized, however, that *in-utero* treatment may shift the natural history, not from death to healthy life, but from death to renal failure in childhood; we have witnessed cases where this seems to have happened. Our scheme for management of dilated renal tract is given in Figure 3.6.

References

Arthur, R.J., Irving, H.C., Thomas, D.F.M. and Watters, J.K. (1989) Bilateral fetal uropathy: What is the outlook? *British Medical Journal*, **298**, 1419–1420

Elder, J.S., Duckett, J.W. Jr and Synder, H.M. (1987) Intervention for fetal obstruction uropathy: has it been effective? *Lancet*, 1007–1010

Gordon, A.C., Thomas, D.F.M., Arthur, R.J. and Irving, H.C. (1988) *Journal of Urology*, **140**, 1231–1234

Greig, J.D., Raine, P.A.M., Young, D.G. *et al.* (1989) Value of antenatal diagnosis of abnormalities of the urinary tract. *British Medical Journal*, **298**, 1417–1419

Irving, H.C., Arthur, R.J. and Thomas, D.F.M. (1987) Percutaneous nephrostomy in paediatrics. *Clinical Radiology*, **38**, 245–248

Lilford, R.J. and Penman, D.G. (1987) The megacystis-microcolon-intestinal hypoperistalsis syndrome; a fatal autosomal recessive condition. *Journal of Medical Ethics*, **26**, 66–67

Longaher, M.T., Adzick, M.S. and Harrison, M.R. (1989) Fetal obstructive uropathy. *British Medical Journal*, **298**, 325–326

Richards, D.S., Seeds, J.W., Katz, V.L. *et al.* (1988) Elevated maternal serum alpha-fetoprotein with oligohydramnios: ultrasound evaluation and outcome. *Obstetrics and Gynecology*, **72**, 337–341

Romero, R., Cullen, M. Grannum, P. *et al.* (1985) Antenatal diagnosis of renal anomalies with ultrasound. *American Journal of Obstetrics and Gynecology*, **151**, 38–43

Smith, D., Egginton, J.A. and Brookfield, D.S.K. (1987) Detection of abnormality of fetal urinary tract as a predictor of renal tract disease. *British Medical Journal*, **294**, 27–28

Thomas, D.F.M. and Gordon, A.C. (1989) Management of prenatally diagnosed uropathies. *Archives of Disease in Childhood*, **64**, 58–63

Thomas, D.F.M., Irving, H.C. and Arthur, R.J. (1985) Pre-natal diagnosis: how useful is it? *British Journal of Urology*, **57**, 784–787

Vintzileos, A.M., Garry, M.D., Turner, W. *et al.* (1985) Polyhydramnios and obstructive renal failure: a case report and review of the literature. *American Journal of Obstetrics and Gynecology*, **152**, 883–885

White, R.H.R. (1989) Fetal uropathy. *British Medical Journal*, **298**, 1408–1409

Chapter 4

Screening for Down's syndrome

H.S. Cuckle and N.J. Wald

Introduction

Down's syndrome is the most common cause of severe mental retardation. In the absence of antenatal diagnosis and therapeutic abortion over 800 infants would be born with this disorder each year in England and Wales. Average life expectancy is now about 60 years and, in addition to associated malformations of the heart, digestive system, eye and ear most affected individuals will eventually develop pathological changes in the brain associated with Alzheimer's disease.

Antenatal diagnosis following amniocentesis or chorionic villus sampling is generally acceptable provided that the group selected for the procedure is at high enough risk of Down's syndrome to warrant the hazards and cost, particularly of producing the karyotype. Until recently such screening has been largely on the basis of advanced maternal age, but now other methods are available, namely the measurement of markers for Down's syndrome in maternal serum and by ultrasound examination of the fetus.

In this chapter we describe the existing and new methods with particular reference to the practical questions arising for the physician who has to interpret the results for an individual patient and to those planning the new service.

Maternal age

The risk of having a term pregnancy with Down's syndrome increases with maternal age, rapidly after age 30 years. The best available estimate of risk is obtained from combining the results of all eight published population studies which included individual years of age (Cuckle, Wald and Thompson, 1987). Figure 4.1 shows this with a curve fitted to overcome statistical fluctuation and allows risk to be calculated more precisely, say using a woman's age in years and months rather than in completed years. A 35-year-old woman's risk will vary between 1:420 and 1:350 depending on whether at her expected date of delivery she is 35 years 0 months or 35 years 11 months (Table 4.1). While all the studies used to produce Figure 4.1 were in largely caucasian populations there is no reason to believe that they cannot be generally applied.

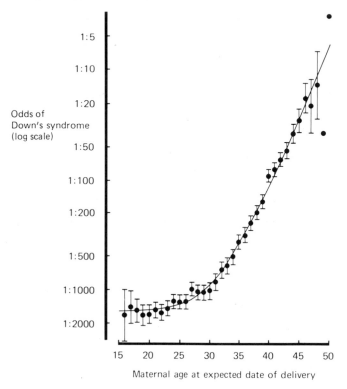

Figure 4.1 The risk of Down's syndrome (expressed as odds) according to maternal age. The fitted curve is compared with the observed value and 95% confidence interval. Derived from data in Table 1 of Cuckle, Wald and Thompson, 1987

Mid-trimester risk

The risk of Down's syndrome is higher in the mid-trimester of pregnancy than at term because of the relatively high miscarriage rate in Down's syndrome pregnancies. Table 4.2 compares the observed risk of a Down's syndrome in women aged 35–46 who underwent amniocentesis with the risk of Down's syndrome term pregnancy in such women. On average the increase in risk at mid-trimester was equivalent to multiplying the right-hand side of the risks in Table 4.1 by 0.77. This is consistent with data on the fetal death rate in pregnancies with Down's syndrome diagnosed at amniocentesis but not ending in a termination of pregnancy, namely 26% in a study of 43 singleton affected pregnancies (derived from Table 1 in Hook, 1983).

Previous Down's syndrome

If a woman has had a previous pregnancy associated with a *non-inherited* Down's syndrome fetus the risk of having a further Down's syndrome pregnancy is still highly dependent on maternal age. Table 4.3 shows that the risk of a recurrence appears to be the age-specific risk plus an additive component (0.42% at

Table 4.1 Risk of a Down's syndrome term pregnancy according to maternal age, in years and months, at the expected date of delivery

Years	Completed months											
	0	1	2	3	4	5	6	7	8	9	10	11
25	1:1376	1:1372	1:1367	1:1363	1:1358	1:1353	1:1348	1:1343	1:1338	1:1333	1:1328	1:1322
26	1:1317	1:1311	1:1306	1:1300	1:1294	1:1289	1:1283	1:1277	1:1271	1:1264	1:1258	1:1252
27	1:1245	1:1239	1:1232	1:1225	1:1219	1:1212	1:1205	1:1198	1:1191	1:1183	1:1176	1:1169
28	1:1161	1:1154	1:1146	1:1138	1:1130	1:1123	1:1115	1:1107	1:1099	1:1090	1:1082	1:1074
29	1:1065	1:1057	1:1048	1:1040	1:1031	1:1022	1:1014	1:1005	1: 996	1: 987	1: 978	1: 969
30	1: 960	1: 951	1: 942	1: 932	1: 923	1: 914	1: 905	1: 895	1: 886	1: 877	1: 867	1: 858
31	1: 848	1: 839	1: 829	1: 820	1: 810	1: 801	1: 791	1: 782	1: 772	1: 763	1: 753	1: 744
32	1: 734	1: 725	1: 716	1: 706	1: 697	1: 687	1: 678	1: 669	1: 660	1: 650	1: 641	1: 632
33	1: 623	1: 614	1: 605	1: 596	1: 587	1: 578	1: 570	1: 561	1: 552	1: 544	1: 535	1: 527
34	1: 518	1: 510	1: 502	1: 494	1: 486	1: 478	1: 470	1: 462	1: 454	1: 446	1: 439	1: 431
35	1: 424	1: 416	1: 409	1: 402	1: 395	1: 387	1: 381	1: 374	1: 367	1: 360	1: 354	1: 347
36	1: 341	1: 334	1: 328	1: 322	1: 316	1: 310	1: 304	1: 298	1: 292	1: 287	1: 281	1: 275
37	1: 270	1: 265	1: 259	1: 254	1: 249	1: 244	1: 239	1: 235	1: 230	1: 225	1: 221	1: 216
38	1: 212	1: 207	1: 203	1: 199	1: 195	1: 191	1: 187	1: 183	1: 179	1: 175	1: 171	1: 168
39	1: 164	1: 161	1: 157	1: 154	1: 151	1: 147	1: 144	1: 141	1: 138	1: 135	1: 132	1: 129
40	1: 126	1: 124	1: 121	1: 118	1: 116	1: 113	1: 111	1: 108	1: 106	1: 103	1: 101	1: 99
41	1: 97	1: 94	1: 92	1: 90	1: 88	1: 86	1: 84	1: 82	1: 81	1: 79	1: 77	1: 75
42	1: 73	1: 72	1: 70	1: 69	1: 67	1: 65	1: 64	1: 63	1: 61	1: 60	1: 58	1: 57
43	1: 56	1: 54	1: 53	1: 52	1: 51	1: 49	1: 48	1: 47	1: 46	1: 45	1: 44	1: 43
44	1: 42	1: 41	1: 40	1: 39	1: 38	1: 37	1: 36	1: 35	1: 35	1: 34	1: 33	1: 32
45	1: 31	1: 31	1: 30	1: 29	1: 29	1: 28	1: 27	1: 27	1: 26	1: 25	1: 25	1: 24
46	1: 24	1: 23	1: 22	1: 22	1: 21	1: 21	1: 20	1: 20	1: 19	1: 19	1: 18	1: 18
47	1: 17	1: 17	1: 17	1: 16	1: 16	1: 15	1: 15	1: 15	1: 14	1: 14	1: 14	1: 13
48	1: 13	1: 13	1: 12	1: 12	1: 12	1: 11	1: 11	1: 11	1: 11	1: 10	1: 10	1: 10
49	1: 9.5	1: 9.2	1: 9.0	1: 8.8	1: 8.5	1: 8.3	1: 8.1	1: 7.9	1: 7.7	1: 7.5	1: 7.3	1: 7.1

Derived from the formula for risk given age in completed years (footnote to Table 1 in Cuckle, Wald and Thompson, 1987) by subtracting 5.5 months from the age in years and completed months and expressing the result as a decimal, before substitution in the formula.

mid-trimester and 0.34% at term). Table 4.4 gives the resultant risk according to age in years and months.

If the previously affected pregnancy was an *inherited* case of Down's syndrome the recurrence risk is high enough to dwarf the age-specific risk at most ages. On average the resultant risk can be approximated by adding 10% to the age-specific risk, but expert genetic advice will be needed in individual cases.

Maternal age screening

Despite the steep increase in risk with maternal age in western countries only a small proportion of affected pregnancies are in women who are relatively old. This is simply because most pregnancies in these countries are among younger women. Table 4.5 shows the estimated proportions of affected and unaffected pregnancies for England and Wales in 1981–85 using different age cut-offs to define advanced age from 30 to 40 years. Using age 40 there is a reasonable detection rate (16%) for a very low false-positive rate (1.1%). The problem arises however when attempts are made to increase detection by lowering the age cut-off. The extra detection can

Table 4.2 Risk of Down's syndrome at the time of amniocentesis, and at the expected date of delivery (EDD)

	At amniocentesis		At EDD		
Age (completed years)	Affected pregnancies	Risk* (a)	Age** (years and decimals)	Risk*** (b)	Ratio† (b)/(a)
35	19	1:285	35.95	1:348	0.82
36	35	1:174	36.95	1:276	0.63
37	47	1:146	37.95	1:216	0.68
38	64	1:122	38.95	1:168	0.73
39	84	1: 91	39.95	1:130	0.70
40	88	1: 80	40.95	1: 99	0.81
41	70	1: 67	41.95	1: 75	0.89
42	69	1: 45	42.95	1: 57	0.79
43	62	1: 30	43.95	1: 43	0.70
44	30	1: 33	44.95	1: 32	1.03
45	23	1: 21	45.95	1: 24	0.88
46	19	1: 11	46.95	1: 18	0.61

   * From Table 2 in Ferguson-Smith and Yates (1984).
  ** Age at amniocentesis in completed years plus 0.5 (average age in decimals) plus 0.45 (average interval from amniocentesis).
 *** From equation in footnote to Table 1 in Cuckle, Wald and Thomspon (1987).
   † Weighted average is 0.77.

detection can only be achieved at the cost of a substantially increased false-positive rate. In economic terms this would be described as indicating a poor marginal return and Table 4.5 shows this quantitatively.

While Table 4.5 describes the maximum detection using maternal age screening, in practice the results are poorer. From the number of women in 1984 having an amniotic fluid karyotype according to the reason for amniocentesis, it can be estimated that less than 14% of affected pregnancies would have been identified (Table 4.6). On the basis of maternities in 1984 only 45% of those aged 40 years or more had an amniocentesis, 48% aged 38–39 and 20% aged 35–37. Several factors may contribute to this shortfall:

1. some older women may not have been offered the procedure
2. termination could be particularly unacceptable to older women for whom this may be their last chance of pregnancy
3. the group may include a disproportionate number from religious subgroups who find antenatal diagnosis and termination of pregnancy unacceptable
4. a higher than average number may have become pregnant following treatment for infertility and would not want to take the risk of miscarriage following amniocentesis.

Maternal serum

Alpha-fetoprotein (AFP)

In Down's syndrome pregnancies second trimester maternal serum AFP levels are, on average, reduced by about one-quarter. The AFP levels vary considerably with

Table 4.3 Recurrence risk of non-inherited Down's syndrome according to maternal age at antenatal diagnosis

Maternal age at prenatal diagnosis	MRC of Canada (1977)		Mikkelsen and Stene (1979)		Stene, Stene and Mikkelsen (1984)		Total observed risk (O)	Expected risk** (E)	Excess risk (O−E)
	Down's syndrome	All pregnancies	Down's syndrome	All pregnancies	Down's syndrome	All pregnancies*			
≤19	0	6	2	199	0	24			
20−	0	45	1	452	3	307	0.86%	0.08%	0.78%
25−	0	96	1	418	7	826			
30−	1	64	3	244	2	734	0.46%	0.14%	0.32%
35−	0	24	0	75	6	343			
40+	1	7			1	119	1.35%	0.85%	0.50%
Total	2	242	7	1388	19	2353	0.70%	0.28%	0.42%***

* Estimated by applying the age distribution at antenatal diagnosis of all 2890 women having an amniocentesis following a child with any non-inherited chromosomal aberration to the 2353 women having the procedure because of a previous Down's syndrome pregnancy.

** The mid-trimester risk at ages 20, 30 and 40 respectively derived from the term risk in Table 1 of Cuckle, Wald and Thompson, 1987 after multiplying the right hand side of the odds by 0.77.

*** Equivalent to an excess risk of 0.34% at term.

Table 4.4 Risk of a Down's syndrome term pregnancy following a previous affected infant with the non-inherited form according to maternal age, in years and months, at the expected date of delivery

Years						Completed months						
	0	1	2	3	4	5	6	7	8	9	10	11
25	1:241	1:241	1:241	1:241	1:241	1:241	1:240	1:240	1:240	1:240	1:240	1:240
26	1:239	1:239	1:239	1:239	1:239	1:239	1:238	1:238	1:238	1:238	1:237	1:237
27	1:237	1:237	1:236	1:236	1:236	1:236	1:235	1:235	1:235	1:235	1:234	1:234
28	1:234	1:233	1:233	1:233	1:232	1:232	1:232	1:231	1:231	1:231	1:230	1:230
29	1:230	1:229	1:229	1:228	1:228	1:227	1:227	1:227	1:226	1:226	1:225	1:225
30	1:224	1:224	1:223	1:223	1:222	1:222	1:221	1:220	1:220	1:219	1:219	1:218
31	1:217	1:217	1:216	1:216	1:215	1:214	1:213	1:213	1:212	1:211	1:211	1:210
32	1:209	1:208	1:208	1:207	1:206	1:205	1:204	1:203	1:203	1:202	1:201	1:200
33	1:199	1:198	1:197	1:196	1:195	1:194	1:193	1:192	1:191	1:190	1:189	1:188
34	1:187	1:186	1:185	1:183	1:182	1:181	1:180	1:179	1:178	1:176	1:175	1:174
35	1:173	1:172	1:170	1:169	1:168	1:166	1:165	1:164	1:162	1:161	1:160	1:158
36	1:157	1:156	1:154	1:153	1:151	1:150	1:149	1:147	1:146	1:144	1:143	1:142
37	1:140	1:139	1:137	1:136	1:134	1:133	1:131	1:130	1:128	1:127	1:125	1:124
38	1:122	1:121	1:119	1:118	1:116	1:115	1:114	1:112	1:111	1:109	1:108	1:106
39	1:105	1:103	1:102	1:100	1: 99	1: 98	1: 96	1: 95	1: 93	1: 92	1: 91	1: 89
40	1: 88	1: 87	1: 85	1: 84	1: 83	1: 81	1: 80	1: 79	1: 77	1: 76	1: 75	1: 74
41	1: 72	1: 71	1: 70	1: 69	1: 67	1: 66	1: 65	1: 64	1: 63	1: 62	1: 61	1: 60
42	1: 58	1: 57	1: 56	1: 55	1: 54	1: 53	1: 52	1: 51	1: 50	1: 49	1: 48	1: 47
43	1: 46	1: 46	1: 45	1: 44	1: 43	1: 42	1: 41	1: 40	1: 40	1: 39	1: 38	1: 37
44	1: 36	1: 36	1: 35	1: 34	1: 34	1: 33	1: 32	1: 31	1: 31	1: 30	1: 29	1: 29
45	1: 28	1: 28	1: 27	1: 26	1: 26	1: 25	1: 25	1: 24	1: 24	1: 23	1: 23	1: 22
46	1: 22	1: 21	1: 21	1: 20	1: 20	1: 19	1: 19	1: 18	1: 18	1: 18	1: 17	1: 17
47	1: 16	1: 16	1: 16	1: 15	1: 15	1: 15	1: 14	1: 14	1: 14	1: 13	1: 13	1: 13
48	1: 12	1: 12	1: 12	1: 11	1: 11	1: 11	1: 11	1: 10	1: 10	1: 10	1: 10	1: 9
49	1: 9	1: 9	1: 9	1: 8	1: 8	1: 8	1: 8	1: 8	1: 7	1: 7	1: 7	1: 7

Derived from Table 4.1 by adding 0.34% to the age-specific probability of a Down's syndrome term pregnancy (*see* Table 4.3)

Table 4.5 Maternal age screening in England and Wales: detection rate (DR) and false-positive rate (FPR) according to age cut-off and marginal effect compared with using a higher cut-off

Maternal age cut-off (years)			Marginal effect compared with					
			1 year older		2 years older		3 years older	
	DR (%)	FPR (%)	DR (%)	FPR (%)	DR (%)	FPR (%)	DR (%)	FPR (%)
40	16	1.1	–	–	–	–	–	–
39	19	1.7	3.1	0.6	–	–	–	–
38	22	2.5	3.5	0.8	6.6	1.4	–	–
37	26	3.7	3.9	1.2	7.4	2.0	11	2.6
36	30	5.3	4.1	1.6	8.0	2.8	12	3.7
35	35	7.4	4.2	2.1	8.3	3.7	12	4.9
34	39	10	4.3	2.6	8.5	4.7	13	6.3
33	43	13	4.3	3.2	8.7	5.8	13	7.8
32	48	17	4.3	3.8	8.7	6.9	13	9.5
31	52	22	4.5	4.5	8.8	8.3	13	11
30	57	27	4.6	5.3	9.0	9.8	13	14

The distribution of maternal ages in Down's syndrome and unaffected pregnancies was derived by applying the age-specific risk (Table 1 in Cuckle, Wald and Thompson, 1987) to the age distribution of maternities in 1981–5 (OPCS, 1984–86).

Table 4.6 Amiotic fluid karyotypes: England and Wales 1984, according to the reason for amniocentesis

Reason for amniocentesis		Karyotypes*	Expected births with Down's syndrome**	
			No.	(%)
1 Maternal age:	35–37	6959	23	(2.8)
	38–39	4490	27	(3.3)
	40 or more	3234	51	(6.3)
	35 or more	14683	101	(12.5)
2 Chromosomal		1697	8	(1.0)
3 Raised maternal serum AFP		2540	0	(0.0)
4 Other		2517	3	(0.2)
Total		21437	110	(13.7)

* Taken from Review of Clinical Cytogenetic Services (1984).
** In the absence of antenatal diagnosis and therapeutic abortion. The numbers for each reason were derived as follows: (1) Table 4.1 taking age to be 36 years 6 months, 39 years 0 months, and 42 years 6 months respectively, (2) Table 4.4 taking age to be 30, (3) Cuckle and Wald, 1986, (4) Table 4.1 taking age to be 25. The percentages were based on an estimated total of 810 derived by applying the age specific risk to the age distribution of maternities in 1984 (OPCS, 1985).

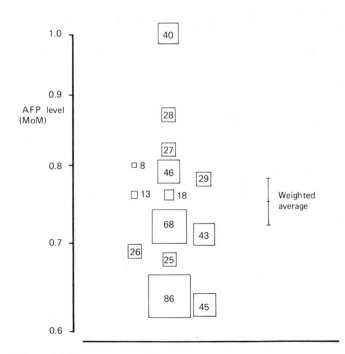

Figure 4.2 The mean or median maternal serum AFP level in Down's syndrome pregnancies in 14 published studies (taken from Wald and Cuckle, 1988). The area of each square is proportional to the number of affected pregnancies which is shown. The weighted average over all studies and its 95% confidence interval are given

gestational age and the laboratory performing the assay, and so they are usually expressed as a multiple of the median (MoM) level for unaffected pregnancies of the same gestation and laboratory. Figure 4.2 shows the mean or median MoM value for Down's syndrome in all 14 published studies on the subject, together with the overall average of 0.75 and its confidence limits, based on a total of 502 affected pregnancies (Wald and Cuckle, 1988).

There does not appear to be a time in the second trimester when the association between low maternal serum AFP levels and Down's syndrome is notably stronger than at any other time (Wald and Cuckle, 1988). Levels also appear to be low in the first trimester (0.78 MoM based on 35 affected pregnancies (Cuckle *et al.*, 1988a; Mantingh *et al.*, 1989)).

Despite the reduction in AFP levels on average, the test by itself is a poor screening test for Down's syndrome. This is because the spread of normal values is wide and so there is substantial overlap in the distribution of values between affected and unaffected pregnancies. However, maternal serum AFP and maternal age are largely independent determinants of the risk of Down's syndrome (since the two are not materially correlated (Wald and Cuckle, 1987)); the use of both together is, therefore, better than either alone. A way of combining the two variables that yields the highest detection rate for a given false-positive rate is to estimate each individual's risk of a Down's syndrome term pregnancy and consider the estimate of risk, itself, a screening variable. This has the advantage of directly providing quantitative risk information that can be used in counselling individual women.

The estimated risk of a woman having a Down's syndrome term pregnancy is derived from the age-specific risk (using Table 4.1) and a factor known as the likelihood ratio (LR). The LR is a measure of the increased likelihood of being affected at a given AFP level. It is calculated from the height of the distribution of AFP in affected pregnancies at the given value divided by the height in unaffected pregnancies at that value. Figure 4.3 illustrates this for 0.40, 0.84 and 2.5 MoM (LR = 3.14, 1.00 and 0.21 respectively) using the AFP distributions found in our study (Cuckle, Wald and Thompson, 1987). Table 4.7 gives the LR according to AFP from 0.40 to 2.9 MoM. The left hand side of the age-specific risk expressed as an odds is multiplied by the LR corresponding to a given AFP level to derive the new risk. For example a woman aged 35 years 0 months has an age-specific risk of 1:420. If her AFP level were 0.40 MoM the risk would become 3.14 × 1:420 or 1:130; if it were 0.84 MoM her risk would be unchanged and if it were 2.5 MoM her risk would be 1:2000 (0.21 × 1:420).

Four sets of formulae or tables providing risk estimates for age and AFP have been published apart from our own. Two used an inappropriate mathematical model – one assumed that the reduction in AFP levels in affected pregnancies was a constant rather than proportional amount (Ashwood, Cheng and Luthy, 1987) and the other assumed that the distributions were Gaussian rather than log Gaussian (DiMaio *et al.*, 1987). The third used our published data and has therefore generated similar risks to our own (Palomaki and Haddow, 1987). The fourth has produced different risk estimates (Tabor *et al.*, 1987) because

1. they were based on a mean AFP value in Down's syndrome of 0.64 MoM which is unusually low (we used 0.72 MoM which is close to the overall median based on the world literature (*see* Figure 4.2))

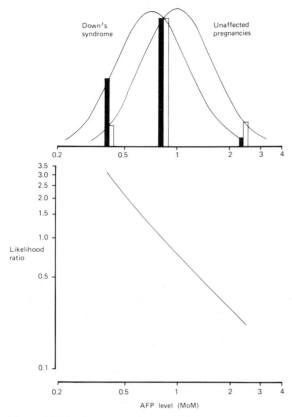

Figure 4.3 Distribution of maternal serum AFP levels in Down's syndrome and unaffected pregnancies together with the likelihood ratio using parameters in Cuckle, Wald and Thompson, 1987. Vertical bars correspond to heights at 0.4, 0.84 and 2.5 MoM

Table 4.7 Likelihood ratio of Down's syndrome according to maternal serum AFP level at 14–20 weeks' gestation

AFP level (MoM)	+0.00	+0.01	+0.02	+0.03	+0.04	+0.05	+0.06	+0.07	+0.08	+0.09
0.40	3.14	3.02	2.91	2.80	2.70	2.61	2.52	2.44	2.36	2.28
0.50	2.21	2.15	2.08	2.02	1.96	1.91	1.86	1.81	1.76	1.71
0.60	1.67	1.63	1.59	1.55	1.51	1.48	1.44	1.41	1.38	1.35
0.70	1.32	1.29	1.26	1.24	1.21	1.19	1.16	1.14	1.12	1.10
0.80	1.08	1.06	1.04	1.02	1.00	0.98	0.97	0.95	0.94	0.92
0.90	0.90	0.89	0.88	0.86	0.85	0.84	0.82	0.81	0.80	0.79

	+0.0	+0.1	+0.2	+0.3	+0.4	+0.5	+0.6	+0.7	+0.8	+0.9
1.0	0.77	0.67	0.59	0.53	0.48	0.43	0.39	0.36	0.33	0.31
2.0	0.29	0.27	0.25	0.24	0.22	0.21	<0.21	<0.21	<0.21	<0.21

Derived from Gaussian distributions with parameters taken from Cuckle, Wald and Thompson, 1987. Select row and column adding up to the nearest AFP level.

Table 4.8 Screening for Down's syndrome using age and AFP or age alone: detection rate (DR) and false-positive rate (FPR) according to risk cut-off*

Risk cut-off	Age and AFP		Age alone	
	DR (%)	FPR (%)	DR (%)	FPR (%)
1:100	17	0.85	13	0.73
1:150	22	1.6	18	1.4
1:200	27	2.6	21	2.3
1:250	30	3.7	25	3.2
1:300	34	5.0	28	4.4
1:350	38	6.4	31	5.5
1:400	41	7.8	33	6.8
1:450	45	9.8	36	8.0
1:500	50	13	38	9.5

* A result is positive if the risk of Down's syndrome term pregnancy based on age and AFP or age alone is more than or equal to specified cut-off risk. The rates were derived using the method given in the Appendix of Wald *et al.* (1988b)

2. the standard deviation in unaffected pregnancies was also small compared with the experience of others.

Table 4.8 shows the detection and false-positive rates associated with different risk cut-offs. Compared to using maternal age alone AFP provides about an extra 5% detection for the same false-positive rate.

Ultrasound gestation

The routine use of ultrasound biparietal diameter measurement to assess gestational age and calculate MoM values will alter the distributions of AFP values. The improved precision will contract the distributions as well as shift them upwards by about 1.5% due to the correction of systematic gestational overestimation in women with doubtful dates (Cuckle and Wald, 1987). While this will have only a small effect on detection and false-positive rates it can alter an individual woman's risk. Table 4.9 compares the LRs for the same MoM based on 'dates' and on scan.

Maternal weight

Maternal serum AFP levels (in MoMs) tend to decrease with increasing maternal weight. To allow for this negative association a woman's AFP level in MoMs is divided by the expected value for her weight. Table 4.10 shows the expected MoM value for a given weight in six studies. Since the average weight will differ between populations it is important for each centre to produce its own expected values for the population being screened. Also, as the data in Table 4.10 show, there may be other between-centre differences which affect the expected values. An Oxford woman weighing 40 kg with an unadjusted AFP level of 2.50 MoM would have an adjusted level of 1.91 MoM (2.50/1.31 using Series II). A woman weighing 90 kg with an unadjusted level of 1.80 MoM would have a level of 2.57 MoM (1.80/0.70) after adjustment. The distribution of adjusted MoM values will have less overlap than unadjusted values since one source of variability in AFP levels is the

Table 4.9 Likelihood ratio of Down's syndrome according to maternal serum AFP level, method of estimating gestational age (dates or scan) and whether or not maternal weight adjustment is carried out

AFP level (MoM)	Not adjusted for weight, gestational age estimated using:		Adjusted for weight, gestational age estimated using:	
	Dates	Scan	Dates	Scan
0.40	3.14	3.40	3.77	4.17
0.45	2.61	2.78	3.05	3.32
0.50	2.21	2.34	2.53	2.71
0.55	1.91	1.99	2.14	2.26
0.60	1.67	1.73	1.83	1.92
0.65	1.48	1.52	1.60	1.65
0.70	1.32	1.34	1.40	1.44
0.75	1.19	1.20	1.25	1.27
0.80	1.08	1.08	1.12	1.13
0.85	0.98	0.98	1.01	1.01
0.90	0.90	0.90	0.92	0.91
0.95	0.84	0.83	0.84	0.83
1.0	0.77	0.76	0.77	0.75
1.5	0.43	0.41	0.40	0.37
2.0	0.29	0.27	0.25	0.23
2.5	0.21	0.19	0.18	0.16

Derived from Gaussian distributions with parameters taken from Cuckle, Wald and Thompson (1987).

Table 4.10 Expected AFP level (MoM) for a given maternal weight in six studies

Study	Number of pregnancies	Maternal weight (kg)							
		30	40	50	60	70	80	90	100
Oxford:									
Series I[1]	902	1.49	1.31	1.16	1.02	0.90	0.79	0.70	0.62
Series II[2]	1725	1.45	1.28	1.13	1.00	0.89	0.79	0.70	0.62
N. Carolina:[3]									
Whites	NR	1.16	1.11	1.06	1.01	0.97	0.92	0.88	0.84
Blacks	NR	1.23	1.17	1.10	1.04	0.99	0.94	0.89	0.84
New York[4]	5740	1.27	1.17	1.09	1.00	0.93	0.86	0.79	0.73
Maine[5]	22 000	1.39	1.26	1.14	1.04	0.95	0.86	0.78	0.71
London[6]	1453	1.32	1.21	1.12	1.03	0.95	0.88	0.81	0.74

NR Not reported
[1] Wald et al., 1981
[2] Cuckle and Wald, unpublished observations
[3] Johnson and Lingley, 1984
[4] Macri et al., 1986
[5] Knight, Palomaki and Haddow, 1988
[6] Cuckle and Wald, unpublished observations

difference in weight within the population. The reduction in overlap is small so there is only a small effect on the false-positive and detection rates (there is no shift in values – maternal weight is similar in affected and unaffected pregnancies). However, given that information on maternal weight is usually readily available, it is probably worth making the adjustments. If values are adjusted the appropriate LR should be used (*see* Table 4.9).

Repeat AFP testing

Because of the effect of regression to the mean a second serum AFP result will tend to be higher than the first if it were repeated because the first was low (Haddow *et al.*, 1986). Consequently, if the second value lies above a given AFP cut-off level this should not necessarily be regarded as a negative screening test and the patient reassured since the risk of a Down's syndrome term pregnancy may still be high. The problem is largely overcome if risk is used as the screening variable since the risk for a second AFP result is contingent on the first result (Table 4.11). There is, however virtually no reduction in the false-positive rate for a given detection rate associated with a policy of routinely offering such women second serum AFP tests. The policy is therefore not justified, particularly since it also has the disadvantage that it will cause extra anxiety by delaying an amniocentesis.

Unjustified as it may be as a general policy, if a woman should happen to have a second AFP test, her risk of having a Down's syndrome term pregnancy should be estimated using both tests, otherwise women are liable to be counselled incorrectly. Table 4.11 gives LRs which permit the appropriate risk to be estimated for individual patients.

Other factors affecting AFP

Maternal serum AFP levels are, on average, high in blacks (about 1.15 MoM (Wald and Cuckle, 1987)) and low in insulin-dependent diabetics (about 0.77 MoM; Table 4.12). They are also high in the presence of a twin pregnancy (2 MoM). In populations with a large black or white minority it may be worthwhile producing race-specific median values for the calculation of MoMs. For insulin-dependent diabetics and twins where the effect is large and the circumstance rare, a different approach is more appropriate. The average MoM value is not known in diabetic pregnancies affected by Down's syndrome or in twin pregnancies in which one of the fetuses is affected. The risk of Down's syndrome cannot, therefore, be estimated. The next best approach is to adopt a screening strategy that would result in the same false-positive rate as in singleton non-diabetic pregnancies and accept that the detection rate is not known. This involves dividing the MoM value by 0.77 for diabetics and by 2 for twin pregnancies, and then calculating a 'pseudo-risk' using the LRs in Table 4.9. This is then compared with the cut-off risk to determine if the screening test is positive.

Other types of aneuploidy and AFP

Down's syndrome screening programmes based on combining information on maternal age and AFP are likely to lead to the incidental detection of trisomy 18 because, as with Down's syndrome, the birth prevalence of trisomy 18 increases with maternal age, and maternal serum AFP levels in pregnancies associated with

Table 4.11 Likelihood ratio of Down's syndrome fetus according to the AFP level in the first and second test

First AFP test (MoM)	No second test	Second AFP test (MoM)																						
		0.40	0.45	0.50	0.55	0.60	0.65	0.70	0.75	0.80	0.85	0.90	0.95	1.00	1.10	1.20	1.30	1.40	1.50	1.60	1.70	1.80	1.90	2.00	2.50
0.40	3.14	3.38	3.08	2.87	2.73	2.63	2.57	2.53	2.50	2.50	*	*	*	*	*	*	*	*	*	*	*	*	*	*	*
0.45	2.61	3.08	2.76	2.53	2.38	2.26	2.18	2.12	2.08	2.06	2.05	2.04	*	*	*	*	*	*	*	*	*	*	*	*	*
0.50	2.21	2.87	2.53	2.30	2.13	2.01	1.91	1.85	1.80	1.76	1.73	1.72	1.71	1.71	*	*	*	*	*	*	*	*	*	*	*
0.55	1.91	2.73	2.38	2.13	1.95	1.82	1.72	1.65	1.59	1.55	1.51	1.49	1.47	1.46	1.45	*	*	*	*	*	*	*	*	*	*
0.60	1.67	2.63	2.26	2.01	1.82	1.68	1.58	1.50	1.43	1.39	1.35	1.32	1.30	1.28	1.26	1.26	*	*	*	*	*	*	*	*	*
0.65	1.48	2.57	2.18	1.91	1.72	1.58	1.47	1.38	1.32	1.26	1.22	1.19	1.16	1.14	1.12	1.10	1.10	*	*	*	*	*	*	*	*
0.70	1.32	2.53	2.12	1.85	1.65	1.50	1.38	1.29	1.22	1.17	1.12	1.09	1.06	1.04	1.00	0.98	0.97	0.97	*	*	*	*	*	*	*
0.75	1.19	2.50	2.08	1.80	1.59	1.43	1.32	1.22	1.15	1.09	1.05	1.01	0.98	0.95	0.91	0.89	0.87	0.87	0.87	*	*	*	*	*	*
0.80	1.08	2.50	2.06	1.76	1.55	1.39	1.26	1.17	1.09	1.03	0.98	0.94	0.91	0.88	0.84	0.81	0.80	0.78	0.78	0.78	*	*	*	*	*
0.85	0.99	*	2.05	1.73	1.51	1.35	1.22	1.12	1.05	0.98	0.93	0.89	0.86	0.83	0.78	0.75	0.73	0.72	0.71	0.70	0.70	*	*	*	*
0.90	0.91	*	2.04	1.72	1.49	1.32	1.19	1.09	1.01	0.94	0.89	0.85	0.81	0.78	0.74	0.70	0.68	0.66	0.65	0.64	0.64	0.64	*	*	*
0.95	0.84	*	*	1.71	1.47	1.30	1.16	1.06	0.98	0.91	0.86	0.81	0.77	0.74	0.69	0.66	0.63	0.62	0.60	0.59	0.59	0.59	0.59	*	*
1.00	0.77	*	*	1.71	1.46	1.28	1.14	1.04	0.95	0.88	0.83	0.78	0.74	0.71	0.66	0.62	0.60	0.58	0.56	0.55	0.55	0.54	0.54	0.54	*
1.10	0.67	*	*	*	1.45	1.26	1.12	1.00	0.91	0.84	0.78	0.74	0.69	0.66	0.61	0.57	0.54	0.52	0.50	0.49	0.48	0.47	0.47	0.46	*
1.20	0.59	*	*	*	*	1.26	1.10	0.98	0.89	0.81	0.75	0.70	0.66	0.62	0.57	0.53	0.49	0.47	0.45	0.44	0.43	0.42	0.41	0.41	*
1.30	0.53	*	*	*	*	*	1.10	0.97	0.87	0.80	0.73	0.68	0.63	0.60	0.54	0.49	0.46	0.44	0.42	0.40	0.39	0.38	0.37	0.36	0.35
1.40	0.48	*	*	*	*	*	*	0.97	0.87	0.78	0.72	0.66	0.62	0.58	0.52	0.47	0.44	0.41	0.39	0.37	0.36	0.35	0.34	0.33	0.31
1.50	0.43	*	*	*	*	*	*	*	0.87	0.78	0.71	0.65	0.60	0.56	0.50	0.45	0.42	0.39	0.36	0.35	0.33	0.32	0.31	0.30	0.28
1.60	0.39	*	*	*	*	*	*	*	*	0.78	0.70	0.64	0.59	0.55	0.49	0.44	0.40	0.37	0.35	0.33	0.31	0.30	0.29	0.28	0.26
1.70	0.36	*	*	*	*	*	*	*	*	*	0.70	0.64	0.59	0.55	0.48	0.43	0.39	0.36	0.33	0.31	0.30	0.28	0.27	0.27	0.24
1.80	0.33	*	*	*	*	*	*	*	*	*	*	0.64	0.59	0.54	0.47	0.42	0.38	0.35	0.32	0.30	0.28	0.27	0.26	0.25	0.22
1.90	0.31	*	*	*	*	*	*	*	*	*	*	*	0.59	0.54	0.47	0.41	0.37	0.34	0.31	0.29	0.27	0.26	0.25	0.24	0.21
2.00	0.29	*	*	*	*	*	*	*	*	*	*	*	*	0.54	0.46	0.41	0.36	0.33	0.30	0.28	0.27	0.25	0.24	0.23	0.20
2.50	0.21	*	*	*	*	*	*	*	*	*	*	*	*	*	*	*	0.35	0.31	0.28	0.26	0.24	0.22	0.21	0.20	0.16

* Cannot be estimated since the higher value is more than double the lower

Derived from Cuckle et al. (1988b)

Table 4.12 Maternal serum AFP levels in insulin dependent diabetics from five studies

Study	Number of women	Median AFP level (MoM)
Oxford		
Series I[1]	27	0.60*
Series II[2]	124	0.81
Boston[3]	322	0.70**
Yale[4]	161	0.91
Boston[5]	164	0.81
Total	798	0.77***

   * Geometric mean
  ** From Figure 1 in reference
*** Weighted geometric mean
[1] Wald *et al.* (1979)
[2] Cuckle and Wald, unpublished observations
[3] Milunsky *et al.* (1982)
[4] Reece *et al.* (1987)
[5] Green *et al.* (1988)

Table 4.13 Maternal serum AFP levels in trisomy 18 pregnancies, from six studies

Study	Number of cases	Median AFP level (MoM)
New York/Cleveland[1]	13	0.65*
Los Angeles[2]	3	0.80*
Toronto[3]	10	0.64
Milan[4]	3**	0.50
Seattle[5]	10	0.72
Oxford[6]	38***	0.60
Madras[7]	3	0.77
Frankfurt[8]	7	0.51
San Diego[9]	3	0.73
Copenhagen[10]	7	0.49
Total	97	0.63†

[1] Merkatz *et al.* (1984)
[2] Hershey, Grandall and Schroth (1985)
[3] Doran *et al.* (1986)
[4] Brambati *et al.* (1986)
[5] Ashwood, Cheng and Lathy (1987)
[6] Lindenbaum *et al.* (1987)
[7] Subramanian *et al.* (1988)
[8] Dix *et al.* (1988)
[9] Bogart *et al.* (1989)
[10] Norgaard-Pedersen *et al.* (1990)
   * Estimated from figure in publication
  ** First trimester cases
*** Excludes cases associated with neural tube defects or exomphalos
†   Weighted geometric mean

trisomy 18 are lower than average (Table 4.13). In a prospective study of combined maternal age and AFP screening for Down's syndrome, out of 807 screen positive women having an amniocentesis, 10 had infants with Down's syndrome and four with trisomy 18 (Palomaki, 1986). The benefits of detecting trisomy 18 antenatally are limited by the fact that most such pregnancies do not reach term and most infants born with the disorder die shortly after birth.

Some reports have suggested that chromosomal abnormalities such as trisomy 13 and Turner's syndrome may also be associated with reduced serum AFP levels but too few data on these have so far been published to enable a judgement to be made on the degree of incidental detection.

Unconjugated oestriol (uE$_3$) and human chorionic gonadotrophin (hCG)

Two studies have shown that second trimester maternal serum uE$_3$ levels are low in pregnancies associated with Down's syndrome (Canick et al., 1988; Wald et al., 1988a; Osathanondh et al., 1989; Norgaard-Pedersen et al., 1990). In the first, among 22 cases and 110 matched controls the median level was 0.79 MoM. In the second including 77 cases and 385 matched controls it was 0.73 MoM. The more recent studies have found medians of 0.66 (26 cases) and 0.74 (42 cases).

Eight studies have shown increased levels of hCG. The first based on 17 cases and 74 controls found that the level in cases was 2.77 times that in controls, but did not allow for changes related to gestational age (Bogart, Pandian and Jones, 1987). The second study used the same 77 cases and 385 controls previously used to study uE$_3$ and found that the median value in the cases was 2.04 MoM (Wald et al., 1988b). Pooling these results with those from other more recent studies (Arab et al., 1988; Bogart et al., 1989; White, Papilia and Magnay, 1989; Osathanondh et al., 1989; Petrocik, Wassman and Kelly, 1989; Norgaard-Pedersen et al., 1990) yields an average of 2.08 MoM in 257 cases. The extent of reduction in uE$_3$ and increase in hCG is not related to maternal age.

A series of samples taken in the first trimester (Cuckle et al., 1988) yielded a low uE$_3$ level of 0.35 MoM (based on 17 cases and 85 controls). This and another study (Bogart et al., 1989) failed to find an increase in hCG (based on 22 cases and 108 controls (Cuckle et al., 1988)).

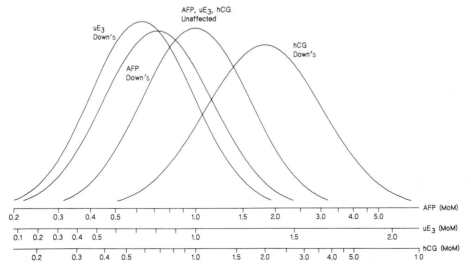

Figure 4.4 Distribution of maternal serum AFP, uE$_3$ and hCG in Down's syndrome and unaffected pregnancies, using parameters in Wald et al., 1988b

Table 4.14 Likelihood ratio of Down's syndrome according to AFP, uE₃ and hCG level at 14–20 weeks' gestation

uE_3 (MoM)	hCG (MoM)	AFP (MoM)					
		0.40	0.70	1.0	2.0	2.5	Not done
0.40	0.50	1.1	0.30	0.14	0.029	0.018	0.34
	0.70	2.1	0.66	0.32	0.074	0.046	0.69
	1.0	4.6	1.6	0.80	0.21	0.14	1.5
	1.5	12	4.5	2.4	0.72	0.49	4.1
	2.0	24	9.8	5.5	1.8	1.3	8.6
	Not done	13	6.0	3.8	1.6	1.3	5.5
0.70	0.50	0.78	0.24	0.12	0.027	0.017	0.23
	0.70	1.4	0.46	0.23	0.061	0.040	0.41
	1.0	2.6	0.96	0.51	0.15	0.10	0.81
	1.5	5.6	2.3	1.3	0.44	0.31	1.9
	2.0	10	4.5	2.7	0.98	0.70	3.5
	Not done	4.7	2.3	1.5	0.65	0.50	1.9
1.0	0.50	0.47	0.16	0.081	0.021	0.014	0.13
	0.70	0.71	0.27	0.14	0.041	0.028	0.20
	1.0	1.2	0.48	0.27	0.087	0.061	0.35
	1.5	2.2	0.98	0.59	0.22	0.16	0.71
	2.0	3.5	1.7	1.1	0.43	0.32	1.2
	Not done	1.6	0.79	0.51	0.23	0.18	0.61
1.2	0.50	0.30	0.11	0.057	0.016	0.011	0.079
	0.70	0.42	0.16	0.091	0.028	0.019	0.12
	1.0	0.62	0.27	0.16	0.054	0.039	0.18
	1.5	1.0	0.49	0.31	0.12	0.090	0.34
	2.0	1.5	0.78	0.51	0.22	0.17	0.54
	Not done	0.73	0.37	0.24	0.11	0.086	0.27
1.4	0.50	0.17	0.067	0.036	0.011	0.007	0.045
	0.70	0.22	0.092	0.053	0.018	0.012	0.061
	1.0	0.30	0.14	0.083	0.031	0.022	0.089
	1.5	0.44	0.22	0.14	0.062	0.047	0.15
	2.0	0.61	0.33	0.22	0.10	0.081	0.22
	Not done	0.32	0.16	0.11	0.050	0.039	0.11
Not done	0.50	0.53	0.16	0.78	0.019	0.012	0.13
	0.70	0.92	0.30	0.14	0.036	0.023	0.23
	1.0	1.7	0.59	0.30	0.081	0.053	0.44
	1.5	3.9	1.4	0.75	0.22	0.15	1.0
	2.0	7.3	2.8	1.5	0.48	0.33	2.0
	Not done	3.2	1.3	0.77	0.28	0.20	1.0

Derived from Gaussian distributions with parameters taken from Wald *et al.* (1988b)

The fact that in some second trimester studies AFP, uE₃, and hCG have been measured on the same samples allows direct comparisons between them. Figure 4.4 gives the distribution of MoM values in affected pregnancies for the three variables appropriately scaled so that the mean and standard deviation for unaffected pregnancies are the same for each variable. This shows that hCG measurement leads to greater separation between affected and unaffected pregnancies than can be achieved using either of the other variables alone.

There is little correlation between the three serum variables so that they each provide considerable independent additional information on the extent of risk

Table 4.15 Detection rates corresponding to specified false-positive rates using maternal age and serumAFP, uE₃ and hCG alone or in combination*

False positive rate (%)	Detection rate (%) using age with:						
	AFP	uE₃	hCG	AFP and uE₃	AFP and hCG	uE₃ and hCG	AFP, uE₃ and hCG
1	18	21	28	23	32	35	38
2	24	27	36	31	41	43	47
3	28	32	41	36	47	49	53
4	32	36	45	40	51	53	57
5	34	40	49	44	55	57	61
6	37	43	52	47	58	60	64
7	39	46	55	50	61	62	66
8	42	48	57	52	63	65	69
9	44	50	59	55	65	67	71
10	46	52	61	57	67	68	72

* Estimated using the method described in the Appendix of Wald *et al.* (1988b)

(Wald *et al.*, 1988b). As with AFP and age, the best screening results are obtained by estimating the age-specific risk from Table 4.1 and multiplying this by the appropriate likelihood ratio. This is derived from the ratio of the heights of a single, bivariate or trivariate distribution for the subset of serum variables considered. Table 4.14 gives the LR for selected values of the three variables.

The detection rate associated with a given false-positive rate using different combinations of the serum variables is shown in Table 4.15. If there are sufficient resources to carry out an amniocentesis and a karyotype on 5% of all pregnant women then the detection achieved by screening using all the tests in combination (61%) is much higher than it is using AFP alone (34%). In trisomy 18, uE₃ and hCG levels appear to be low (Arab *et al.*, 1988; Bogart *et al.*, 1989; Norgaard-Pedersen *et al.*, 1990) but it is not yet possible to estimate the impact of serum screening on their incidental detection.

Ultrasound

Two distinct methods of screening for Down's syndrome using ultrasound have been proposed. The first is the identification of associated abnormalities such as duodenal atresia and cardiac defects. Although such abnormalities can be demonstrated late in pregnancy there is little information available on which to assess the value of second trimester ultrasound screening to identify them. The second method is based on quantitative measurement of different parts of the fetus. Three such measures have been suggested: namely the ratio of the biparietal diameter (BPD) to the occipitofrontal diameter of the fetal skull (the cephalic index), nuchal thickness and femur length.

Cephalic index

Since Down's syndrome fetuses early in pregnancy have BPD measurements that are similar to unaffected fetuses (Cuckle and Wald, 1987) and brachycephaly is a feature of Down's syndrome infants, it was speculated that the cephalic index might

Table 4.16 Cephalic index* in Down's syndrome and unaffected pregnancies, results from four studies

Study	Down's syndrome			Unaffected pregnancies		
	No.	Mean	(s.d.)	No.	Mean	(s.d.)
Australia[1]	1	0.93	(–)	53	0.81**	(NR)
Canada[2]	8	0.83	(0.03)	308	0.82	(0.04)
New Haven[3]	16	0.81	(0.04)	180	0.80	(0.04)
Detroit[4]	12	0.80	(0.07)	16	0.77	(0.04)
Alabama[5]	15	0.81	(0.03)	45	0.79	(0.02)

[1] Buttery (1979)
[2] Perry *et al.* (1984)
[3] Lockwood *et al.* (1987)
[4] Sacks *et al.* (1988)
[5]Brumfield *et al.* (1989)
* Occipitofrontal diameter (OFD) divided by biparietal diameter (BPD)
** The mean of the BPD/OFD was reported (1.24); 0.81 is the inverse of this mean
NR Not reported

be increased in affected pregnancies. Five studies have been published on cephalic index including measurements on a total of 52 affected pregnancies (Table 4.16). All indicate a tendency for the index to be increased in affected pregnancies though none reach statistical significance and on the basis of these results a large effect can be excluded.

Nuchal thickness

Infants with Down's syndrome can have an excess of skin or soft tissue at the back of the neck. This observation prompted Benacerraf and her colleagues to investigate the nuchal thickness of fetuses measured by ultrasound in the second trimester; 43% (12/28) of affected and 0.1% (4/3804) of unaffected pregnancies had an occipital soft tissue thickness of 6 mm or more (Benacerraf, Frigoletto and Cramer, 1987). In an attempt to verify these findings Toi and colleagues reviewed the autopsies from 11 Down's syndrome fetuses that were aborted following an amniocentesis, but were not macerated and did not have hydrops fetalis; two (18%) had neck thickening (Toi, Simpson and Filly, 1987). The ultrasound results relating to 28 unaffected control pregnancies (that had raised amniotic fluid AFP levels) demonstrated nuchal thickening of 6 mm or more in six (21%), virtually the same

Table 4.17 Likelihood ratio of Down's syndrome according to femur length expressed as a multiple of the value expected for the biparietal diameter and centre

Femur length	+0.00	+0.01	+0.02	+0.03	+0.04	+0.05	+0.06	+0.07	+0.08	+0.09
0.8	28	21	16	12	9.2	7.2	5.7	4.6	3.6	2.9
0.9	2.4	2.0	1.7	1.4	1.2	1.0	0.92	0.81	0.73	0.65
1.0	0.60	0.55	0.55	0.48	0.46	0.44	0.42	0.4	0.41	0.41
1.1	0.42	0.42	0.44	0.46	0.48	0.51	0.55	0.68	0.66	0.73

Derived from Gaussian distributions with parameters taken from Cuckle *et al.* 1989. Select row and column adding up to the nearest femur length.

proportion that was found in the affected autopsy series. It was also found that it was possible to produce an artefactually increased nuchal thickness on the ultrasound image by inclining the image plane so that it included the cerebellum and occiput.

The discrepancy between the estimates of the false-positive rate in the two studies together with the demonstration of how artefact can so easily be introduced means that, on present evidence, screening for Down's syndrome by ultrasound nuchal thickness measurement is not justified.

Femur length

There is a possibility that the short stature associated with children with Down's syndrome is reflected *in utero* by short second trimester femur lengths measured by ultrasound. Ten studies including information on femur length in affected and unaffected pregnancies have been published. The first two showed marked effects (Benacerraf, Gelman and Frigoletto, 1987; Lockwood *et al.*, 1987), as did only one of the subsequent studies (Brumfield *et al.*, 1989). The remainder either found no material effect on similar numbers of observations (Platt *et al.*, 1988; Porto *et al.*, 1988; Sacks *et al.*, 1988; Winston and Horger, 1989; Lynch *et al.*, 1989) or found that the magnitude of the effect was relatively modest (Peters, Lockwood and Miller, 1989; Cuckle *et al.*, 1989).

In the first report the median femur length of 28 pregnancies with Down's syndrome was 88% of that expected from 192 unaffected pregnancies (Benacerraf, Gelman and Frigoletto, 1987a). The second report based on 33 cases and 277 control pregnancies found that the mean femur length was reduced to 88–91% of the mean value for the controls at each of three gestational periods between 16 and 21 weeks (Lockwood *et al.*, 1987). The other confirmatory study yielded results in 15 affected pregnancies which were 91% of those in 45 controls.

All of the studies except our own (Cuckle *et al.*, 1989) include too few cases to draw reliable conclusions. In our own study of 83 affected and 1340 control pregnancies from 27 centres, femur length was expressed as a multiple of the expected value for BPD measured at the same centre. Expected values were based on linear regression of femur length and BPD. The median value in affected pregnancies was 0.94 and the extent of reduction was independent of BPD (and hence gestation) and maternal age. Values fitted a Gaussian distribution and Table 4.17 gives the LRs for different femur lengths between 0.80 and 1.19 multiples of the expected value. Using these LRs to estimate risk from maternal age and femur length would lead to a 34% detection rate for a 5% false-positive rate, a similar benefit over using age alone to that achieved by AFP. Until correlation studies have been carried out between femur length and AFP, uE$_3$ and hCG levels in both Down's syndrome and unaffected pregnancies, information on femur length cannot be used in serum screening programmes for Down's syndrome.

Planning a screening programme

There are a number of practical issues involved in setting up a screening programme for Down's syndrome that need to be considered. These affect the choice of tests, the choice of assay method, how to derive normal medians, when to screen, what special arrangements are needed for women of advanced maternal age, whether women with a previously affected pregnancy should be screened, how to estimate risk and the choice of risk cut-off level.

Which tests to use

In centres using AFP to screen for neural tube defects there is no extra assay cost associated with using AFP for Down's syndrome screening. Screeners at such centres may want to test the same sample for uE_3 and hCG, but if resources were available only for one of these tests, hCG is the one of choice since it gives the higher rate of detection. If AFP were not already being measured and only two tests could be carried out then hCG and uE_3 would be the tests of choice. However, since AFP has the major advantage of being able to screen for neural tube defects and hCG and uE_3 do not, the 'best' pair of tests are hCG and AFP particularly as the Down's syndrome detection rate using hCG and AFP is not much less than that of hCG and uE_3.

The economic argument for performing all three tests is strong, especially if an AFP test is being performed routinely as part of an antenatal screening programme for neural tube defects. At any level of detection the extra cost of the hCG test and the uE_3 tests would be much less than the cost of the amniocenteses and karyotypes that would otherwise be needed to obtain the same detection rate. For example, to achieve 60% detection, out of every 1000 women screened using age and all three serum tests, 48 (47 unaffected and about one affected) would need an amniocentesis and a karyotype, compared with 201 (200 unaffected and about one affected) using age and AFP alone. The cost of 153 amniocenteses and karyotypes saved would exceed the cost of 1000 hCG and uE_3 tests by about fivefold.

Centres which do not have the resources for serum screening but have routine ultrasound examination of the fetus will be able to improve maternal age screening by incorporating information on femur length as described above.

Which assay to use

AFP assays based on radio-immunoassay (RIA) and enzyme-linked immunosorbent assay (ELISA) which are in current use have been optimized to measure high AFP levels (for neural tube defect screening) rather than low AFP levels. An immunoradiometric assay (IRMA) system is likely to have a wider operating range and so be suitable for both neural tube defect and Down's syndrome screening. However, an existing RIA or ELISA system is adequate for Down's syndrome screening. There are three reasons for this. First, most of the published results use these assay systems and the predicted performance can therefore be achieved with such assays. Secondly, a woman can have a positive screening result over a wide range of AFP levels not with only low values. For example a 33-year-old woman with moderate AFP, uE_3 and hCG levels of 0.70, 0.60 and 1.50 MoM respectively will have a risk greater than 1 in 200. Thirdly, assay imprecision represents only a small proportion (about 10–20%) of the variance of AFP, so that even if it were halved, the overlap in the distributions between affected and unaffected pregnancies would not alter much.

Existing uE_3 and hCG assays have been optimized for third and first trimester pregnancies respectively. These assays can be readily modified for use in the middle trimester of pregnancy; the uE_3 assay can be made more sensitive by increasing the volume of sample used (and diluting the standards accordingly) and the hCG assay modified by diluting the sample about 500-fold.

Derivation of normal medians

In order to calculate accurate MoM values for the serum tests, a normal median is required for each day of gestation. Such values can be obtained by performing regression analysis on the medians for each completed week of gestation ideally weighted by the number of women tested. For AFP, linear regression of the logarithms of the medians should be used; for uE_3 a linear regression on the unlogged medians, and for hCG a more complicated regression is required based on an exponential plus a constant term (Wald *et al.*, 1988b). The hCG regression can however be simplified by transforming the gestation in days, x, to $e^{-0.06814x}$ and using linear regression on the result.

The use of medians in the regression rather than the individual values is to avoid the necessity of using data relating exclusively to unaffected pregnancies. (The occasional outlying value from an affected pregnancy will not greatly influence a median.)

When in pregnancy to screen

In centres with AFP screening programmes for neural tube defects a serum sample is normally taken as close as possible to 16–18 weeks' gestation when there is the least overlap between the distributions of AFP values in affected and unaffected pregnancies. With Down's syndrome screening the limiting factor is the 3 weeks needed to produce a fetal karyotype from an amniotic fluid sample. This necessitates screening tests being carried out as early as possible in the second trimester. If AFP is used in both neural tube defect and Down's syndrome screening these considerations lead to 16 weeks' gestation as the optimal time for the test.

Maternal age

Serum screening for Down's syndrome should be offered to all women irrespective of their age. Some older women who previously would have been offered an amniocentesis because of their age will no longer have positive screening results. Table 4.18 shows that, for example, when using a 1:250 risk cut-off only 22% of woman aged 35 or more would be considered positive though this would include 86% of the affected pregnancies in the group. The loss of detection by not including all women aged 35 or more is 4.9% ([100-86%] × 35% – the proportion of affected pregnancies in the group; *see* Table 4.5) but it is more than compensated for by the increased detection of 31% (48% × 65%) by including younger women and this is achieved with a reduction in the false-positive rate from 7.4% (*see* Table 4.5) to 5.0%.

Until serum screening is generally accepted it may be necessary to provide resources for some 'older' women with negative screening results having an amniocentesis.

Previous Down's syndrome

Some women with a history of a Down's syndrome pregnancy may have a low risk based on biochemical findings. Unlike the older women it would be reasonable still to regard such women as having positive screening results. The numbers involved are not great and any woman who has had an affected pregnancy is likely to want to have the opportunity of choosing whether to have an amniocentesis regardless of any prior screening procedure.

How to estimate a woman's risk

When using maternal age and serum AFP alone the likelihood ratios in Table 4.7 will provide an estimate of risk for a MoM value derived from gestational age based

Table 4.18 Maternal serum screening for Downs syndrome using age, AFP, uE₃ and hCG in combination: detection rate (DR) and false-positive rate (FPR) in different maternal age groups, according to cut-off*

Maternal age at EDD (years)	Risk cut-off					
	1:200		1:250		1:300	
	DR (%)	FPR (%)	DR (%)	FPR (%)	DR (%)	FPR (%)
≥35	83	19	86	22	88	26
<35	43	2.7	48	3.6	52	4.6
≥38	90	31	92	36	94	40
<38	47	3.2	52	4.2	56	5.2
≥40	94	42	96	48	96	53
<40	50	3.5	54	4.5	58	5.6
Any	57	3.9	61	5.0	64	6.1

*A result is positive if the risk of a Down's syndrome term pregnancy based on age, AFP, uE₃ and hCG is greater than or equal to the specified risk cut-off. The rates were derived using the method given in the Appendix of Wald *et al.* (1988b).
EDD = Expected date of delivery

on dates. For MoM values derived from estimates of gestational age based on ultrasound or MoM values adjusted for maternal weight the likelihood ratio can be obtained from Table 4.9. If a second test is performed on a fresh sample the likelihood ratio can be obtained from Table 4.11 for gestational age based on dates or from published formulae for gestational age based on ultrasound and maternal weight adjusted values (Cuckle *et al.*, 1990).

When using maternal age and any combination of the three serum screening variables the LR can be obtained by interpolating from Table 4.14 or using the published formulae (Wald *et al.*, 1988b) which are for MoM values based on dates with AFP values unadjusted for maternal weight. If the LRs in Table 4.14 or the published formulae are used for MoM values based on ultrasound or AFP values adjusted for maternal weight, the result will be conservative in the sense that those designated screen positive will have on average a greater risk of Down's syndrome than estimated and those who are screen negative will have a lower risk than estimated.

Which cut-off risk to use

The choice of risk cut-off will be determined mainly by the expected workload in terms of number of amniocenteses and karyotypes that would result from any particular screening policy. It can be chosen to reduce the workload associated with an existing maternal age screening programme while maintaining the same detection rate. Alternatively, it can be chosen to increase the detection rate while maintaining the same workload.

The amniocentesis rate with most reasonable risk cut-off levels is almost the same as the false-positive rate. These rates have been published using data on the maternal age distribution for England and Wales in 1981–85 (Wald and Cuckle, 1987; Wald *et al.*, 1988a, b). For populations with a different age structure the amniocentesis rate can be estimated empirically by estimating the risk in say, 200 women and determining the number of women whose risk exceeds the chosen risk cut-off level.

An additional consideration is the need to weigh the risk of having an affected term pregnancy against the hazards of amniocentesis or chorionic villus sampling (CVS). Randomized clinical trials are currently evaluating the efficacy and safety of CVS. The hazards of amniocentesis have been investigated in four non-randomized studies, three of which did not reveal any particular risks (National Institute for Child Health and Development, 1976; Medical Research Council of Canada, 1977; Crandall *et al.*, 1980), while the fourth suggested a 1.3% excess risk of miscarriage as well as an increased risk of congenital dislocation of the hip, talipes and neonatal respiratory problems (Working Party on Amniocentesis, 1978). The suggestion that amniocentesis is a cause of congenital dislocation of the hip and talipes has been discounted by a large case-control study (Wald *et al.*, 1983), but an excess risk of miscarriage has been confirmed by a randomized trial (Tabor *et al.*, 1986; 1988). This showed in those randomized to amniocentesis compared with the controls a 0.8% excess risk of miscarriage.

This risk of miscarriage is undoubtedly important in counselling women and in selecting a cut-off risk of Down's syndrome in screening programmes. However, there is no way of balancing values such as those of a Down's syndrome pregnancy and an amniocentesis-induced miscarriage for patients in general. Different people will assess each differently (*see* Chapter 11). In general, and resources permitting, it is probably best to choose a cut-off risk of Down's syndrome that is numerically lower than the risk of an amniocentesis-induced miscarriage and accept that following counselling some may not want the amniocentesis.

Another approach is to use a cut-off risk equivalent to the maternal age cut-off used before the introduction of serum screening. The previous acceptability of screening at this risk level would then justify the new policy. This argument is not a strong one. Previous practice could not have been influenced by knowledge of the risks of amniocentesis which have only become reliably quantified recently and the approach ignores the resource implications of the policy.

Conclusion

Using maternal age to select women for an amniocentesis and make an antenatal diagnosis of Down's syndrome is associated with a low detection rate. It is a poor method of screening. New methods are needed that can distinguish affected from unaffected pregnancies in a simple, safe and inexpensive way; the recently described use of maternal serum markers offers this opportunity. Such screening has a much higher detection rate and is likely to be generally acceptable. From the point of view of the patient, it involves no additional inconvenience (the tests can be performed on a blood sample that is already routinely collected) and from the point of view of the laboratory it involves the performance of two additional tests that are already available for other purposes. Computer software is needed to interpret the screening data and this is now available commercially for use either in the laboratory or in the doctor's clinic. There are therefore no reasons to delay the general introduction of Down's syndrome screening using the new maternal serum methods.

References

Arab, H., Siegel-Bartelt, J., Wong, P.Y. and Doran, T. (1988) Maternal serum beta human chorionic gonadotropin (MSHCG) combined with maternal serum alpha fetoprotein (MSAFP) appears superior for prenatal screening for Down syndrome (DS) than either test alone. *American Journal of Human Genetics*, **43**, A225

Ashwood, E.R., Cheng, E. and Luthy, D.A. (1987) Maternal serum alpha-fetoprotein and fetal trisomy-21 in women 35 years and older: implications for alpha-fetoprotein screening programs. *American Journal of Medical Genetics*, **26**, 531–539

Benacerraf, B.R., Frigoletto, F.D. and Cramer, D.W. (1987) Down syndrome: sonographic signs for diagnosis in the second trimester. *Radiology*, **163**, 811–813

Benacerraf, B.R., Gelman, R. and Frigoletto, F.D. (1987) Sonographic identification of second-trimester fetuses with Down's syndrome. *New England Journal of Medicine*, **317**, 1371–1376

Bogart, M.H., Golbus, M.S., Sorg, N.D. and Jones, O.W. (1989) Human chorionic gonadotropin levels in pregnancies with aneuploid fetuses. *Prenatal Diagnosis*, **9**, 379–384

Bogart, M.H., Pandian, M.R. and Jones, C.W. (1987) Abnormal maternal serum chorionic gonadotropin levels in pregnancies with fetal chromosome abnormalities. *Prenatal Diagnosis*, **7**, 623–630

Brambati, B., Simoni, G., Bonacchi, I. and Pecini, L. (1986) Fetal chromosome aneuploidies and maternal serum alpha-fetoprotein levels in the first trimester. *Lancet*, **ii**, 165–166

Brumfield, C.G., Hauth, J.C., Cloud, G.A., Davis, R.O., Henson, B.V. and Cosper, P. (1989) Sonographic measurements and ratios in fetuses with Down syndrome. *Obstetrics and Gynecology*, **73**, 644

Buttery, B. (1979) Occipitofrontal-biparietal diameter ratio: an ultrasonic parameter for the antenatal evaluation of Down's syndrome. *Medical Journal of Australia*, **2**, 662–664

Canick, J.A., Knight, G.J., Palomaki, G.E., Haddow, J.E., Cuckle, H.S. and Wald, N.J. (1988) Low second trimester maternal serum unconjugated oestriol in pregnancies with Down's syndrome. *British Journal of Obstetrics and Gynaecology*, **95**, 330–333

Crandall, B.F., Howard, J., Lebherz, T.B., Rubinstein, L., Sample, W.F. and Sarn, D. (1980) Follow-up of 2000 second trimester amniocenteses. *Obstetrics and Gynecology*, **56**, 625–628

Cuckle, H.S. and Wald, N.J. (1986) Amniotic fluid alpha-fetoprotein levels in Down syndrome. *Lancet*, **ii**, 290–291

Cuckle, H.S. and Wald, N.J. (1987) The effect of estimating gestational age by ultrasound cephalometry on the sensitivity of alpha-fetoprotein screening for Down's syndrome. *British Journal of Obstetrics and Gynaecology*, **94**, 274–276

Cuckle, H.S., Wald, N.J., Barkai, G. *et al.* (1988a) First trimester biochemical screening for Down's syndrome. *Lancet*, **ii**, 851–852

Cuckle, H.S., Wald, N.J., Nanchahal, K. and Densem, J.W. (1988b) Repeat maternal serum testing in antenatal screening programmes for Down syndrome. *British Journal of Obstetrics and Gynaecology*, **96**, 52–60

Cuckle, H.S., Wald, N.J., Quinn, J., Royston, P. and Butler, L. (1989) Ultrasound fetal femur length measurement in the screening for Down's syndrome. *British Journal of Obstetrics and Gynaecology*, **96**, 1373–1378

Cuckle, H., Wald, N. and Thompson, S. (1987) Estimating a woman's risk of having a pregnancy associated with Down syndrome using her age and serum alpha-fetoprotein level. *British Journal of Obstetrics and Gynaecology*, **94**, 387–402

DiMaio, M.S., Baumgarten, A., Greenstein, R., Saal, H. and Mahoney, M. (1987) Screening for fetal Down syndrome in pregnancy by measuring maternal serum alpha-fetoprotein levels. *New England Journal of Medicine*, **317**, 342–346

Dix, U., Grams, M., Grubisic, A., Derick-Tan, J.S.E. and Langenbeck, U. (1988) Alpha-Fetoprotein im mutterlichen Serum bei Schwangerschaften mit Trisomie 18. *Z. Gerburtsh. U. Perinat.*, **192**, 231–233

Doran, T.A., Cadesky, K., Wong, P.Y., Mastrogiacomo, C. and Capello, T. (1986) Maternal serum alpha-fetoprotein and fetal autosomal trisomies. *American Journal of Obstetrics and Gynecology*, **154**, 277–281

Ferguson-Smith, M.A. and Yates, J.R.W. (1984) Maternal age specific rates for chromosome aberrations and factors influencing them: report of a collaborative European study on 52 965 amniocenteses. *Prenatal Diagnosis*, **4**, 5–44

Greene, M.F., Haddow, J.E., Palomaki, G.E. and Knight, G.J. (1988) Maternal serum alpha-fetoprotein levels in diabetic pregnancies. *Lancet*, **ii**, 345–346

Haddow, J.E., Palomaki, G.E., Wald, N.J. and Cuckle, H.S. (1986) Maternal serum alpha-fetoprotein screening for Down syndrome and repeat testing. *Lancet*, **ii**, 1460

Hershey, D.W., Crandall, B.F. and Schroth, P.S. (1985) Maternal serum alpha-fetoprotein screening of fetal trisomies. *American Journal of Obstetrics and Gynecology*, **153**, 224–225

Hook, E.B. (1983) Chromosome abnormalities and spontaneous fetal death following amniocentesis: further data and associations with maternal age. *American Journal of Human Genetics*, **35**, 110–116

Johnson, A.M. and Lingley, L. (1984) Correction formula for maternal serum alpha-fetoprotein. *Lancet*, **ii**, 812

Knight, G.J., Palomaki, G.E. and Haddow, J.E. (1988) Use of maternal serum alpha-fetoprotein measurements to screen for Down's syndrome. *Clinical Obstetrics and Gynaecology*, **31**, 306–327

Lindenbaum, R.H., Ryynanen, M., Holmes-Siedle, M., Puhakainen, E., Jonasson, J. and Keenan, J. (1987) Trisomy 18 and maternal serum and amniotic fluid alpha-fetoprotein. *Prenatal Diagnosis*, **7**, 511–519

Lockwood, C., Benacerraf, B., Krinsky, A. *et al.* (1987) A sonographic screening method for Down syndrome. *American Journal of Obstetrics and Gynecology*, **157**, 803–808

Lynch, L., Berkowitz, G.S., Chitkara, U., Wilkins, I.A., Mehalek, K.E. and Berkowitz, R.L. (1989) Ultrasound detection of Down syndrome: is it really possible? *Obstetrics and Gynecology*, **73**, 267–270

Macri, J.N., Kasturi, R.V., Krantz, D.A. and Koch, K.E. (1986) Maternal serum alpha-fetoprotein screening, maternal weight, and detection efficiency. *American Journal of Obstetrics and Gynecology*, **155**, 758–760

Mantingh, A., Marrink, J., de Wolf, B., Breed, A.S.P.M., Beekhuis, J.R. and Visser, G.H.A. (1989) Low maternal serum alpha-fetoprotein at 10 weeks gestation and fetal Down's syndrome. *British Journal of Obstetrics and Gynaecology*, **96**, 499–500

Medical Research Council of Canada (1977) Diagnosis of genetic disease by amniocentesis during the second trimester of pregnancy. A Canadian Study. *Report No. 5*. Supply Services, Ottawa, Canada

Merkatz, I.R., Nitowsky, H.M., Macri, J.N. and Johnson, W.E. (1984) An association between low maternal serum alpha-fetoprotein and fetal chromosomal abnormalities. *American Journal of Obstetrics and Gynecology*, **148**, 886–894

Mikkelsen, M. and Stene, J. (1979) Previous child with Down syndrome and other chromosome aberration. In *Prenatal Diagnosis, Proceedings of the 3rd European Conference on Prenatal Diagnosis of Genetic Disorders* (Eds J. Murken, S. Stengel-Rutkowski and E. Schwinger). Enke, Stuttgart, pp.22–29

Milunsky, A., Alpert, E., Kitzmiller, J.L., Younger, M.D. and Neff, R.K. (1982) Prenatal diagnosis of neural tube defects. VIII The importance of serum alpha-fetoprotein screening in diabetic pregnant women. *American Journal of Obstetrics and Gynecology*, **142**, 1030–1032

National Institute for Child Health and Development (1976) National Registry for amniocentesis study group. Mid-trimester amniocentesis for prenatal diagnosis. Safety and accuracy. *Journal of the American Medical Association*, **236**, 1471–1476

Norgaard-Pedersen, B., Larsen, S.O., Arends, J., Svenstrup, B. and Tabor, A. (1990) Maternal serum markers in screening for Down syndrome. *Clinical Genetics*, **37**, 35–43

Office of Population Censuses and Surveys (1984–1986) *Birth Statistics*. Series FM1, no. 8–12. HMSO: London

Osathanondh, R., Canick, J.A., Abell, K.B. *et al.* (1989) Second trimester screening for trisomy 21. *Lancet*, **ii**, 52

Palomaki, G. (1986) Collaborative study of Down syndrome screening using maternal serum alpha-fetoprotein and maternal age. *Lancet*, **ii**, 1460

Palomaki, G.E. and Haddow, J. (1987) Maternal serum alpha-fetoprotein, age and Down syndrome risk. *American Journal of Obstetrics and Gynecology*, **156**, 460–463

Perry, T.B., Benzie, R.J., Cassar, N., *et al.*, (1984) Fetal cephalometry by ultrasound as a screening procedure for the prenatal detection of Down's syndrome. *British Journal of Obstetrics and Gynaecology*, **91**, 138–143

Peters, M.T., Lockwood, C.J. and Miller, W.A. (1989) The efficacy of fetal sonographic biometry in Down syndrome screening. *American Journal of Obstetrics and Gynecology*, **161**, 297–300

Petrocik, E., Wassmanm, E.R. and Kelly, J.A. (1989) Prenatal screening for Down syndrome with maternal serum human chorionic gonadotropin levels. *American Journal of Obstetrics and Gynecology*, **161**, 1168–1173

Platt, L.D., Medearis, A.L., Horenstein, J.M., Devore, G.R., Beall, M. and Wassman, R. (1988) Sonographic screening for Down's syndrome: does it really work? *The Society of Perinatal Obstetricians*, 8th Annual Meeting, Las Vegas, Nevada, February 3–6, 1988 (abstract)

Porto, M., McCulloch, B.P., Grade, M. *et al.* (1988) Is the BPD/FL ratio a useful screening test for Down's syndrome? *The Society of Perinatal Obstetricians*, 8th Annual Meeting, Las Vegas, Nevada, February 3–6, 1988 (abstract)

Reece, E.A., Davis, N., Mahoney, M.J. and Baugarten, A. (1987) Maternal serum alpha-fetoprotein in diabetic pregnancy: correlation with blood glucose control. *Lancet*, **ii**, 275

Review of Clinical Cytogenetic Services (1984) Association of Clinical Cytogeneticists, London, 1986

Sacks, A.J., Drugan, A., Zador, I.E., Evans, M.I. and Sokol, R.J. (1988) Sonographic biometry does not identify the structurally normal, karyotypically abnormal fetus. *The Society of Perinatal Obstetricians*, 8th Annual Meeting, Las Vegas, Nevada, February 3–6, 1988 .abstract)

Stene, J., Stene, E. and Mikkelsen, M. (1984) Risk for chromosome abnormality at amniocentesis following a child with a non-inherited chromosome aberration. A European Collaborative Study on Prenatal Diagnosis 1981. *Prenatal Diagnosis*, **4**, 81–95

Subramaniam, R., Sadasivan, T., Rao, M.R. and Reddy, S.B. (1988) An association between maternal serum alpha-fetoprotein and fetal autosomal trisomies. *American Journal of Human Genetics*, **43**, A250

Tabor, A., Larsen, S.O., Nielsen, J. *et al.* (1987) Screening for Down syndrome using an iso-risk curve based on maternal age and serum alpha-fetoprotein level. *British Journal of Obstetrics and Gynaecology*, **94**, 636–642

Tabor, A., Madsen, M., Obel, E.B., Philips, J., Bang, J. and Norgaard-Pedersen, B. (1986) Randomised controlled trial of genetic amniocentesis in 4606 low-risk women. *Lancet*, **i**, 1287–1293

Tabor, A., Philip, J., Bang, J., Madsen, M., Obel, E. and Nogaard-Pedersen, B. (1988) Needle size and risk of miscarriage after amniocentesis. *Lancet*, **i**, 183–184

Toi, A., Simpson, G.F. and Filly, R.A. (1987) Ultrasonically evident fetal nuchal skin thickening: is it specific for Down syndrome? *American Journal of Obstetrics and Gynecology*, **156**, 250–253

Wald, N. and Cuckle, H. (1987) Recent advances in screening for neural tube defects and Down syndrome. In *Prenatal Diagnosis*, (ed. C. Rodeck). Bailliere Tindall: London

Wald, N.J. and Cuckle, H.S. (1988a) AFP and age screening for Down syndrome. Proceedings of the American Society of Human Genetics Conference, October 1987. *American Journal of Human Genetics*, **31**, 197–209

Wald, N.J., Cuckle, H., Boreham, J., Stirrat, G.M. and Turnbull, A.C. (1979) Maternal serum alpha-fetoprotein and diabetes mellitus. *British Journal of Obstetrics and Gynaecology*, **86**, 101–105

Wald, N., Cuckle, H., Boreham, J., Terzian, E. and Redman, C. (1981) The effect of maternal weight on maternal serum alpha-fetoprotein levels. *British Journal of Obstetrics and Gynaecology*, **88**, 1094–1096

Wald, N.J. Cuckle, H.S. Densem, J.W. *et al.* (1988a) Maternal serum unconjugated oestriol as an antenatal screening test for Down's syndrome. *British Journal of Obstetrics and Gynaecology*, **95**, 334–341

Wald, N.J., Cuckle, H.S., Densem, J.W. *et al.* (1988b) Maternal serum screening for Down syndrome in early pregnancy. *British Medical Journal*, **297**, 883–887

Wald, N.J., Terzian, E., Vickers, P.A. and Weathrall, J.A.C. (1983) Congenital talipes and hip malformation in relation to amniocentesis: a case-control study. *Lancet*, ii, 246–249

White, I., Papiha, S.S. and Magnay, D. (1989) Improving methods of screening for Down's syndrome. *New England Journal of Medicine*, **360**, 401–402

Winston, Y.E. and Horger, E.O. (1988) Down syndrome and short femur length. *American Journal of Obsterics and Gynecology*, **159**, 1018

Working Party on Amniocentesis: an assessment of the hazards of amniocentesis. (1978) *British Journal of Obstetrics and Gynaecology*, **85**, (suppl. 2), 1–4

Chapter 5

Chromosomes in prenatal diagnosis

R.J. Lilford and C. Gosden

Structure

The chromatin of the human nucleus is arranged as 46 chromosomes (22 pairs of autosomes and one pair of sex chromosomes (XX in the female and XY in the male)). Pairs of chromosomes are called homologous chromosomes. The autosomes are numbered in order of total size from 1 to 22 (with occasional exceptions, e.g. chromosome 22 is larger than chromosome 21). Before chromosomal banding methods were available, the chromosomes were only identifiable in groups. The A group consisted of chromosomes 1,2,3, B 4 and 5, C 6−12+X, D 13−15, E 16−18, F 19, 20, G 21, 22 and Y.

When the centromere is centrally placed the chromosome is described as metacentric; if it is off centre the chromosome is submetacentric and if it is near the end of one arm it is called acrocentric.

Metacentrics   Submetacentrics   Acrocentrics
e.g. 3 and X   e.g. 4,5,11 and 12   e.g. 13,14,15,21 and 22

Each chromosome contains double helical deoxyribonucleic acid (DNA) complexed with structural proteins and histones. The DNA of the chromosome adjacent to the centromere consists largely of genetically inert 'heterochromatin' which contains highly repeated copies of simple sequences of DNA which remain densely coiled during interphase (euchromatin only becomes coiled during mitosis or meiosis). The short arm of each chromosome is called the p arm (from the French petit) and the long arms are q arms. Non-homologous chromosomes which are similar in size and shape may be distinguished by means of banding techniques with dyes such as quinacrine and Giemsa (G banding). Chromosome bands are numbered from the centromere outwards towards the telomeres. There are variable regions of certain chromosomes where the banding patterns show genetic polymorphism (i.e. they differ between individuals) and it is sometimes possible to trace fetal autosomes to a specific parent. The variable areas are shown cross-hatched on idiograms of human chromosomes. Variable regions show different staining characteristics with chromosomal banding techniques such as fluorescence or centromeric heterochromatin banding (C-banding).

Chromosomes 13, 14, 15, 21 and 22 have small terminal regions called cytological satellites. The nucleolar organizer regions adjacent to these satellites contain ribosomal DNA and are incorporated into the nucleolus during interphase. The size and shape of the satellites, and of the distal part of the long arm of the Y chromosome can vary greatly between normal individuals.

Females have an XX sex chromosome complement and males an XY pair. The X chromosome is much larger than the Y chromosome and contains many more genes, thus one of the X chromosomes is inactivated during development in every female as a method of dosage compensation (Lyon hypothesis). In the female (XX), the inactivated X chromosome exists in a tightly coiled form which in interphase cells after staining with basic dyes, can be seen as the sex chromatin or Barr body. Only the terminal portion of the short arm of this chromosome remains active in all cells.

As X chromosome inactivation takes place at random, the female carrier of an X-linked deficiency (for all regions of the X chromosome other than the tip of the short arm) has about 50% of the normal amount of the deficient substance, e.g. a carrier of haemophilia will have about 50% of the normal levels of Factor VIII (but *see* Chapter 7). After quinacrine staining the long (q) arm of the Y chromosome can be identified by brilliant fluorescence of the distal two-thirds. This can be seen in interphase cells as the brightly fluorescent Y body. The genes for testes determining factor are situated on the short arm of the Y chromosome. In 1 in 3000 people, the fluorescent heterochromatin on the distal part of the long arm of the Y chromosome is translocated onto an autosome, usually an acrocentric chromsome such as 15 or 22 and may thus be present, albeit very rarely, in phenotypically normal females. Some males (about 1 in 5000 individuals) have a Y chromsome which lacks the fluorescent portion. This fluorescent part contains only highly repeated non-coding DNA sequences. Because these Y chromosomes still have all the normal genes (such as testes determining factor) on the short arm and proximal long arm these individuals with a variant of the Y chromosome are normal males.

Mitosis and meiosis

Mitosis

The cell cycle can be divided into a sequence of phases: G1, S, G2 M. M is the phase of mitosis, S the phase of nucleic acid synthesis (and DNA replication), while G1 and G2 are 'resting' phases as far as cell division is concerned. Most of the variation between cell dividing times is in G1 and if the cell is not dividing then G1 is prolonged – sometimes called G0.

During the S phase, the two DNA strands in each chromosome separate. Each strand then acts as a template for the formation of a complementary strand: the resulting double strand is thus identical with parental DNA. During prophase, the duplicated chromatin condenses into well-defined chromosomes joined at the centromere, and the centrioles and their associated microtubules form the mitotic spindle. In metaphase the chromosomes assemble at the midpoint of the spindle – the metaphase plate. This is the plate at which chromosomes are at their shortest and can be visualized for karyotyping and identified by banding.

At anaphase the new sets of chromosomes separate to opposite poles of the nucleus guided by the mitotic spindle. The nucleus reforms in telophase. Finally the cytoplasmic contents are divided (cytokinesis).

Meiosis

Meiosis is the process by which the 46 chromosomes of a normal diploid cell are reduced to 23 chromosomes and this occurs only in the germ cells in the ovary and the testes. It involves two divisions, an initial meiotic reduction division followed by 'mitotic division' of these cells, giving rise to four haploid cells. During the first stage each of the 46 chromosomes duplicates and assembles side-to-side in homologous pairs, except for the X and Y chromosomes in the male, which assemble end-to-end. Crossing-over and recombination at 'chiasmata' lead to exchanges of DNA.

Chromosome abnormalities

The most common type of chromosomal abnormality is the presence of an extra chromosome – trisomies. An individual with a normal complement of 46 chromosomes is called euploid; variations in number (those individuals with 45, 47, 48 or 69 chromosomes) are termed aneuploid. The majority of autosomal trisomies are lethal, and result in failure of implantation or early spontaneous abortion. The three commonest surviving autosomal trisomies are those for relatively small chromosomes: trisomy 21 (Down's syndrome) (Figure 5.1), 13 (Patau's syndrome), and 18 (Edwards' syndrome) (Figure 5.2). Even in these cases, most affected embryos abort; e.g. only 20% of Down's syndrome embryos attain viability. The best known trisomy of sex chromosomes is XXY (Klinefelter's syndrome). Only one form of monosomy is consistent with development to term, that of monosomy X (45,X Turner's syndrome). This is the commonest abnormality at conception.

The most common cause of chromosomal abnormality is non-disjunction; this is a failure of the relevant chromosome pair to separate at meiosis, usually during the first meiotic division. After fertilization by a normal gamete the zygote either has an extra chromosome (e.g. XXY), or a missing chromosome (e.g. XO). In 80% of cases of autosomal trisomy, the causative non-disjunction takes place in the mother and this becomes increasingly common with advancing maternal age. The incidence of these trisomies therefore rises with maternal age to peak at age 45. It then decreases because older mothers selectively abort non-euploid fetuses very efficiently.

Non-disjunction in the father is not related to paternal age. In 60% of cases of Turner's syndrome it is the paternal X which is lost. In some cases this is due to a meiotic error in the father, in others to an early mitotic non-disjunction in the embryo. The incidence of Turner's syndrome is inversely related to maternal age.

There are two other much less common mechanisms by which a trisomy may arise: mosaics or chimaeras and translocation.

Mosaics or chimaeras

A mosaic is an individual whose body is composed of cells of different chromosome constitution arising from the same zygote. This may be due to non-disjunction during early divisions of the zygote or to anaphase lag. In the latter abnormality, the chromosome is delayed in its movement on the spindle and does not reach the appropriate daughter cell before the nuclear membrane closes. This, too, gives rise to mosaicism but only in the descendants does it form an abnormal cell line; other cells in the embryo are normal.

A chimaera also has cells of different genetic constitutions, but here the two cell lines result from two separate zygote lineages, e.g. fertilization of both the polar

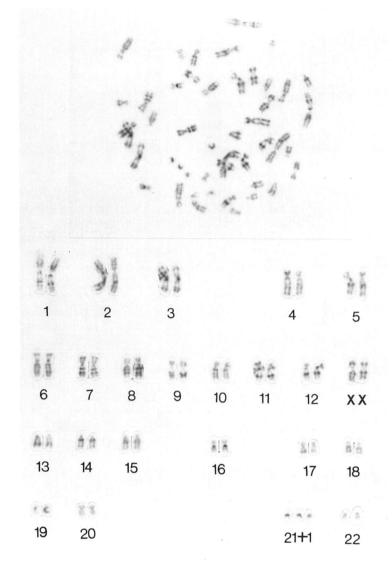

Figure 5.1 Banded karyotype showing non-disjunction Down's syndrome

body and the ovum, which subsequently fuse, or fertilization of two ova, which then fuse. The rare XX/XY form of gonadal dysgenesis may arise in this way.

Translocation

This involves the transfer of a segment of one chromosome to another and often a reciprocal exchange takes place. If the total chromosomal complement is unchanged and the chromosomal material merely rearranged, this is usually

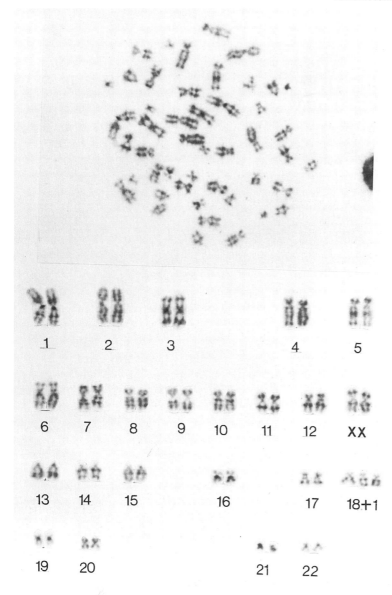

Figure 5.2 Non-disjunction trisomy 18

harmless and described as 'balanced'. Sometimes when translocations arise *de novo*, the chromosomal breaks occur in important gentic segments or important genetic material is deleted and there are phenotype consequences of this, usually in the form of mental handicap in the individual with the *de novo* rearrangements. Since such individuals seldom reproduce, these deletion translocations are usually lost in a single generation. Such an individual is, however, a 'carrier'.

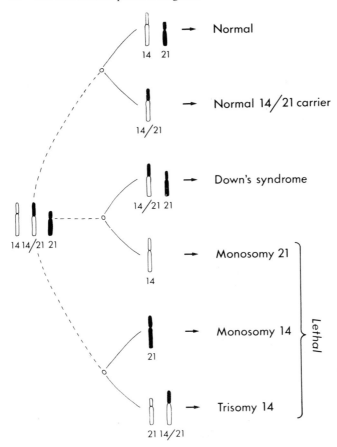

Figure 5.3 Possible gametes in a Robertsonian translocation carrier

If the breakage and rejoining occur at the centromere of two acrocentric chromosomes, however, the tiny short arm fragments are usually lost and the centromeres and attached long arms joined together; this is known as a Robertsonian translocation or centric fusion (Figure 5.3).

The carrier of this translocation does not suffer any ill-effects as the short arms consist only of repeated DNA sequences. The most common Robertsonian translocation occurs between chromosomes 13 and 14, and is described in short form as t(13q14q) and occurs in 1 in 600 persons. Robertsonian translocations which can give rise to Down's syndrome include all those rearrangements including chromosome 21, i.e. 13/21, 14/21, 15/21, 21/21 and 21/22 of which 14/21 is the most common D/G translocation and 21/22 the most common G/G translocation. There are six possible chromosomal patterns after recombination (Figure 5.3), three of which are immediately lethal. Theoretically, one in three of the viable offspring of such parents should be affected with trisomy. In reality the risk is 10% if the mother is a carrier, as many affected embryos abort. If the father is a carrier, the risk is 5%, due to poor functional capacity of affected sperm. With the extremely rare 21/21 translocation 100% of viable pregnancies of a carrier parent are affected.

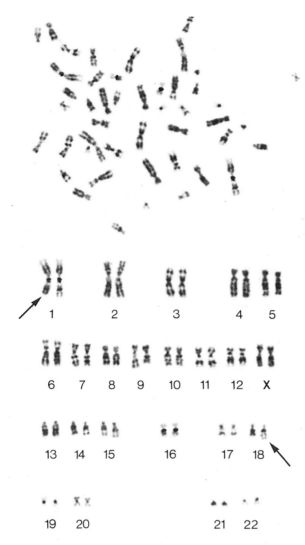

Figure 5.4 Reciprocal translocation between chromosomes 1 and 18. The zygote will be either: 1. completely normal; 2. carrier (and clinically normal); 3. monosomic for a portion of chromosome 1 and trisomic for a portion of 18; 4. trisomic for a portion of 1 and monosomic for a portion of 18. The clinical effects will depend on: (*a*) the relative frequency of the above – this varies and is very difficult to predict; and (*b*) the extent to which 3. and 4. are 'lethal' to the embryo. If they are always or nearly always lethal, then recurrent miscarriage will occur. If not, then abnormal children will occur. The latter is much more likely if the family is ascertained through an abnormal child

Reciprocal translocations do not involve loss of short arm material and can involve any chromosome (Figure 5.4). Recurrence risks are very variable (*see* Chapter 6).

Polyploidy

Another common chromosomal abnormality is triploidy (i.e. three complete sets of chromosomes, as opposed to two) so that the fetus has 69 chromosomes. About 2%

of all human conceptions are triploid but the vast majority abort very early in pregnancy, especially those with an XYY sex chromosome complement, only 1 in 10 000 surviving to birth. In about 50% of cases triploidy is associated with hydatidiform change in the placenta, and this occurs when 46 of the 69 chromosomes are from the father (diandry).

This either arises from fertilization of an egg which has 46 chromosomes due to failure to eject a polar body either at meiosis 1 or meiosis 2, or to a diploid sperm with 46 chromosomes (arising as a failure of disjunction at meiosis 1 or 2 in the father) fertilizing an egg with 23 chromosomes, or in some cases to dispermy (two sperm fertilizing a single egg). All result in embryos with 69 chromosomes.

Rare syndromes have been described in which chromosomes, show an excessive number of breaks or fagile sites in culture, chromosome instability syndrome and this may be associated with severe clinical effects. In the fragile X syndrome of mental retardation there is a fragile site at band Xq27.3 on the X chromosome; in certain inherited chromosomal breakage syndromes such as ataxia telangiectasia (AT), Fanconi's anaemia (FA), xeroderma pigmentosa (XP) and Bloom's syndrome (BS), chromosome breaks occur at a very high frequency and their presence can be enhanced by certain culture conditions.

Partial deletions and duplications

Rare partial deletions of the short arm of chromosomes 4 and 5 lead to mental deficiency. 4p- is called the Wolff-Hirschhorn syndrome and 5p- is the cri-du-chat syndrome. Small partial deletions of chromosome 13 have been associated with congenital retinoblastoma and of chromosome 15 with the Prader-Willi syndrome.

Pericentric and paracentric inversions

There are two types of inversion:

1. pericentric (pii) where the centromere is included in the inverted segment (Figure 5.5) and
2. paracentric (pai) in which a segment of only one arm of the chromosome is involved (Figure 5.6).

Some pericentric inversions are associated with a high risk of giving unbalanced recombinants. In contrast, other pericentric inversions are associated with a very low risk and are clinically less significant. Pericentric inversions of the extensive heterochromatic material in chromosome 9 are common and harmless.

High risk of unbalanced recombinants	*Low risk of unbalanced recombinants*
inv(8)(p23q22)	inv(1)(p13q21)
inv(3)(p25q21)	inv(2)(p11.2q13)
inv(13)(p13q21)	inv(5)(p13q13)
inv(18)(p11q21)	inv(10)(p11.2q21.2)
inv(4)(p14q35)	inv(Y)(p11.1q11.2)

An inversion involves two chromosomal breaks and reinsertion of the intercalary chromosomal segment after rotating through 180°. There are two principal clinical consequences of an inversion.

1. When the inversion occurs *de novo*, if either or both the breaks involve critical genetic regions then this might have adverse consequences for the individual. To

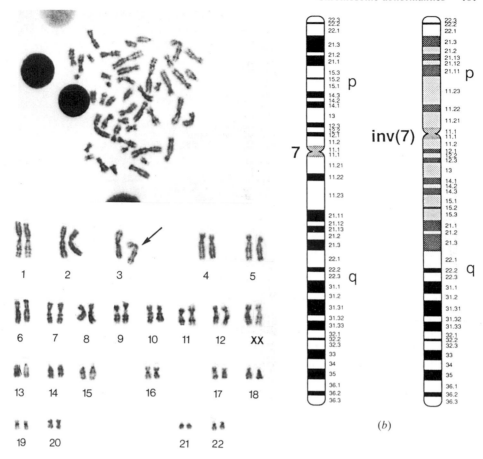

(a)

(b)

Figure 5.5 (a) Banded preparation showing pericentric inversion chromosome 3. (b) Idiogram of banded chromosomes showing pericentric inversion chromosome 7

what extent the changed polarity of the DNA strands (change from 5′ to 3′) may have an effect is not yet known.

2. When meiosis occurs in individuals who are heterozygous for an inversion, crossing over in the inverted segment may generate chromosomally unbalanced gametes. In general, the risk of imbalance depends on the probability of crossing over in the inverted segment. This is not a simple correlation with the length of the segment, but depends both on the cross-over frequency of the particular region and the effects of genetic imbalance in the recombinant. This is reflected in the risks for pericentric inversion carriers where the overall spontaneous abortion rate is about 10% although for some inversions it may rise to over 30% where there is a large inversion involving regions where the frequency of crossing over is high.

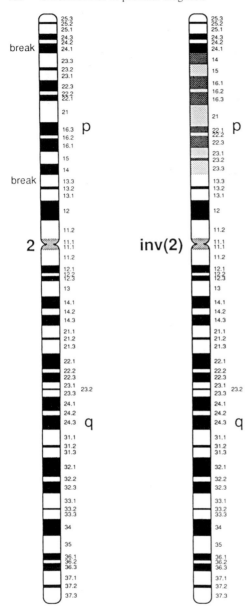

Figure 5.6 Idiogram of paracentric inversion chromosome 2

Pericentric inversions have been described for all chromosomes with a total frequency in the population of about 1.3 to 1.4% (Kaiser, 1988). They occur much more frequently in some chromosomes than others and among the most frequent in order of occurrence are those on 9, 2, 8, 3, Y, 1, 5, 10, 11, 18, 4, 13 and 6. The genetic risk for pericentric inversion carriers is highest if ascertained through a recombinant individual and is approximately 10% for a female carrier, although in some exceptional cases this may be as high as 50%, and 5% for a male carrier.

Reference

Kaiser, P. (1988) Pericentric inversions: their problems and clinical significance. In *The Cytogenetics of Mammalian Autosomal Rearrangements* (ed. A. Daniel). Alan R. Liss, New York, pp. 163–247

Chapter 6

Prenatal diagnosis of chromosome anomalies

C. Gosden

Introduction

There are two principal aims to this chapter: the first is to consider which couples or pregnancies are at high risk of a major fetal cytogenetic disorder; the second is to attempt to help to predict the significance of a chromosome abnormality found in an initial amniotic fluid or chorionic villus sample (CVS), and determine the extent to which this is associated with significant risk of handicap for the fetus. Avoidance of births of infants with major handicapping cytogenetic disorders can only be achieved when the majority of those at risk can be offered early, accurate prenatal diagnosis while minimizing the possibility that non-significant abnormalities might be misinterpreted.

Who is at risk?

The first approaches to prenatal diagnosis with amniocentesis in the early 1970s had, as their initial target, detection of fetal chromosome disorders. Today, risk for cytogenetic disorder is still the most frequent indication for prenatal diagnosis. The increase in range of the cytogenetic conditions amenable to diagnosis in addition to those for advanced maternal age, parental chromosome abnormality and previous abnormal child now include fragile X syndrome, microdeletion syndromes and chromosomal breakage syndromes. Cytogenetic developments have paralleled the development of powerful new methods of obstetric imaging by ultrasound, fetal assessment and sampling. Developments in the ability to perform rapid karyotyping on different fetal tissues such as chorionic villi early in gestation, are being combined with new screening techniques for cytogenetic disorders (such as structural malformations detected on ultrasound scan or the association of altered levels of fetoplacental products in maternal serum with Down's syndrome; *see* Chapter 4), and therefore radically altering the perspectives and indications for prenatal karyotyping.

Specific associations are beginning to pinpoint high risk of a chromosomal anomaly. These include low maternal serum alpha-fetoprotein (AFP), low unconjugated oestriols and raised maternal human chorionic gonadotrophin (HCG) levels (Chapter 4) combined with factors such as advanced maternal age, fetal nuchal skin thickening and decreased fetal femur length, all of which indicate an increased risk of trisomy 21. Fetal anomalies such as omphalocoele, cystic hygromata, cardiac and renal anomalies (which can be detected on detailed ultrasound scan) indicate a high risk of certain abnormal karyotypes such as trisomies 13, 18 and 45,X (Nicolaides, Rodeck and Gosden, 1986). Older mothers are the major group currently recognized as being of increased risk for chromosomal non-disjunction at meiosis. Although the overall risk of Down's syndrome may be only 1 in 100 there are important questions about whether there is a small subgroup of older mothers at a higher risk and whether hormonal, environmental or teratogenic factors havge significant roles. The identification of groups at high risk is important for this reason. Recognition of parents with a chromosome abnormality (such as translocations or mosaicism) is important. Although it is a small group, the recurrence risks are high.

The maternal age related risks for Down's syndrome are well established, but it is important to recognize that other types of aneuploidy such as autosomal trisomies 13 and 18, sex chromosome aneuploidy (47,XXY, 47,XXX) and supernumerary marker chromosomes also show maternal age related trends and will be detected in a significant number of pregnancies when the primary purpose of screening is the detection of fetuses with Down's syndrome. For example, at the age of 35, the risk of Down's syndrome at amniocentesis is 3.5 per 1000, but the risks for trisomies 13 and 18, together with those for supernumerary markers, autosomal mosaicism, unbalanced rearrangements XXY, XXX, XYY, 45,X and other sex chromosome anomalies give a figure of 5.4 per 1000 amniocenteses. This is cumulatively greater than the risk of Down's syndrome (see Table 6.1).

Trends seen in the amniocentesis data are also seen in more recent figures from chorionic villus sampling (CVS). In the collaborative CVS series of 4481 cases reported by Hook et al. (1988), there were 48 cases of trisomy 21 and 51 other chromosomal anomalies which included 39 cases of major non-lethal chromosome abnormalities and 12 lethal cytogenetic abnormalities, which highlights the problems of pregnancy counselling and management when abnormalities other than trisomy 21 are detected prenatally. For autosomal rearrangements alone detected in prenatal diagnostic samples, there is a total frequency of 1 in 250 cases (Robertsonian translocations 0.11%, reciprocal translocations 0.17% and inversions 0.12%) giving a total of 0.4%. This is twice that seen in newborn surveys which have frequencies of only 0.19% or 1 in 526 (Hook and Hamerton, 1977; Neilsen et al., 1986). The mutation rate is thus 4.3 per 10000 gametes per generation, just for rearrangements (Van Dyke et al., 1983) and this gives an idea of the scale of the problem.

The major target of prenatal studies lies not only in the identification of clinically significant chromosome abnormalities but also in contributing to the understanding of the aetiology of the different cytogenetic disorders, so that primary prevention becomes a realistic goal.

Unexpected abnormalities in prenatal diagnosis

At present, the major focus of cytogenetic prenatal diagnosis is the detection of autosomal trisomies. However, much more difficult decisions must be made when chromosome abnormalities other than trisomies are found in prenatal diagnostic specimens, either from amniotic fluid or chorionic villus samples. These include de novo chromosomal translocations, rearrangements, fragile X, or chromosomal mosaicism. The difficulties in counselling, prediction of the fetal phenotype and resolution of the dilemmas of mosaicism in these cases may cause major problems, particularly because of the urgency due to advancing gestation. Abnormalities detected early in pregnancy by CVS show the same trends as those seen at amniocentesis, but the problems of mosaicism and confined placental anomalies are even greater, so that counselling when abnormalities are discovered in CVS samples is an important part of the obstetrician's or geneticist's responsibility. For *de novo* rearrangements, in the absence of a previous affected child, parental abnormality or family history, it is often difficult to assess the possible phenotype and prognosis. The problems of confined placental abnormalities and the risks associated with certain abnormal karyotypes will be discussed in later sections.

In prenatal testing, a balance must be achieved between effective and rapid screening of large numbers of samples for fetal aneuploidy (which is numerically the greatest risk for a pregnancy) and examining sufficient cells in detail so that small chromosomal rearrangements, deletions and true mosaicism are not missed. Failure to examine adequate numbers of prenatal samples means that women who are at relatively high risk of having trisomic offspring are not offered prenatal testing. The dangers of failing to detect rarer, but clinically significant and serious abnormalities in pregnancies which have been subjected to prenatal testing may result in the births of children with profound handicaps, and create crises of confidence in the patients, obstetricians and laboratories.

Indications for prenatal diagnosis and risks of chromosome anomaly

Advanced maternal age

The increasing risks of fetal aneuploidy with advancing maternal age are given for the collaborative amniocentesis studies in Table 6.1. These figures show that the risks associated with advanced maternal age are not restricted to Down's syndrome alone, but include a variety of other clinically significant chromosome abnormalities (Ferguson Smith and Yates, 1984). Data from CVS studies show even higher frequencies of abnormalities (Hook *et al.*, 1988).

Table 6.1 Maternal age specific rates per 1000 amniocenteses for chromosome abnormalities in pregnancies monitored for maternal age >35 years

Maternal age	No. of pregnancies monitored	Autosomal						Sex chromosome				Total
		+21 +18 +13	+mar	mosaic+ unbalanced	Balanced including +t(13;14)	XXX	XXY XYY	XO	Balanced +mosaic+ unbalanced			
35	5409	3.5 0.7 0.4	0.5	0.6	3.3	1.6	0.5	0.6	0.5			12.2
36	6103	5.7 0.8 0.3	0.3	0.5	3.0	1.6	0.2	1.0	0.7			14.1
37	6956	6.8 0.9 0.3	0.7	1.1	2.3	1.1	0.3	0.6	0.9			15.0
38	7926	8.1 1.5 0.4	0.3	0.6	2.6	1.5	0.3	0.6	0.6			16.5
39	7682	10.9 2.0 0.7	0.5	0.8	1.8	2.7	0.4	0.3	0.9			21.0
40	7174	12.3 2.5 1.3	0.8	1.0	2.2	2.1	0.3	0.4	0.7			23.6
41	4763	14.7 3.6 1.7	0.6	0.6	1.9	4.4	0.4	–	0.4			28.3
42	3156	21.9 6.3 1.9	0.6	1.3	2.6	6.3	0.3	0.3	0.3			41.8
43	1912	32.4 7.9 0.5	1.0	1.6	0.5	6.3	–	–	0.5			50.7
44	1015	29.5 4.9 –	–	–	1.0	8.9	–	–	–			44.3
45	508	45.3 3.9 0.2	3.9	2.0	–	13.7	2.0	–	–			71.0
46	232	81.9 4.3 –	–	–	–	17.2	–	–	–			103.4
>46	129	23.3 7.8 –	–	–	7.8	30.9	–	–	–			69.8

Maternal biochemical screening (abnormal maternal serum AFP, oestriol and hCG levels)

See Chapter 4

Previous child with a chromosome abnormality

There are three major groups in which there is relatively high risk of parental chromosome abnormality (such as translocations, rearrangements or parental mosaicism); these include those with a chromosomally abnormal child, couples with a family history of chromosome disorder or mental retardation and those with recurrent abortions.

For those with a child with a suspected chromosome disorder, karyotyping the child establishes the diagnosis and indicates whether there is a probability of there being a parental chromosome abnormality, e.g. risk of parental chromosome abnormality is high if a child has translocation Down's syndrome rather than simple

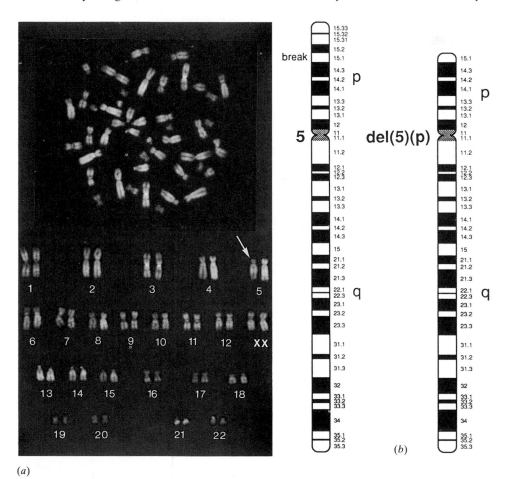

(a)

Figure 6.1 (a) Karyotype showing deletion of 5p (short arm of chromosome 5). (b) Idiogram to show breakpoint and deletion

Table 6.2 Maternal age and origin of chromosome abnormalities

---

Abnormalities with advanced maternal age effect and probable maternal non-disjunctional error at meiosis
aneuploidy, e.g. trisomy 47,+21, 47,+18, 47,+13
sex chromosome abnormalities 47,XXX, 47,XXY
supernumerary markers especially inverted duplication of 15p and cat eye syndrome (partial duplication of 22q)
Abnormalities without a maternal age effect and possible paternal origin or post-zygotic error
47,XYY (error in paternal meiotic non-disjunction at second meiotic division)
45,X (60% of all cases have lost paternal X)
some rearrangements, deletions, inversions, *de novo* translocations
supernumerary markers, mosaic abnormalities (post-zygotic error)
polyploidy; triploidy – 50–60% of cases due to errors at meiosis 1 or 2 in father or dispermy
At present recurrence risks for abnormalities other than trisomy 21 are difficult to asses as there are few data relating to these conditions. In the absence of abnormal parental karotypes general risks of recurrence appear to be less than 1% for mothers under 35

---

trisomy 21. Parental karyotyping should be undertaken in all cases of chromosomal rearrangements, e.g. when the child has a chromosomal deletion such as 5p- (cri-du-chat) (Figure 6.1) and 4p- (Wolf-Hirshhorn syndrome), to ensure that these are not secondary to a parental translocation, inversion or other anomaly (Niebuhr, 1978). If, however, the abnormality has arisen *de novo* (as a new mutation) this may have originated either as a maternal or as a paternal meiotic error or it may be due to a mitotic error in the zygote (Table 6.2). Those conditions which are due to a maternal meiotic error, e.g. autosomal trisomies, have an association with advanced maternal age. The overall risk of recurrence for mothers under 35 is about 1–2% (Stene, Stene and Mikkelsen, 1984). At maternal ages over 35, the risks of recurrence increase with advancing maternal age and an indication of the overall risk is shown in Table 6.1. It is important to recognize that this is a general risk of recurrence of a chromosomal disorder; a mother of a child with trisomy 21 may have a fetus with trisomy 13 (Figure 6.2), or a supernumerary marker chromosome in a subsequent pregnancy. Identifying the parental origin of an abnormality either by chromosomal, DNA or other genetic markers (Mattei and Mattei, 1988), may help in the future to determine groups at high risk for cytogenetic disorders and give more accurate recurrence risks.

Family history of chromosome disorder

This is a heterogeneous group; it includes women with a family history of Down's syndrome because their mothers had children with trisomy 21 associated with advanced maternal age. It also includes those with mentally handicapped relatives where the aetiology of the retardation is unknown and fragile X testing has not been undertaken. In order to try to determine whether there is a specific cytogenetic or genetic component involved, the following studies should be carried out:

1. karyotype the affected individual, or try to determine the aetiology of the mental handicap
2. assess the carrier status of potential carriers (such as that involved in translocation Down's syndrome and especially females at risk for fragile X; *see* fragile X section)

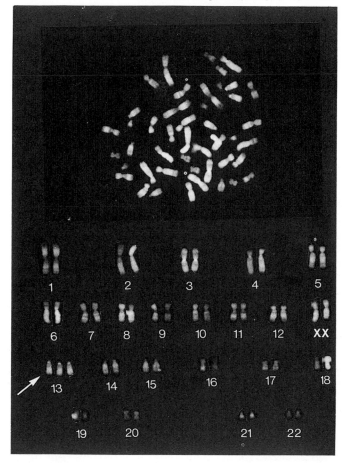

Figure 6.2 Trisomy 13, female, karyotype – Q banded = quinacrine stain

3. construct a family tree and undertake pedigree studies and testing to assess risks for relatives.

In some cases, a parent will be found to be a carrier – the specific risks for each of the anomalies are given in the section on parental chromosome anomalies (Tables 6.5 and 6.6).

Abnormalities on ultrasound scan

Fetal structural abnormalities detected on ultrasound scan may indicate the presence of major chromosomal abnormalities in the fetus. Some anomalies may be associated with a very high risk of chromosomal disorder (Table 6.3) and the possibility of rapid prenatal karyotyping should be considered. The risks of chromosome abnormality vary according to the type of fetal anomaly, but are often in the region of 5–25% for major anomalies such as exomphalos, obstructive uropathy or cardiac defects (Nicolaides, Rodeck and Gosden, 1986). Detailed ultrasound scanning can be of help in screening for anomalies such as nuchal fatty

Table 6.3 Chromosome abnormalities associated with structural abnormalities in the fetus

Fetal abnormality on ultrasound scan	Chromosome abnormalities
Non-immune hydrops, oedema, ascites	45,X
Cystic hygromata	45,X; trisomy 21
Increased nuchal skin thickness	trisomy 21; 45,X
Abnormal head shape, dolicocephaly	trisomy 18; 21
Microcephaly	4p-; 5p-; 18q; trisomy 4p
Hydrocephalus	triploidy
Holoprosencephaly	trisomy 13q; 18; 1q; 3p; 5q; 22q
Choroid plexus cysts	trisomy 18
Agenesis of corpus callosum	trisomy 18
Facial clefting	trisomy 13; 4p-
Duodenal atresia (double bubble)	trisomy 21
Omphalocoele	trisomy 13; 18
Cardiovascular defects e.g. ASD/VSD	trisomy 13; 18; 21; triploidy
Pleural effusion	trisomy 21
Renal anomalies particularly obstructive uropathy	trisomy 18; 13
Syndactyly/polydactyly	triploidy, trisomy 13
Aplasia thumb/radius	Fanconi's syndrome, 13q
Clasped/overlapping fingers	trisomy 18
Intrauterine growth retardation	4p-; 5p-; trisomy 18; triploidy
Diaphragmatic hernia	trisomy 18; isochromosome 12p

pad and shortening of the fetal fumur which are associated with Down's syndrome (Bennacerraf and Frigoletto, 1987), although the sensitivity and specificity of these screening parameters is controversial.

Some structural anomalies detected on ultrasound scan indicate a much higher risk of chromosome disorder than the risks for advanced maternal age or a previous child with trisomy. In most centres, amniocentesis would be offered to a woman on the basis of her maternal age related risk of aneuploidy of about 1%, but often, karyotyping would not be considered a priority even if the fetus had a structural disorder, such as exomphalos, which is associated with a risk of karyotypic abnormality up to 25 times higher than the maternal age associated risk. This is because the changes of chromosome abnormalities in populations other than those of advanced maternal age, previous child or parental karyotypic abnormality are not well recognized. Furthermore, the role of rapid karyotyping (taking only 2–4 days) has not yet been accepted as an adjunct to detailed anomaly scanning at 18–20 weeks. Conventional amniocentesis would often not be appropriate at late gestations if the results routinely take 3 weeks or more, but more rapid methods are available if the risks are high. Advances in the accuracy of ultrasound scanning for the detection of structural anomalies has improved greatly over the past 5 years (Sabbagha et al., 1985) and it would be regrettable if the contribution that scanning could make to the recognition of major chromosome anomalies prenatally was not effective solely because definitive karyotyping was not implemented.

Rapid fetal karyotyping is important when prenatal fetal therapy is being considered for those fetal anomalies where there may be a good prognosis, provided the defect is an isolated one and it is not associated with a major chromosome abnormality. Prenatal therapy is feasible for some structural anomalies (Manning, Harrison and Rodeck, 1985), might soon become a reality for some single gene disorders (Anderson, 1984), but is unfortunately still only a very distant prospect for chromosome abnormalities because of the devastating early effects the thousands of genes carried by a single chromosome have on all the major organ systems. For example vesico-amniotic shunting might be undertaken for obstructive uropathy in the fetus provided that fetal renal function is adequate. However, the risk of chromosome disorder, particularly that of trisomy 18 is high and karyotypic abnormalities may be found in about 20–25% of cases (Nicolaides, Rodeck and Gosden, 1986). Rapid karyotyping from fetal blood takes only 1–3 days and it is thus possible to obtain the fetal karyotype before shunting is carried out. Fetal blood karyotyping offers speed and accuracy over amniotic fluid cell culture but is only available in a limited number of centres and may be associated with a slightly higher fetal loss rate (about 1–2%) than amniocentesis. It does however have a special role to play in urgent cases at late gestations, particularly for those anomalies such as trisomy 18 and 45,X which have a substantial danger of giving false-positive or false-negative results in second trimester CVS cell lines. False-negative results have been found for trisomy 18 in placental biopsy, even when there is true trisomy 18 in the fetus, because one of the three copies of chromosome 18 is often lost in trophoblastic cell lines. It has been suggested that normal (non-trisomic) placental cell lines might favour fetal survival in fetuses with trisomies 13 and 18 (Kalousek, Barret and McGillivray, 1989).

In certain fetal conditions, such as non-haemolytic hydrops or intrauterine growth retardation, the growth of fetal cells (particularly fetal blood lymphocytes or CVS preparations), may be very poor; karyotyping in these circumstances is difficult, (Gosden, 1984). Other diagnostic problems may be found in anomalies, such as diaphragmatic hernia (which may be found in the Pallister Killian syndrome

Table 6.4 Particular problems in prenatal diagnosis of intrauterine growth retardation and diaphragmatic hernia

Fetal abnormality	Possible chromosome disorder	Problems/tissues
Intrauterine growth retardation	Trisomy 18	CVS may give false-negative results AFC and fetal blood more accurate
Diaphragmatic hernia	Trisomy 18	CVS may give false-negative results AFC and fetal blood more accurate
	Pallister Killian syndrome, iso(12p)	Fetal blood may give false-negative results AFC or CVS more accurate

CVS: chorionic villus sampling
AFC: amniotic fluid cells

(isochromosome 12p) or trisomy 18 (Table 6.4)). Pallister Killian syndrome (Figure 6.3) is known to be associated with false negative results in fetal blood because the isochromosome 12p is expressed only in fibroblastic cell lines.

Parental chromosome anomalies

There are differences in the frequency of maternal and paternal non-disjunctional errors occurring at meiosis, because the underlying biological processes in male and female meiosis are very different. For Robertsonian translocations (particularly 13, 14 or 15/21) (Figure 6.4) the maternal and paternal risks of the translocation

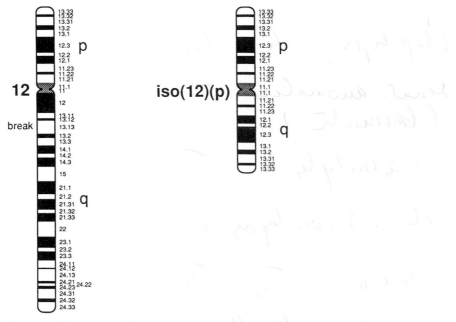

Figure 6.3 Idiogram of Pallister Killian syndrome – isochromosome for short arm chromosome 12. The arm designated q on the isochromosome is actually a duplicated short arm

leading to a chromosomally unbalanced conceptus differ markedly (Daniel and Lam-Po-Tang, 1976; Daniel, Williams and Lam-Po-Tang, 1980; Gosden, Lawrie and Gosden, 1981). Male carriers have a very high chance (about 60%) of having children with a balanced rearrangement like themselves but, in contrast, they have only a very small chance (1–3%) of having children with unbalanced forms of the translocation. Mothers carrying the translocation have a very much higher chance (about 12–15%) of having a child with an unbalanced form of the translocation (Stene and Stengel-Rutkowski, 1988). Some supernumerary marker chromosomes confer infertility on males carrying them; transmission thus occurs more frequently from the mother. For reciprocal translocations, the risks for paternal and maternal carriers are approximately equal, but the overall risks depend on the mode of ascertainment (Daniel, Hook and Wulf, 1988).

Risks for parents with reciprocal translocations

Analysis of data for parents with reciprocal translocations (Daniel, Hook and Wulf, 1988) (Figure 6.5), shows that the major factor which governs the risks of a child or fetus inheriting an unbalanced form of the translocation is the mode of ascertainment. The underlying explanation for this comes from the sizes of the genetic imbalances which result from the translocation. The unbalanced gametes from reciprocal translocation carriers usually arise by adjacent – 1 segregation at meiosis (*see* Chapter 5), so that there is a duplication of one chromosomal interchange segment and a deficiency of the other. The extent of the duplication/deficiencies which occur obviously depends on the chromosomes and

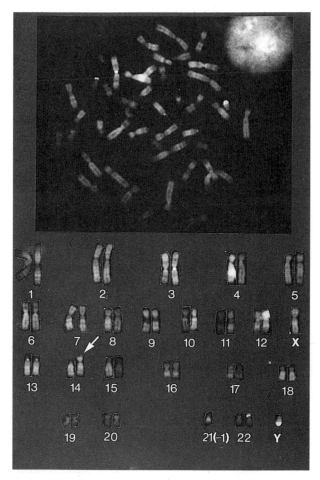

Figure 6.4 Fluorescent (Q banded) karyotype of male carrier of 14/21 Robertsonian translocation. He has a single free chromosome 21, the other being attached to a chromosome 14

individual breakpoints involved, and whether the larger chromosomal segment occurs in trisomic or monosomic form. If the imbalances are very great (and involve chromosomal regions which in trisomic or monosomic form are lethal), then the parents will tend to have repeated miscarriages because of the large amounts of genetic material causing problems from the unbalanced forms of the translocation (Jalbert, Sele and Jalbert, 1980). In such cases, the greatest risk for any future pregnancy is of miscarriage, rather than a viable but unbalanced child. However, when smaller chromosomal regions are involved, particularly when the imbalance involves segments which are known to be tolerated as viable trisomies, (e.g. those involving partial trisomy 13, 18, 21, 12p or monosomy 4p, 5p, 13q, 18p; Schinzel, 1984; Borgaonkar, 1989). Parents who have already had a pregnancy with a chromosomally unbalanced child have a much higher recurrence risk of a surviving child with an unbalanced form of the translocation (Table 6.5).

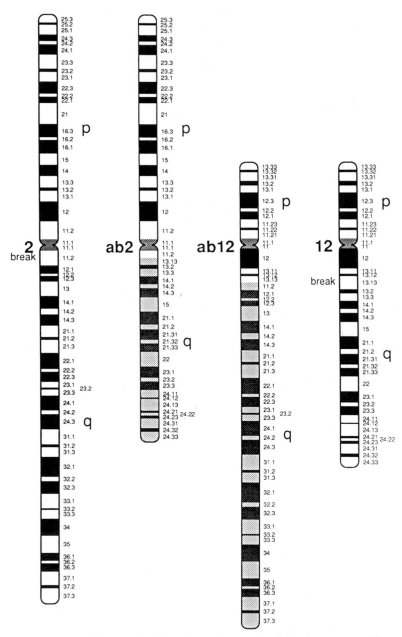

Figure 6.5 Idiogram of reciprocal translocation involving chromosomes 12 and 2

Table 6.5 Risk of unbalanced progeny for parental reciprocal translocation carriers according to the mode of ascertainment

Ascertainment	Risk (%)
Previous, fullterm unbalanced child	Maternal 20
	Paternal 24
Recurrent miscarriage	Maternal 5
	Paternal 2
Incidental, unrelated to rearrangement	Maternal 7
	Paternal 5

Risks for parents with Robertsonian translocations

The highest genetic risk for a parent carrying a Robertsonian translocation is the 100% risk of recurrence for a 21;21 translocation carrier (Figure 6.6). These carriers do not have a free chromosome 21, so that all their children must inherit the translocation chromosome (with the two chromosomes 21 joined together). Since the other parent will contribute a gamete which also has a chromosome 21, this will inevitably lead to trisomy 21 in all conceptuses of such couples. For other Robertsonian translocations, the risks vary according to the specific translocations involved (Table 6.6) and whether the chromosomes are monocentric or dicentric (i.e. whether the breaks in the formation of the Robertsonian translocation occurred in the short arms of both acrocentric chromosomes, giving rise to a dicentric translocation chromosome, or whether in only one short arm and a long arm giving a translocation chromosome with only one centromere (monocentric). For example, Daniel, Williams and Lam-Po-Tang (1980) found that there was a higher risk for dicentric t(13,21) carriers than for dicentric t(14,21) carriers.

Inversions and other rearrangements (excluding heterochromatic inversions of 1,9,16,Y)

Some inversions are associated with a high risk of having handicapped children who survive with chromosomal imbalance due to duplications and deficiencies resulting from crossing over within a pericentric inversion loop formed at meiosis in a carrier parent. Others are either stable, or lethal at an early stage of gestation and lead to early pregnancy loss (Sherman, Iselius and Galliano, 1986; Groupe de Cytogeneticiens Français, 1987; Kaiser, 1988). This is because the underlying genetic risk is similar for both reciprocal translocations and for pericentric inversions. It depends upon the length and the genes carried by the chromosomal segments involved; if this involves large chromosomal regions (or those carrying genes essential for early development), then this may result in early spontaneous abortions (Johnson et al., 1988). The section on inversions in Chapter 5 describes the risks for inversion carriers more fully.

Supernumerary marker chromosomes (SMC)

Small additional marker chromosomes (supernumerary or accessory chromosomes) are not only heterogeneous with regard to the chromosomal material involved, but

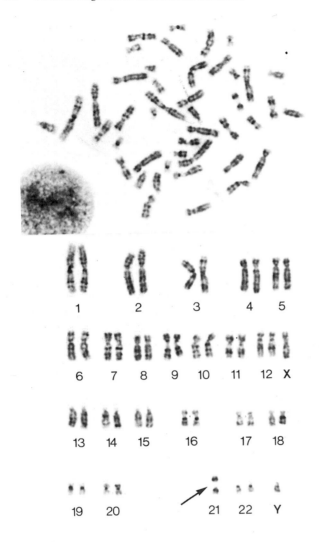

Figure 6.6 Karyotype of parental male carrier of a 21/21 Robertsonian translocation. This man had two children with Down's syndrome

some are associated with a high risk of abnormality while others are benign in their effects. In some families they are transmitted from generation to generation without problems. Some people may carry the SMC in all cells, but in a substantial number of cases, the SMC has arisen as a result of a new mutation either as a non-disjunctional error in a parent or as a post-zygotic error in the zygote (Benn and Hsu, 1984; Buckton *et al.*, 1985; Sachs *et al.*, 1987). In the latter case the individual will be a mosaic.

    Parents who themselves carry an SMC in all cells have a 50% risk that a child will inherit the marker. This risk tends to be greater for maternal transmission of the

Table 6.6 The risk for parental Robertsonian translocation carriers of having children or fetuses with unbalanced forms of the translocation

The only unbalanced forms of these translocations giving rise to a viable fetus at the time of sampling are those involving trisomies 13 and 21, so only translocations involving these chromosomes are given.

1. D/D TRANSLOCATIONS t(13;14) and t(13;15)
   D/D maternal 2–3%
   D/D paternal 3–4%

2. D/G TRANSLOCATIONS t(14;21), t(15;21) and t(13;21)
   D/G maternal 12–15%
   D/G paternal 3%

3. G/G TRANSLOCATIONS t(21;22) and t(21;21)
   21/22 maternal 12–15%
   21/22 paternal 3%
   21/21 maternal 100%
   21/21 paternal 100%

marker, since some markers (but not all) are associated with infertility in males. If the parent carries the marker in all cells, then the predicted phenotype of the child is expected to be similar to that of the parent. It is, however, important to ensure that the marker has not arisen *de novo* in the parent, who carries it only in mosaic form and therefore may show a dilution of the full phenotypic effects. If a mosaic parent carries the SMC in germ cells (germ line mosaicism), then there is a risk of transmitting it to a child, who will then carry the SMC in all cells. There are a large number of examples described (e.g. in Buckton *et al.*, 1985) of mentally normal parents who are mosaic for SMCs who have children who have inherited the marker, but who, without the ameliorating effects of a normal cell line, particularly in the brain, are severely mentally handicapped. This emphasizes the importance, wherever possible, of studying the parents and siblings of a patient with a marker chromosome in order to try to ascertain the origin and risks.

Parental trisomic mosaicism or other mosaicism

A proportion of parents may show the trisomic cell line in their peripheral blood cells, but it is important to recognize that a significant number of true mosaics may have the abnormal cell line only in certain restricted tissues (including the germ cells) but not show the mosaicism in blood. The differences between the newborn figures for trisomic mosaicism (less than 1%) and estimates for the proportions of cases of trisomies where a parent shows trisomic mosaicism vary from 1 to 8%, and probably reflect the proportion of people who may have 'cryptic' germ line mosaicism. Trisomic mosaicism for some anomalies, e.g. trisomy 13 and trisomy 21 may be more frequent than in other trisomies.

Fragile X syndrome

Down's syndrome (trisomy 21) is recognized as the most frequent and major genetic cause of mental handicap (occurring in 1 in 700 births). However, there is now increasing recognition of the role of other genetic or chromosomal contributions to mental handicap. Fragile X syndrome is second only to Down's syndrome in its prevalence among all ethnic groups in causing mental handicap with prevalence rates of 1 in 1100 for males. The prevalence rates for females too are high but estimates are complicated by the fact that about one-third of the females show mild to moderate mental handicap, but a sizeable proportion of carrier females do not show the fragile X, although they may have several affected sons and carrier daughters who do.

There are significant differences in the aetiology and modes of inheritance of these genetic forms of mental handicap. These have major implications for screening programmes, prenatal diagnosis and prevention. The vast majority of cases of Down's syndrome occur as a result of a non-disjunctional event in a parent; in 70–80% of cases this is a first meiotic error in the mother. Mothers under 35 years old have only the population risk of having a child with Down's syndrome (i.e. about 1 in 700) and even for a mother of 40, the risk is only 1.23% (*see* Table 6.1). In contrast, fragile X shows a Mendelian X-linked mode of inheritance, so that carrier mothers have a 50% risk of having affected sons or carrier (and often mildly affected) daughters. In the fragile X syndrome, affected males and about two-thirds of carrier females have a fragile site at Xq27.3 when cells are cultured in low folate media. Affected males have moderate to severe mental retardation. Macro-orchidism is the other most consistent diagnostic feature and 80% have a high forehead, large jaw and long ears (Turner and Jacobs, 1986). Diagnosis in male patients is confirmed by finding the fragile X chromosome in 5–50% of cells cultured in appropriate culture conditions (low folate medium, or with folate antagonists or thymidylate stress; Sutherland, 1979; Glover, 1981). About 10–20% of males who are positive for fragile X function at the low to normal range of intelligence.

The situation in females is much more complicated. About one-third of carrier females are mildly mentally handicapped and the vast majority of these handicapped females (about 90%) are positive for the fragile X, but usually a lower proportion of cells are fragile site positive than for affected males. Some of these females have lowered fertility. Unfortunately, the carrier status of a female 'at risk' who has normal intelligence is difficult to determine since only about one-third of true carriers are fragile X positive. Thus although screening female relatives of affected males will identify carriers in a proportion of cases, it is clear that many women who have a 50% risk of having affected sons show no fragile sites themselves and so they cannot, at present, be identified as being at risk by cytogenetic testing. The use of DNA probes to study linkage polymorphisms in fragile X syndrome using probes for the distal part of the long arm of the X chromosome may help in carrier detection, but at present this technique gives problems because there is a very high frequency of recombination in the distal part of Xq, affecting linkage disequilibrium (Davies *et al.*, 1985).

Laird (1987) has produced a hypothesis to explain these phenomena which suggests that expression of the fragile site depends on the cycle of X chromosome inactivation and reactivation in females. The fragile X mutation blocks reactivation just at the fragile site, creating a partially reactivated chromosome which is said to be imprinted. This imprinting is a second chromosomal event which follows an initial fragile X mutation. Transmitting males (Fryns and Van den Berghe, 1982) have inherited a non-imprinted fragile X chromosome from their mothers, and transmit the non-imprinted fragile X chromosome to their daughters in whom this X chromosome is imprinted by inactivation and then partially reactivated during oogenesis in their mothers. Males who inherit this imprinted fragile X from their mothers are affected with the fragile X syndrome and are mentally retarded, and daughters of carrier mothers who inherit the imprinted fragile X may be mentally retarded. Major questions still remain about the risks for unaffected carrier females.

Prenatal diagnosis in families at risk for fragile X syndrome

The fragile X syndrome may be recognized in those families where there is a mentally handicapped male or in those families where there is moderate to severe mental handicap in a number of family members. The high frequency of this condition and the severity of the mental handicap in affected males suggests that more general screening for the disorder might be of value. Screening mentally handicapped males (either in the community, or in mental handicap hospitals) would identify affected males and their female relatives at risk could then be identified and counselled. A combination of factors including the severity and frequency of fragile X syndrome and the high (50%) risk of a female carrier having an affected son, indicate that there is a need for reliable and accurate prenatal diagnosis. Prenatal diagnosis using cytogenetic methods should be offered to all proven female carriers expressing the fragile site at Xq27.3 and obligate carriers (who may or may not show expression of fragile Xq27.3). The situation is more difficult for those with a high probability of being carriers (although fragile X negative), who have a previous affected child, or are relatives of affected males. Before undertaking prenatal diagnosis it is crucial to know the proportion of cells showing the fragile X in affected males in the family and the culture conditions which give the best expression of the fragile X in order to minimize errors and maximize confidence limits.

The most accurate method for prenatal diagnosis of fragile X is fetal blood karyotyping with growth of the fetal lymphocytes in appropriate culture conditions (low folate media, use of folate antagonists and thymidylate stress). Fetal blood cultures give more accurate results than other techniques since cell synchronization and conditions of folate deprivation can be readily achieved (Webb et al., 1987; Jenkins et al., 1988; McKinley et al., 1988). Expression of the fragile X in at least 4% of cells (with analysis of a minimum of 300–400 cells) should be seen before a positive diagnosis of fragile X is considered. Although amniocentesis is more readily available than fetal blood sampling, amniotic fluid cells have a greater risk of giving false-negative results. Amniocentesis at 16 weeks with a cell culture time required to provide sufficient mitoses from cells grown in stringent culture conditions for analysis may take 3–4 weeks, so that women with a 50% chance of having an affected male may have to face the prospect of a late (18–21 week) termination if the fetal cells are positive for fragile X. Fetal blood sampling cannot be undertaken until 17–18 weeks' gestation, but fetal blood cell culture takes only 3–4 days and appears to be associated with the lowest risk of error. If the amniotic fluid or CVS cells give an equivocal result, the possibility of confirmatory fetal blood sampling should be considered.

Early prenatal diagnosis of fragile X was initially restricted to fetal sexing of CVS samples in the first trimester, with selective termination of males. More recently, attempts have been made to detect fragile X in first and second trimester CVS. Accuracy of diagnosis between fetal blood, amniotic fluid and CVS is not simply a matter of false-negative results, although, of course, definitive diagnosis is crucial

(McKinley *et al.*, 1988; Purvis-Smith *et al.*, 1988; Shapiro *et al.*, 1988). If 4% is taken as the lower limit for positive samples, then sufficient cells are required to determine this with adequate confidence limits and under the rather cytotoxic culture conditions required for fragile X expression, and insufficient cells for analysis are sometimes found either from amniocentesis or CVS. Fetal blood analysis at present seems to offer the greatest chance of accuracy and speed. The opportunity of undertaking karyotyping studies in parallel with a fetal blood and CVS or amniotic fluid sample should be undertaken wherever possible in fragile X cases in order to assess the diagnostic accuracy achieved with the different tissues. Our studies (McKinley *et al.*, 1988) indicate that fetal blood analysis has the greatest accuracy and that neither amniotic fluid cells nor CVS samples give such satisfactory results. It is at present rather difficult to give confidence limits for the sensitivity of the three different methods (fetal blood, amniotic fluid and CVS) since there have been insufficient continuing pregnancies after prenatal diagnosis to monitor false-negative rates, but there are indications that CVS samples carry the greatest risk of false-negative findings.

Discovery of fragile sites at Xq27.3 in CVS, amniotic fluid cells (AFC) or fetal blood samples (FBS) in a pregnancy not known to be at risk for fragile X

The problems of detecting cells with a fragile X in CVS, amniotic fluid cells or fetal blood cells in a pregnancy not previously recognized as being at risk for fragile X syndrome creates a dilemma. Provided that at least 4% of the cells show the fragile X, full family studies, cytogenetic analysis and DNA marker studies should be undertaken.

Chromosomal instability syndromes

Chromosomal instability syndromes are individually rare, but they have severe effects in affected individuals (mental handicap, immunodeficiency and childhood malignancy), and because they are due to single gene defects with an autosomal recessive mode of inheritance have a high (1 in 4) risk of recurrence (McKusick, 1988). The principal reason for including details of the syndromes here is that sometimes very high rates of chromosomal breakage are observed in amniotic fluid cells, CVS samples or fetal blood cultures and in such circumstances a chromosomal breakage syndrome may be suspected. The fragile X syndrome which involves a single fragile site on the X chromosome was described above. In certain inherited chromosomal instability syndromes such as ataxia telangiectasia (AT), Fanconi's anaemia (FA), xeroderma pigmentosa (XP) and Bloom's syndrome, chromosomal breaks occur at a very high frequency and their presence can be enhanced by specific culture conditions (Auerbach, Sagi and Adler, 1985; Auerbach, Min and Ghosh, 1986; Llerena *et al.*, 1989). Each syndrome has a characteristic pattern of chromosomal damage and response of cells to specific clastogens (e.g. a high frequency of chromosomal breaks occurs if diepoxybutane is used in cultures of those affected by Fanconi's anaemia). These breakage syndromes all have autosomal recessive modes of inheritance so that both parents are heterozygous carriers and for some instability syndromes the heterozygous carriers may show characteristic chromosomal changes.

   If the pregnancy is at risk for a specific chromosomal breakage syndrome, prenatal diagnosis may be possible with appropriate conditions and controls. If, however, the pregnancy is not known to be at risk but shows a high frequency of

Table 6.7 Culture conditions and chromosomal instability or fragility syndromes

Chromosomal syndrome	Abnormalities	Conditions for expression
Fragile X	Mental retardation, macro-orchidism	Low folate levels, folate antagonists and thymidylate stress
Ataxia telangiectasia	Progressive cerebellar ataxia, predisposition to malignancy	Hypersensitive to gamma radiation and radiomimetic chemicals, impaired response to phytohaemagglutinin
Bloom's syndrome	Intrauterine growth retardation, short stature, photosensitivity immune defect	Increased levels of SCE. Homologous chromosome interchanges
Fanconi's anaemia	Pancytopenia, hypoplastic radius/thumb	High frequency spontaneous chromosome breaks. Sensitive to mitomycin C and diepoxybutane
Xeroderma pigmentosa	Photosensitivity, multiple skin cancers	Deficient UV repair

chromosomal breakage in cultured cells, it is possible to take a rational approach and carry out systematic testing on cultured fetal cells and the parents (Table 6.7).

Ataxia telangiectasia (AT)

There is progressive cerebellar ataxia, telangiectases especially of the conjunctiva and a strong predisposition to malignancy (Cleaver, 1986). Patients and their cultured cells are sensitive to gamma radiation and radiomimetic chemicals such as bleomycin because of defective DNA repair and they show chromosomal breakage. T cells have impaired responsiveness to phytohaemagglutinin (PHA). Many AT patients develop T-cell malignancies and show chromosomal rearrangements involving the alpha, beta and gamma T-cell receptor genes on chromosomes 7 and 14, the TCL oncogene and the immunoglobulin heavy chain gene on chromosome 14.

Bloom's syndrome

In an affected fetus there is intrauterine growth retardation and post-natal growth too is affected. Other problems in childhood include photosensitivity, telangiectatic erythema and severe immune defect. Cellular abnormalities are characterized by chromosome interchanges between homologous chromosomes (in contrast, in Fanconi's anaemia exchanges usually occur between non-homologous chromosomes). Cells show very large numbers of sister chromatid exchanges (SCE). This increase can be reduced by a factor produced when Bloom's syndrome cells are co-cultivated with normal cells. Heterozygous parents have normal frequencies of SCEs.

Fanconi's anaemia

Pancytopenia with congenital abnormalities (radial hypoplasia/absent thumbs, heart defects), hyperpigmentation and a predisposition to leukaemia are the most characteristic features of this syndrome. Spontaneous chromosomal aberrations occur at a high frequency and are more numerous than those seen in Bloom's syndrome. Fibroblasts from affected individuals have an impaired capacity to remove DNA interstrand cross links induced by mitomycin C (MMC) and Auerbach *et al.* (1985, 1986) have attempted prenatal diagnosis in 30 fetuses at risk using increased baseline and diepoxybutane (DEB) induced chromosome damage in Fanconi's anaemia cells.

Xeroderma pigmentosa (XP)

Affected individuals have sensitivity to sunlight with the development of carcinomas at an early age. Cells from patients with XP lack the capacity to repair UV-induced DNA damage, but there are a number of different complementation groups, i.e. mutations at a number of different loci cause defective DNA repair leading to the XP phenotype.

Miscellaneous

There are a number of conditions which might be associated with a slightly increased risk of chromosome abnormalities, but where the extent of the risk has not been quantified and where the existence of the association is often controversial or speculative. These include patients with recurrent spontaneous abortion (especially missed abortions) or a family history or previous child with neural tube defect.

Tissues for karyotyping

Amniotic fluid cells (AFC)

Genetic amniocentesis was first undertaken in the early 1970s and the experience from hundreds of thousands of cases has permitted risk tables to be compiled for all the different chromosome abnormalities for each maternal age. Amniocentesis undertaken solely for advanced maternal age has been shown to be a relatively safe and accurate procedure. The risks of cytogenetic abnormality are comparatively low, culture success rates are high (usually exceeding 98%) and the error rates are usually less than 1%. Factors contributing to error rates include mosaicism in culture, confined placental anomalies, maternal cell contamination and errors involved in mislabelling cultures and incorrectly transcribing results. For each different abnormal karyotype there is excellent documentation of the general risks, but for each individual case, it may be difficult to determine whether or not there is a clinically significant abnormality in the fetus.

Problems of prenatal karyotyping amniotic fluid cells

Maternal cell contamination
When the amniotic fluid sample is blood stained, there is a substantial risk of maternal cell contamination in culture when the number of blood cells exceeds 5×10^6 cells (Gosden and Brock, 1978). When a female karyotype is obtained in such cases it is essential to ensure that this is from the fetus and distinct from the

mother by comparing fetal polymorphisms, either chromosomal, enzyme or DNA, with those of the mother. The general problems of maternal cell contamination for AFC, CVS and FBS and methods of exclusion testing are covered above.

Low viable cell numbers
If the viable cell count is inappropriate for the gestational age, a detailed ultrasound scan should be performed to confirm gestation, fetal viability and to detect abnormalities such as polyhydramnios or oligohydramnios which are associated not only with alterations in the viable cell counts but also with fetal malformations such as oesophageal atresia, obstructive uropathy, omphalocoele, or exstrophy of the cloaca (Gosden and Brock, 1978; Gosden, 1983). In these cases there may be a high risk of chromosome abnormality. Low viable cell counts are one of the principal reasons for failure of the cell culture and thus failure to obtain a fetal karyotype. If there is a significant risk of chromosomal anomaly (e.g. 30% of cases of duodenal atresia are associated with trisomy 21 but involve polyhydramnios and consequently low cell numbers), then other methods of rapid fetal karyotyping should be considered.

Detection of small deletions and rearrangements
An increasing number of serious fetal and childhood syndromes are now recognized as being due to chromosomal microdeletion syndromes. These are known to be attributable to the absence of a number of contiguous genes on the chromosome which gives rise to a small chromosomal deletion, but this is frequently below the level of detection if conventional chromosomal banding is used (ISCN, 1981). Some of these small deletions can however be recognized when high resolution banding at the 800 band level is used. In order to carry out high resolution banding, synchronous cell divisions in culture permit relatively large numbers of cells to be collected in the prophase of mitosis before the chromosomes have fully condensed, so that prometaphase chromosome preparations can be prepared for high resolution banding. These conditions are relatively difficult to achieve in both AFC and CVS but are much easier in fetal blood cultures. Thus the recognition of small chromosomal deletions or duplications may be comparatively difficult in amniotic fluid cells.

Fragile X and chromosomal breakage syndromes
Specialized techniques such as those involving low folate levels and thymidylate stress for fragile X syndrome or special conditions for chromosomal breakage syndrome can be carried out most successfully in fetal blood cultures. They are more difficult in amniotic fluid cells in that less mitotic figures are usually available for analysis and there is a danger of false-negative results if the culture conditions are not correct. Positive control samples from an affected family member (preferably amniotic fluid cells from an affected fetus in the same family) but certainly fibroblast cultures which have greater similarities to AFC than peripheral blood cells should be studied where possible.

Confined placental anomalies and mosaicism
Confined placental anomalies and mosaicism do occur in AFC (Bui, Iselius and Lindsten, 1984; Hsu and Perlis, 1984; Worton and Stern, 1984), but occur to a much greater extent in CVS samples. The problems associated with all the different fetal tissues will therefore be discussed in greater detail below.

Chorionic villus sampling

Chorionic villus sampling is a recent introduction; there are certain problems of karyotyping trophoblast which occur at a greater frequency than those found with amniotic fluid cells. The particular problems for amniotic fluid cells described in the sections above all apply to CVS samples, and those points which are of special significance in CVS are those involving maternal cell contamination (especially for cultured CVS preparations where it is a major problem), confined placental anomalies, including mosaicism, false-negative results and hypodiploidy or monosomy especially for 45,X. Each of these points will be considered in detail.

Problems with CVS

Maternal cell contamination

Maternal cell contamination is a major problem for cultured CVS samples and has been reported at frequencies of 12–14% (Therkelsen *et al.*, 1988; Roberts, Duckett and Lang, 1988; Canadian Collaborative CVS-Amniocentesis Clinical Trial Group, 1989). It is important to develop rational plans of approach, with analysis of cellular markers, other confirmatory tests and further sampling if necessary. These are discussed in more detail below.

In cases of XX/XY mosaicism or more complex forms of mosaicism involving 46,XX cells, maternal contamination is a much more likely source of error than true hermaphroditism in the fetus. In some cases the levels of 46,XX cells are so high that the parents are often warned of the possible dangers of an intersex fetus. This causes a great deal of anxiety and more than 99% of these cases are due to maternal cell contamination.

Confined placental anomalies

Confined placental anomalies and mosaicism occur frequently in CVS. Mosaicism may arise as a result of pseudomosaicism (culture artefact), or because the karyotypes of placental cells are genuinely different from the fetus (confined placental anomalies) (Kalousek and Dill, 1983; Kalousek *et al.*, 1987; Kalousek, Barret and McGillivray, 1989). Both of these problems arise in AFC but the latter problem, genuine difference in karyotype between placenta and fetus, occurs more commonly with CVS. Discrepancies exist between the karyotypes obtained from direct and cultured preparations of chorionic villi and between the trophoblastic tissues and the fetus itself; this is called extra embryonic/fetal karyotypic discordance (Crane and Cheung, 1988) or confined placental anomaly. It can involve a number of different types of chromosome abnormality. These include mosaicism for autosomal trisomy, polyploidy (triploidy and tetraploidy), chromosomal rearrangements, supernumerary markers and sex chromosome mosaicism.

Direct CVS chromosomal preparations involve the epithelial cells of the cytotrophoblast which is derived from trophectoderm and mural trophoblast (Watanabe *et al.*, 1978). Cultured cells represent a cell lineage derived from the inner cell mass rather than that of the trophoblast divergence (Luckett, 1978). Cultured CVS preparations are thought to be from extra embryonic mesenchymal cells. An early mitotic error in a cell destined to form the placenta will result in chromosome abnormalities confined to trophoblast. Hogge, Schonberg and Golbus (1986) found a frequency of mosaicism of 1.7%, Simoni *et al.* (1983, 1984, 1986) and Brambati, Lanzani and Oldrini (1988) found a 1% discrepancy between placental and fetal lines and a number of cases have shown discrepancies between direct preparations from cytotrophoblast and cultured cells. Considerable differences in the levels of mosaicism may be observed between centres. In the three large series of first trimester CVS diagnoses reported by Hook *et al.* (1988), the rate of mosaicism in the Milan cases (47 karyotypic abnormalities were found among 922 chorionic villus samples, of which 12 were mosaic) was 0.13% compared with one mosaic case among the 22 abnormalities found in 1424 cases in Chicago and two cases of mosaicism among 43 chromosome abnormalities found among the 2132 samples karyotyped by the Philadelphia group.

False-negative results have been described

False-negative results have been described especially for trisomy 13 and 18, (Eichenbaum *et al.*, 1986; Linton and Lilford, 1986; Martin *et al.*, 1986; Leschot, Wolf and Weenink, 1988).These may become an even greater problem for second and third trimester CVS than for first trimester samples. It has been suggested that survival of fetuses with pure trisomies 13 and 18 is much greater if there are normal (non-trisomic) cells in the placenta and it has been reported that over 75% of cases of trisomies 13 and 18 do exhibit high levels of normal cells which explains the risk of these false-negative results (Kalousek, Barret and McGillivray, 1989).

The presence of hypodiploidy

Hypodiploidy, (usually involving 45,X with loss of X or Y) is a major problem in CVS but also occurs in amniotic fluid cells especially when cell growth and spreading are poor. In cases of XX/XY or more complicated types of mosaicism, maternal contamination may be the greatest problem.

In CVS, hypodiploidy and chromosome loss are common and it is difficult to get satisfactory chromosome banding in direct preparations. Inability to distinguish the different chromosomes in a group (especially the C group) leads to problems. 45,X cell lines constitute a major problem, and the fact that loss of any of the C group chromosomes (which include 6,7,8,9,10,11,12 and X) may be attributed to X loss confounds the problem. Mikkelsen and Aymé (1986) reporting the European Collaborative Data showed that at least 30% of pure 45,X cases are discrepant and the majority of 45,X mosaics represent confined placental anomalies. Culture gives more reliable cytogenetic results but the danger of maternal contamination is great, even with the most careful cleaning and dissection of the villi. Enzyme treatments particularly with proteolytic enzymes trypsin and protease may increase the risks of maternal cells being cultured.

Fetal blood karyotyping

Rapid karyotyping from cultured fetal blood cells may be particularly helpful in cases of mosaicism in culture because fetal blood is a true fetal tissue and results can be obtained in 2–4 days (Gosden, 1984; Gosden *et al.*, 1985; Gosden, Nicolaides and Rodeck, 1988). It is also important for specialized culture techniques and high resolution banding such as those involved in the fragile X syndrome, detection of small deletions and rearrangements, chromosomal breakage syndromes and where rapid karyotyping is important, where the gestational age is advanced or where fetal treatment *in utero* might be necessary. Each of these and its associated problems will be examined in greater detail.

Certain specific fetal anomalies such as non-immune fetal hydrops (NIH), or severe intrauterine growth retardation (IUGR), may be associated with very poor growth of the fetal blood cells in culture. Special culture techniques must be used to optimize growth in these circumstances. It is essential to use a purified mitogen such as phytohaemagglutinin (PHA) for lymphocyte stimulation and medium with a variety of special growth supplements may be necessary. Some conditions, e.g. fragile X, or breakage syndromes, require control samples or samples from affected family members so that the pattern of chromosomal abnormalities in culture can be characterized. Maternal blood cell contamination may be monitored by Kleihauer testing and if maternal cells are detected, comparison of fetal and maternal heteromorphisms, either cytogenetically, or using DNA or enzyme markers, should be undertaken. Specialized banding techniques such as high resolution banding can be used to detect small chromosomal deletions or rearrangements and identify the specific chromosomal regions and breakpoints involved. Studies of sufficient fetal cells to give adequate confidence limits will help to exclude mosaicism.

Problems in the interpretation of prenatal karyotypes

Does the prenatal diagnostic karyotype indicate the true karyotype of the fetus?

Two questions arise each time an abnormal karyotype is detected prenatally. The first is whether this indicates the possibility of a true chromosomal abnormality in the fetus, or whether this simply indicates a confined placental abnormality and the fetus is cytogenetically normal. The second problem is what are the risks of mental and physical handicap in the child if the chromosome abnormality is shown to be real. For each of these different types of abnormality there are two major problems. The first is in assessing whether or not the abnormality is likely to be associated with true mosaicism in the fetus. If the fetus does indeed have the chromosome abnormality, then the risks of phenotypic abnormality and handicap must be evaluated for each individual chromosome disorder but the underlying biological process is that fetus and placenta have a common origin but may diverge during development.

Maternal cell contamination

The problem of maternal cell contamination, particularly in chorion villus cultures, may be considerable. Frequencies of 10–14% are often reported even by the most careful and experienced laboratories (Therkelsen et al., 1988; Roberts, Duckett and Lang, 1988), although there is a very low frequency in direct CVS preparations (Blakemore et al., 1985). Maternal cell contamination is usually seen as 46,XX/46,XY mosaicism but, in more extreme form, is seen as a 46,XX karyotype where the true fetal karyotype is 46,XY or an abnormal karyotype.

Confined placental abnormalities

There is now a substantial number of studies indicating the scale of the problems of confined abnormalities and demonstrating that this is greater for CVS than for amniocentesis. The Canadian MRC randomized controlled trial of CVS versus amniocentesis showed the extent of the problem. Of the 1391 women randomized to the CVS group (of whom 932 were actually eligible for CVS), 45 were found to have chromosome abnormalities, but 19 of the 45 were subsequently demonstrated to have only confined placental anomalies which were not present in the fetus. There were 22 chromosomal abnormalities in the 1396 patients randomized to amniocentesis (of whom 929 were eligible) and of these, three had confined placental anomalies. Thus 42% of all the chromosomal abnormalities in the CVS series and 13.6% of the chromosome anomalies in the amniocentesis series were confined abnormalities and serious diagnostic errors would have occurred if further confirmatory testing had not been carried out. The confined abnormalities were non-mosaic and mosaic aneuploidy, polyploidy in mosaic form and unbalanced translocations also in mosaic form. It is not possible to achieve greater levels of confidence simply by analysing larger numbers of cells from different cultures from the same initial sample. It is important to recognize that, although it is possible to demonstrate a major karyotypic abnormality in non-mosaic form in several hundred cells from three different cultures, this still may not indicate that the fetus itself has a chromosome anomaly. Sheer weight of numbers of abnormal cells in culture and predominance of the abnormality in all culture flasks does not guarantee that the fetus is chromosomally abnormal.

There are eight different types of confined placental anomalies:

1. trisomies for clinically recognized chromosomal syndromes
2. trisomies for non-clinically recognized syndromes
3. sex chromosome abnormalities particularly 45,X in non-mosaic and mosaic forms and deletions of the X
4. chromosomal rearrangements (including balanced and unbalanced translocations, duplications and deletions or partial trisomies and monosomies, inversions and ring chromosomes)
5. supernumerary marker chromosomes
6. polyploidy
7. normal cell lines in the placenta when the fetus has a major chromosomal abnormality (false-negative result)
8. discrepancies between the direct chromosomal preparations in CVS and cultured cells.

All the eight types of abnormality described above may also be seen in mosaic form. Chromosomal mosaicism occurs when two or more cell lines with different karyotypes are present. True chromosomal mosaicism occurs when different lines may have originated during early post-zygotic development, and more than one line is present in the fetus (Hall, 1988). This has been reported in a large number of cases involving autosomal trisomies, sex chromosome anomalies, chromosomal rearrangements and polyploidy. Mosaicism is usually found in multiple tissues; the clinical manifestations depend upon the chromosomes involved, and the proportion of cells in individual tissues (Hoehn et al., 1978). For those conditions where mental handicap is involved, the crucial factor appears to be the proportion of abnormal cells in the brain. In some cases of true mosaicism, the zygote may have had an abnormal karyotype at conception, but the abnormal chromosome or set of chromosomes is lost during an early cell division, and this leads to a normal cell line in the fetus. The origin of such mosaic abnormalities can sometimes be determined using chromosomal markers. This has been used in cases of mosaic trisomy 21 where the child has three different chromosomes 21 (Mikkelsen et al., 1980).

Mosaicism is a very frequent and serious problem in prenatal diagnosis (Gosden, Nicolaides and Rodeck, 1988). It may indicate:

1. the presence of true mosaicism for a major chromosome abnormality in the fetus as described above
2. contamination with maternal tissue
3. post-zygotic non-disjunction restricted entirely to trophoblast and extra-embryonic membrane (called confined placental mosaicism)
4. *in vitro* changes in cultured amniotic fluid or CVS cells (culture artefact)
5. unrecognized dizygotic twin pregnancy with early death of an abnormal twin, but persistence of its trophoblast (Landy *et al.*, 1986).

Autosomal trisomies

Autosomal trisomies can be subdivided into those trisomies which are seen in living children and are thus associated with a risk of a surviving handicapped child (clinically significant trisomies), and those where there is a very high risk of pseudomosaicism which is not true in the fetus; this includes trisomies 2, 3, 14, 16, 20 and 22, which are almost exclusively limited to trophoblast and extra-embryonic membrane cells. In cases of mosaicism for chromosomes 2, 3, 14, 16, 20 and 22 it may be inappropriate to carry out further investigations other than detailed follow-up of the infant and studies of the placenta at delivery.

Trisomy for clinically recognized syndromes (trisomies 13, 18 and 21 and mosaic trisomies 7, 8, 9)

For those trisomies associated with clinically recognized syndromes (because genuine cases of mosaicism exist), the risk is often thought to be high; fetal blood sampling has shown that these abnormalities in particular have a very high chance of representing only pseudomosaicism and are not present in the fetus (Gosden, Nicolaides and Rodeck, 1988). Precipitate action in these cases might lead to the termination of a normal fetus. Pseudomosaicism has been demonstrated for pure trisomies 13 (Malin *et al.*, 1987), trisomy 18 (Mikkelsen and Ayme, 1986), and for mosaic trisomies 7, 8, 9, 13, 18 and 21 (Simoni *et al.*, 1983, 1984; Mikkelsen and Ayme, 1986; Delozier-Blanchet *et al.*, 1988; Gosden, Nicolaides and Rodeck, 1988).

Trisomies 2, 3, 14, 15, 16, 17, 19, 20 and 22

These trisomies occur relatively frequently in prenatal diagnostic samples. Trisomies 2 and 20 occur frequently in AF cell cultures and 3, 14, 16 and 22 in CVS samples. Taking trisomy 20 as an example, 85% of cases where trisomy 20 mosaicism has been found in amniotic fluid cells have been associated with a fetus or infant with grossly normal fetal phenotype. In those with an abnormal phenotype the patterns of malformation have been varied and non-specific. No trisomy 20 cells have been detected in blood samples of the fetuses or infants, although some cells with trisomy 20 have been detected in specific fetal tissues such as kidney, rectum, oesophagus and placenta (Bardinger *et al.*, 1987; Hsu, Kaffe and Perlis, 1987). This suggests that trisomy 20 is confined to certain specific fetal organs and particularly extra-embryonic tissues. Whether there is an association between an abnormal phenotype or pregnancy complications when there is a high percentage of trisomy 20 cells has not yet been established. However, no causal relationship between trisomy 20 and a specific malformation syndrome has so far been established and many hundreds of cases have now been studied in detail. There is a need to collect more data in collaborative international trials in order to provide more accurate information for counselling and pregnancy management in these circumstances (Mikkelsen and Ayme, 1986).

Sex chromosome mosaicism

A large number of surveys of newborns and surveys of adults with abnormalities of genitalia or secondary sexual development has demonstrated that true mosaicism for sex chromosome abnormalities does exist (Simpson, 1982). The most frequently observed form of sex chromosome mosaicism in prenatal diagnosis is 46,XX/46,XY mosaicism. However, the vast majority of these cases are due simply to maternal cell contamination and can in some cases be resolved by careful studies of maternal and fetal markers (Williams *et al.*, 1987). True 46,XX/46,XY mosaicism is often suspected, either because a large proportion of 46,XX cells are present or because attempts to demonstrate that this was due to maternal contamination were unsuccessful. The vast majority of these cases are ultimately shown to involve a normal male fetus with maternal cell contamination. This can happen even if the original amniotic fluid sample did not appear to be bloodstained or the chorionic villus sample showed no microscopic evidence of maternal decidua. If the possibility of termination is being considered, then further sampling should be undertaken. However, the phenomenon of anaphase lag may also take place in placental tissue or in cultured amniotic cells so that daughter cells lose either an X or Y chromosome by this mechanism and X chromosome monosomy is the result.

45,X karyotypes occur in chorionic villus samples, but in 75% of cases this is due to confined placental anomalies and in such cases does not reflect the true karyotype of the fetus (Mikkelsen and Aymé, 1986; Wheeler *et al.*, 1988). It may also occur to a more limited extent in amniotic fluid samples where it also reflects confined placental anomalies and in many cases may not indicate the presence of a true 45X line in the fetus (Gosden, Nicolaides and Rodeck, 1988). It is often assumed that when a 45,X line occurs this is the result of loss of an X chromosome and that the fetus will be female; frequently though, it is associated with loss of a Y chromosome and the pregnancies where a 45,X karyotype is seen are often terminated. There is a relatively high probability that 45,X mosaicism or even a pure 45,X karyotype may occur solely because of confined placental mosaicism and serious diagnostic errors can be made unless the possibility of confirmatory studies is considered.

The phenotype/karyotype correlations for individuals with true 45,X/46,XX or 45,X/46,XY mosaicism are complex because they depend not principally upon the proportion of 45,X cells in peripheral blood, but on the proportion of cells with two functional X chromosomes or an X and Y in the gonads. For 45,X/46,XX mosaics both the germ cells and a certain proportion of somatic cells (usually a minimum of 40–45%) must have two X chromosomes in order to ensure that the germ cells do not atrophy in early fetal development and the female develops some of the stigmata of Turner's syndrome. When germ cell atrophy does occur, menopause precedes menarche. For 45,X/46,XX mosaics, those with relatively few 45,X cells may appear to be phenotypically normal females. Individuals with a greater proportion of 45,X cells may be similar to females with full Turner's syndrome; having short stature, primary amenorrhoea and neck webbing. The vast majority of true mosaics are found as part of the spectrum in between the two extremes (Ferguson-Smith, 1965; Sarkar, 1983; Hook and Warburton, 1983; Rosenberg *et al.*, 1987; Hsu, 1989).

For true 45X/46,XY mosaics three different phenotypes are found; these are normal male, intersex or pseudohermaphrodite, and Turner's syndrome female. Even when the proportion of 45,X cells in peripheral blood approaches 45%, the mosaic individual may still have a normal male phenotype and even be fertile. This demonstrates the powerful effect of the testis determining gene on the Y chromosome. In other mosaics, however, a slight increase in the proportion of 45,X cells leads to a female Turner-like phenotype, in spite of the fact that a considerable number of cells have a 46,XY karyotype. Perhaps in these cases there are insufficient cells containing the Y chromosome for proper testis organization; in some cases ovaries develop which, in the absence of a second X chromosome in embryonic life, regress and become streak gonads by the time of birth. When more complicated admixtures of germ cells occur, ovotestes or streak gonads develop and intersex phenotypes with pseudohermaphroditism are seen. True hermaphroditism is usually only observed when an XX line is present to influence true ovarian development in an ovotestis in addition to the 46,XY cell line.

Other more complex forms of sex chromosome mosaicism may occur such as 45,X/46,XX/47,XXX or 45,X/46,XY/47,XYY. Some of these may involve true fetal mosaicism or chimaerism (Freiberg *et al.*, 1988), but others may simply be the consequence of abnormal mitotic non-disjunction as a confined placental abnormality restricted to trophoblastic cells. Counting very large numbers of cells may indicate the different cell lines present (Hook, 1977), but will not increase the accuracy if the anomaly is due to confined placental mosaicism and further fetal sampling may be necessary.

Chromosomal rearrangements

This is a complex group because it consists of many different types of rearrangements. These include translocations, deletions, pericentric and paracentric inversions and ring chromosomes. Some of these may be unique and a literature search may not reveal even a single living individual with the same chromosomal breakpoints. In other cases there may be a number of people with the same chromosome abnormality as for example in the 11q;22q translocation (Fraccaro *et al.*, 1980). The phenotypes may vary from normal to severely handicapped, so the prognosis in an individual case is very difficult to predict (Boué *et al.*, 1982; Schinzel, 1984).

The suggested methods of approach are:

1. check parental karyotypes and confirm paternity
2. try to identify and delineate the chromosomal segments involved and the breakpoints
3. a literature search to find individuals with similar karyotypes. It must be remembered that data from many surveys especially those of the mentally handicapped or those with dysmorphic features are biassed
4. further sampling to confirm that the karyotype does not reflect a confined placental anomaly and permit high resolution banding, genetic marker studies (such as DNA probe mapping) and other studies.

Supernumerary marker chromosome mosaicism

The prognosis for cases of *de novo* supernumerary marker chromosomes is very difficult. The first and most crucial task is to ensure that this is a true fetal anomaly and exclude confined placental mosaicism. Provided familial cases have been excluded, the prediction of what the additional material will do in *de novo* cases is complex. In a large proportion of cases it may have no phenotypic effect if it involves the short arms and cytological satellite regions of short arms of acrocentric chromosomes. However, even in mosaic form, markers which involve euchromatin often have serious consequences.

There are a number of investigations which should be initiated when a supernumerary marker chromosome is discovered in prenatal diagnosis:

1. is the marker familial or *de novo* (confirm paternity)?
2. is the marker present only in mosaic form or in every cell in the parent?
3. is the marker in mosaic form in the fetus?
4. size (smaller than a G-group chromosome?)
5. composition (G,C,R,Q,AgNOR and kinetochore staining)
6. derived from chromosome 15? (DA/DAPI technique)
7. literature search for risks of particular marker.

Detailed cytogenetic testing needs to be carried out in all cases where a supernumerary chromosome is found in order to determine whether euchromatic material is present (this contains active genetic material) or whether only genetically inert heterochromatin is present. This can be done by a combination of G-banding and C-banding (C-banding is a technique for centromeric heterochromatin; Sumner, 1972), quinacrine fluorescence or spermidine bisacridine (Van De Sande, Lin and Deugau, 1979) and reverse (R) banding (Verma and Lubs, 1975). The use of a staining technique using the antibiotic Distamycin A combined with DAPI (DA/DAPI) (Schweitzer, Ambros and Andrle, 1978) is useful because it distinguishes those markers derived from chromosome 15 from those derived from other chromosomal segments (*see* Table 6.9). Centromeric heterochromatin may be present usually as one or two blocks demonstrated by C-banding but the number of centromeres present (that is whether the supernumerary marker is monocentric or dicentric) should be determined by kinetochore staining.

Much of the behaviour of a supernumerary marker chromosome at mitosis is determined by whether or not it contains ribosomal DNA and thus whether it participates in satellite associations with other acrocentric chromosomes (Figure 6.7). The presence of active ribosomal regions (that is nucleolar organizer regions (NORs)) actively transcribing can be determined by silver staining (the AgNOR technique; Bloom and Goodpasture; 1976). However, this only distinguishes active NORs; NOR regions which are present but inactive can be demonstrated with *in situ* hybridization using probes for ribosomal DNA (Gosden, Lawrie and Gosden, 1981). The short arms of the acrocentric chromosomes are usually heteromorphic (i.e. there is recognizable variation between individuals) and it is sometimes possible to determine the parental origin of a supernumerary marker chromosome using a combination of techniques such as Q, C, R, AgNOR and DA/DAPI staining. Most markers originate from *de novo* rearrangements of the short arms of maternal acrocentric chromosomes (Figure 6.8) which is consistent with the maternal age effect. Karyotypes of two different individuals with marker chromosomes are shown; one has a large supernumerary marker and is severely

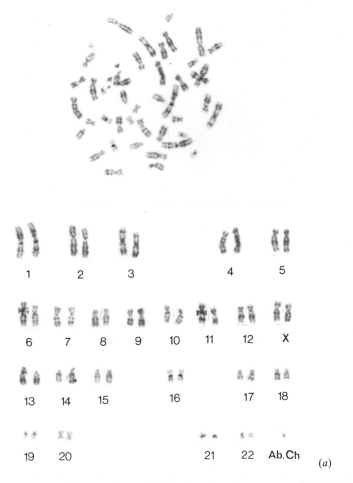

Figure 6.7 (*a*) A small non-15 derived marker chromosome which the female carrier of normal intelligence had inherited from her mother. G banding suggests a small fragment composed mainly of heterochromatic short arm material from around the centromere and this was confirmed by C, R, Q and DA/DAPI banding.

handicapped and the other person with a marker is in the general population and has an average IQ, (*see* Figure 6.7). However, even in mosaic form, markers which involve chromosomal regions carrying unique DNA sequences may be associated with malformation syndromes such as the cat eye syndrome duplication 22q. Many other cases involve neurological problems, mental retardation or behavioural problems. The risks for supernumerary markers are given below where data are included which show that even in mosaic form some markers can have severe effects.

Polyploidy

Diploid/triploid mosaicism may sometimes occur as a result of post-zygotic error but is often associated with an initial twin pregnancy in which there has been death

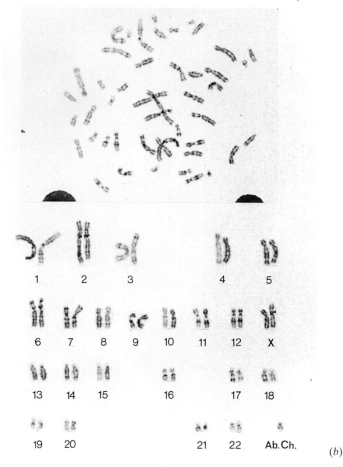

1	2	3	4	5	

6	7	8	9	10	11	12	X

13	14	15	16	17	18

19	20	21	22	Ab.Ch.

(b)

Figure 6.7 (b) A large asymmetric marker in a mentally retarded girl containing euchromatic sequences

of the co-twin: this can be established using chromosomal markers. Triploidy occurs very frequently in the first trimester of pregnancy (Jacobs *et al.*, 1982) and more rarely triploid fetuses survive to the second trimester (Nicolaides, Rodeck and Gosden, 1986). There is a risk that it can represent true mosaicism in the fetus and that a handicapped child might survive as a result of the mosaicism, but there is a very substantial chance that it represents a false-positive result from a confined placental anomaly or twin pregnancy; further sampling preferably with fetal blood karyotyping to avoid placental cells and identification of markers for a twin pregnancy should help to resolve the problem.

An even greater danger of a culture artefact or confined error is encountered in diploid/tetraploid mosaicism (either 46,XX/92,XXXX or 46,XY/92,XXYY). This occurs very frequently and in over 95% of cases signals a false-positive result. It probably occurs as a form of endoreduplication (i.e. the chromosomes replicate without a subsequent cell division) giving rise to a tetraploid cell. Careful further

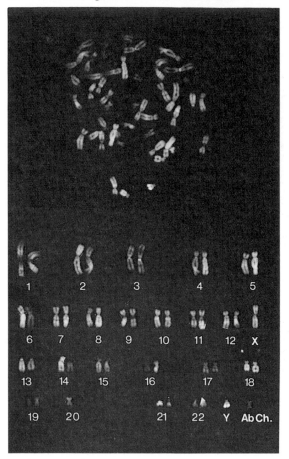

Figure 6.8 Symmetric 15p/15p *de novo* marker. Note the fluorescent cytological satellites at both ends, characteristic of short arm markers derived from chromosomes 13, 14, 15, 21 and 22

testing is important in such cases, but it is mandatory to undertake complex testing to ensure that the same unusual form of 'endoreduplication' does not also occur in a different tissue. The highest levels are seen in CVS, but not infrequently tetraploidy is observed in amniotic fluid cultures where every cell is tetraploid with 92 chromosomes, but the fetus has a diploid karyotype. Amniotic fluid cells do not provide a good means of confirmation for tetraploidy in CVS because cell cycle studies are difficult. Fetal blood too can show erroneous false-positive tetraploid lines if the cultured fetal blood cells are allowed to proceed beyond a first division *in vitro*. In order to prevent this, cells must be harvested after only one round of replication after 24–48 h in culture, and bromodeoxyuridine incorporation patterns can be used to ensure that the cells are only in first division. It is also possible to measure nuclear volumes in an unstimulated blood smear. In tissues such as chorion or amniotic fluid, the cells may be in active cell division so that tetraploid

(4n) cells cannot be distinguished from replicating or mitotic 4n cells; this therefore constitutes a major problem in trying to establish whether true tetraploidy is present. In many cases every cell examined in CVS and amniotic fluid may have a tetraploid karyotype, but this may still indicate culture artefact or confined placental anomalies (Mikkelsen and Ayme, 1986). Tetraploidy occurs with greater frequency if cells are left for protracted periods in culture at very high cellular densities without subculture.

False negatives for true trisomy in the fetus

There are both biological and technical explanations for the occurrence of false-negative results. The biological explanation of the enhanced survival of chromosomally abnormal fetuses if there are normal cell lines in the placenta is one which must be taken into account when considering the indications for karyotyping. For example, if the fetus has abnormalities such as holoprosencephaly, facial clefting, polydactyly, renal cysts or heart defects suggesting possible trisomy 13, or growth retardation, choroid plexus cysts, renal or cardiac anomalies suggesting trisomy 18, then the dangers of a false-negative result from CVS should be recognized and the possibility of rapid karyotyping from other fetal tissues should be examined.

Technical artefacts, too, can contribute to false-negative results. The problems of hypodiploidy have been mentioned previously in the context of chromosome loss from a normal fetus, but if the fetus actually has 47 chromosomes then cell breakage with chromosome loss might lead to the erroneous conclusion that the fetus has a normal karyotype when it is abnormal. The dangers of this are greatest when the preparations and banding are poor and there are very few mitotic figures for analysis. Paradoxically cellular growth and the mitotic indices are always poorest when the fetus is karyotypically abnormal.

Direct chromosomal preparations are derived from cells of the cytotrophoblastic layer, while those of the cultured villi are from the mesenchymal core. This does not simply reflect a difference between epithelial cells and mesodermally derived ones, but has a much more profound implication about the stage of embryological development at which the two different cellular layers diverged from the embryo itself. According to Luckett (1978), the cytotrophoblastic layer is derived from the trophoblast which separated from the cells of the inner cell mass very early in development, at about the 64 cell stage, but the mesenchymal core of the villi is derived from the extra-embryonic mesenchymal layer which did not diverge from the embryo itself until the delamination of the hypoblast from the epiblast at 11–12 days of embryonic development. The mesenchymal layer would thus be expected to have greater karyotypic similarity to the fetus than the cytotrophoblastic layer. In practice the results of many centres which undertake both direct and cultured CVS karyotyping indicate that cultured chorionic villus preparations give more accurate results than those from the direct preparations. In cases of karyotypic abnormality in direct preparations, the initial step should thus be to ensure that the cultured cells show the same abnormality. If there is any discrepancy between the two, the scientific evidence favours the greater accuracy of the cultured cell results.

Frequency of mosaicism

Mosaicism is not rare, excluding cases of level 1 mosaicism (single abnormal cell), level 2 mosaicism (multiple cells with the same abnormality in a single flask or colony) has a frequency of 0.7% and level 3 mosaicism (multiple cells in multiple flasks/colonies) has a frequency in 0.2% of all amniotic fluid samples. These data are derived from the Canadian, European and USA collaborative surveys of levels of mosaicism in over 50 000 amniotic fluid cell samples (Bui, Iselius and Lindsten, 1984; Hsu and Perlis, 1984; Worton and Stern, 1984). There are figures which indicate that the levels of type 2 and type 3 mosaicism in CVS samples are about 3–10-fold higher than for amniotic fluid samples (Simoni *et al.*, 1984; Callen *et al.*, 1988; Hogge, Schonberg and Golbus, 1986; Wolstenholme, Crocker and Jonasson, 1988). Maternal cell contamination (which may manifest as potential intersexuality or hermaphroditism, (giving 46,XX/46,XY mosaicism if the fetus is male) occurs in some 3–14% of CVS cultures from some centres (Therkelson *et al.*, 1985), and this is one reason why direct preparations (where maternal contamination is not a problem) can be valuable.

In prenatal diagnosis two different problems must be considered. The first of these is the probability that a particular kind of mosaicism will occur exclusively in chorionic villus samples, or amniotic fluid, reflecting confined chorionic/placental mosaicism or pseudomosaicism but where no abnormal cells are present in the fetus. Secondly there are the risks for a child if a particular form of chromosomal mosaicism turns out to be real. These differ according to the proportion of abnormal cells in those tissues crucial for development.

Methods of resolving problems of confined anomalies and mosaicism

It is important to recognize that the majority of amniotic fluid cells, (perhaps over 60–70% in early second trimester pregnancy), are trophoblastic and are derived from placenta and extra-embryonic membranes. There is thus a small but significant danger that the same abnormality might arise in the amniotic fluid cell culture as in the CVS, but that the fetus would be normal. In later gestations (from 17–18 weeks onwards), fetal swallowing, urination and skin cell desquamation increase the contribution of fetal dermal, respiratory and gastrointestinal tract cells to the amniotic fluid. If it is considered essential that confirmatory testing must avoid fetal membranes and trophoblastic cells, then only fetal blood or fetal tissue samples will give access to fetal tissues which contain no placental elements (Gosden, Nicolaides and Rodeck, 1988).

The risks for each of the five different types of true fetal mosaic chromosome abnormality (trisomy, sex chromsomes, rearrangements, markers and polyploidy) are covered in the next section. However, the risks that a mosaic on CVS or AFC is real are summarized in Table 6.8. There are several general points which are applicable to all the types of mosaicism.

1. The risks derived here for the probabilities of confined placental abnormalities observed in amniotic fluid or CVS culture are derived from a large series where fetal blood karyotyping was undertaken to resolve problems of mosaicism in the AFC or CVS; other similar cases are derived from the literature. Only those cases where the initial mosaicism involved many cells with the same abnormal karyotype in multiple flasks or colonies (level 3 mosaicism), or in very rare cases (usually where cell growth was poor and there was only one flask) with multiple cells with the same abnormality in a single flask are included. No cases of level 1 mosaicism (single abnormal cells) were included in risk calculations as this occurs frequently and is not itself an indication for further sampling, unless some

Table 6.8 Mosaicism in AFC and CVS

Type of mosaicism	Estimated proportion which are true mosaics (%)	Particular problems
Autosomal trisomies including +21, +18, +13, +8, +9	0–15	Do not assume trisomies 21,13,18 are real
Sex chromosome mosaicism 45,X/46,XX or XY, 46,XX/46,XY	0–15	Exclude maternal contamination
Chromosomal rearrangements translocations, deletions, rings	45–60	Even bizarre anomalies may be real
Supernumerary markers e.g. 47,+mar(15p15p)	60–70	Risk varies from normal to severe mental handicap
Diploid/tetraploid mosaicism 46,XX/69,XXX or 46,XY/69,XXY	0–15	Exclude confined placental anomalies, and twin pregnancy
Diploid/triploid mosaicism 46,XX/92,XXXX or 46,XY/92,XXYY	0–5	Exclude polyploidy or endoreduplication and confined placental anomalies

other risk factor (such as a significant abnormality on ultrasound scan) is present. Similarly, those cases where 'confirmatory' studies of mosaicism were undertaken only with placental tissue, extra-embryonic membrane or villi were excluded because of the inherent errors in this approach.

2. In order to try to determine whether there is true mosaicism in the fetus, or merely confined placental mosaicism, confirmatory sampling on a different fetal tissue should be undertaken. Fetal blood karyotyping gives rapid results in 2–3 days and gives access to a different fetal tissue where there is no danger of trophoblastic cell lines. The risk to the pregnancy of cordocentesis in centres experienced in the technique is only 1–3%. Although amniocentesis offers a similar sampling technique which is widely available with marginally less risk to the pregnancy, there are several problems. Culture takes 10–14 days and the pregnancy is usually quite advanced at the stage at which confirmatory sampling is required. The most significant problem though is that some 60–70% of amniotic fluid cells are derived from trophoblast. Thus if two sequential amniocenteses reveal mosaicism, they may both be wrong and repeat only confirms placental mosaicism. Thus in some cases a second amniocentesis result may differ from the first, but it is difficult to predict which is correct. As the greatest risk of error in these cases arises from confined placental mosaicism, second trimester placental biopsy is not ideal in most cases of mosaicism since it only samples trophoblastic tissue with relatively high levels of spurious mosaicism and maternal contamination in culture.

Although ultrasound scanning plays a very important role in the identification of fetal abnormality, it is important to recognize the limitations that detailed ultrasound scanning has in cases of mosaicism. The greatest probability of true mosaicism is with chromosomal rearrangements such as translocations, rings or supernumerary markers. The major handicap associated with these abnormalities, even in mosaic form, is moderate to severe mental handicap and any dysmorphic features are usually only minor and would not be detectable on scan.

In true mosaicism, the finding of a normal ultrasound scan and the exclusion of major structural anomalies may give a sense of false reassurance. The fact that there may be a high risk of having a child who survives with an IQ of less than 20 may be obscured by over-reliance on imaging which at present cannot yet detect the effect of chromosomal imbalance on neurological development. Furthermore, for those chromosomal anomalies where structural malformation might be expected in the fetus, mosaicism for a normal cell line usually has the effect of diluting the abnormal fetal phenotype so that although abnormalities may be present, they are frequently not identifiable even with the highest resolution ultrasound scanning available. It is important however to delineate the chromosome abnormality and its associated anomalies so that detailed scanning can help in the evaluation of risks. For example, true 45,X/46,XY mosaicism is associated with three different phenotypes. Those fetuses with a very high proportion of 45,X cells may show a Turner-like phenotype; with rather fewer 45,X cells and an increasing proportion of 46,XY cells, hermaphroditism may result and, if 46,XY cells predominate over the 45,X (even with ratios of 55% 46,XY to 45% 45,X), there may be a normal male phenotype. Clearly in these circumstances detailed ultrasound scanning of the genitalia can be of help.

What is the prognosis if the abnormality is real?

The major focus of prenatal cytogenetic screening has been the detection of autosomal trisomies, particularly trisomy 21, but also trisomies 13 and 18. Counselling the parents when one of these trisomies is diagnosed is demanding because difficult decisions have to be taken, but a wealth of information is available so that most of the relevant facts can be given. However, the data for maternal age risks in Table 6.1 showed that in a substantial number of cases, the abnormality is not an autosomal trisomy, but either a sex chromosome anomaly where decisions whether or not to terminate are controversial, or a rare chromosomal rearrangement in which prediction of the probable phenotype is difficult. The difficulties of prognosis for the unusual abnormalities occur because many of these chromosome rearrangements are rare or unique and, there are few such cases from which risks can be derived. Unfortunately many of the figures are available only from biassed sources of ascertainment. There are thus great dangers that these data might erroneously be construed as indicating a high risk of fetal anomaly when the risks are actually quite low. Conversely, grouping similar but not identical cases in order to give more 'general' risks might lead to the conclusion that the prognosis is good when, in fact, there are very substantial dangers of severe mental handicap. Reliance on the outcome of previous reported cases is not always helpful as they have often resulted in termination of pregnancy. Data, particularly those for mental and behavioural effects of many of these abnormalities, are very sparse. For this reason, although some comparatively small data sets are reported here, they include long-term follow-up of the patients and are provided to give a foundation on which more detailed risks can be assembled when faced with the dilemma of an unusual or rare abnormality in prenatal diagnosis.

When a chromosome abnormality such as translocation, inversion, supernumerary marker or other rearrangement is found either in AF culture, CVS or fetal blood, it is essential to determine whether this has arisen *de novo* (as a new mutation), or is an inherited abnormality and one of the parents is a carrier (Aurias *et al.*, 1978; Jacobs, 1981). If a parent carries the same abnormality, then, provided that the parent does not carry it in mosaic form (so that there is a 'dilution' of the abnormalities by normal cells) there is a general expectation that the fetus would have a phenotype similar to that of the parent for a 'familial' rearrangement. If, however, the parents have normal karyotypes, then the abnormality has usually arisen *de novo* (except in rare cases of germinal mosaicism) and prediction of the possible fetal phenotype may be more difficult.

   Thus full parental karyotyping should be carried out as a matter of urgency in all cases where a chromosomal rearrangement is detected prenatally. It is important to confirm paternity since non-paternity can be an important source of error occurring at a frequency of 8–15%. It is sometimes possible by studying chromosomal or genetic markers to determine the parental chromosomal origin of the new mutation (*see* Table 6.2).

Risks for *de novo* rearrangements

Chromosomal rearrangements include Robertsonian and reciprocal translocations, paracentric and pericentric inversions, ring chromosomes, deletions, insertions, isochromosomes and supernumerary marker chromosomes.

De novo *apparently balanced rearrangements*

The greatest problem occurs with apparently balanced chromosomal rearrangements which have arisen as a new mutation, i.e. *de novo*. Eighty-five per cent of people who have a *de novo* apparently balanced rearrangement have a normal phenotype, but they do occur more often than expected among the mentally handicapped. Funderburk, Spence and Sparkles, (1977) and Warburton (1984) found that an apparently balanced *de novo* rearrangement substantially increases the risk of mental retardation. This is because a submicroscopic deletion may affect gene function. Since the rearrangement has occurred *de novo*, there is no parent or relative carrying it to indicate its possible effects. It is important to try to ensure that such arrangements appear to be truly balanced, and to exclude the presence of small deletions and duplications, so that high resolution banding is necessary although this may not exclude a deletion at submicroscopic level.

   The most valuable sources of data for deriving risks for *de novo* rearrangements (occurring in those cases where both parents have normal karyotypes and paternity is confirmed) are those whose ascertainment is not from a biassed source. The principal sources here are the large surveys of the newborn or those children identified at amniocentesis in a low risk group (e.g. that for advanced maternal age) where termination was not carried out. Data from full follow-up of these children and normal controls to monitor morbidity and mortality are obviously the most valuable for assessing risks but because of the vast resources required for a task of this magnitude, there are only relatively small numbers in a series. The MRC Human Genetics Unit Registry in Edinburgh is one such source of data.

   The risks for this unbiassed group are:

Nine cases identified in newborn/amniocentesis survey (unbiassed source)
3 children   very bright, above average
3 children   average
3 children   slow or handicapped

1 at 10th centile for growth, hypospadias, IQ75
1 child IQ80
1 severely retarded and epileptic, died at 4 years
1 pregnancy terminated for risk of abnormality after amniocentesis

In those cases with biassed ascertainment such as those with mental handicap, congenital anomalies or infertility, it is important to carry out serial follow-ups to detect all significant complications for the overall morbidity and mortality and to detect positive trends such as growth spurts in small for dates infants, or conceptions and births among the infertile.

10 cases identified through biassed sources of ascertainment
5 individuals subnormality hospitals all with IQs<30
4 individuals infertility, 3 normal, 1 slow with special schooling
1 individual   routine survey nuclear workers, normal with 2 children

In some cases, the chromosomal rearrangements may only occur in a single individual in a large family where all the other relatives are normal, but if one or both parents are dead or unavailable, there is no proof that the abnormality has arisen *de novo*, although many of these are probably new mutations.

18 cases of translocations of unknown origin (potentially de novo)
9 people normal
3 people normal but infertile
4 people intelligent but antisocial behaviour, in maximum security hospitals
2 people mentally handicapped

It is reasonable to conclude from these data and from those of other authors (Warburton, 1984) that the risk of mental handicap is between 10 and 30%. Parents' perceptions of the risks differ and are also dependent upon the way in which they are counselled about the risks and types of handicap.

Unbalanced chromosomal rearrangements

These occur where there is duplication and/or deficiency of euchromatic chromosomal material. Absence or addition of euchromatic chromosomal material tends to disrupt the genetic and metabolic control involved in developmental pathways and this often leads to serious abnormality. Unbalanced chromosomal rearrangements include unbalanced forms of Robertsonian and reciprocal translocations, recombinant forms of pericentric inversions, ring chromosomes in which formation of the ring involves a deletion of chromosomal material, isochromosomes, deletions, insertions, duplications and supernumerary marker chromosomes. In these cases there is loss or gain of crucial genetic material and phenotypic consequences of this are usually severe.

The diagnostic problems here are the least difficult, since the presence of deletion or duplication for certain chromosomal regions usually predicts the possibility of serious physical or mental handicap. If the chromosome anomaly can be identified and the breakpoints defined, some idea of risks can be ascertained from the catalogues of chromosomal abnormalities (Schinzel, 1984; Borgaonkar, 1989) and by undertaking literature searches for the appropriate chromosome abnormalities. Occasionally, there will be associated fetal abnormalities detectable on ultrasound scanning, such as microcephaly, which make prediction of abnormality more certain. In some cases, identification of the precise chromosomal segments (and breakpoints involved) may not be possible. These pose the greatest problems for prognosis because in certain rare instances small duplications or deficiencies without apparent phenotypic effect have been described.

The only exceptions to the generally poor prognosis are when heterochromatic regions or those involving only repeated sequences such as the short arms of acrocentric chromosomes (non-coding) are involved (as for example in certain supernumerary markers) and the risks are covered specifically in a subsequent section.

Estimates for the frequency of *de novo* rearrangements have been given by Warburton (1984). One-fifth of all chromosomal rearrangements in the newborn arise *de novo*, with a prevalence of 0.37 per 1000, this figure increases to 0.56 per 1000 in amniotic fluid samples demonstrating that there is an increasing risk of rearrangements occurring with advanced maternal age.

Ring chromosomes

Ring chromosomes are relatively rare, occurring in only about 1 in 50 000 newborns (Hook and Hamerton, 1977). Ring chromosomes have been reported for each human chromosome but they do not all occur with equal frequency. Ring chromosome 13 (Figure 6.9) occurs more frequently (about 20% of all rings), than rings 18, 21, 22, 15, 14 and 9 (Wyandt, 1988; Borgaonkar, 1989). In a few cases, the ring chromosome is familial and inherited from a parent (usually for rings 9, 14, 18, 21 and 22), but the vast majority occur as *de novo* rearrangements.

The major clinical significance of ring chromosomes is that, in the formation of the ring, a deletion of chromosomal material may occur and, as ring chromosomes

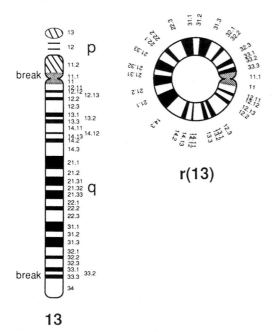

Figure 6.9 Ring chromosome 13, idiogram, involving a break on long arm 13, with loss of terminal band

tend to be unstable at mitosis, this results in the formation of other abnormal cell lines. In these, either the ring chromosome is lost altogether (resulting in monosomy), or products of broken rings such as deleted chromosomes, acentric or centric fragments or additional rings may occur. It is often very difficult to determine the breakpoints in ring chromosomes (especially for small rings) because the ring tends to have an unusual morphology, chromosomal contraction and straining properties and is refractory to detailed banding studies and high resolution banding (HRB). Mosaicism for ring chromosomes occurs frequently, and it is difficult to determine whether this is primarily due to instability of certain ring chromosomes, or whether post-zygotic errors with ring formation have occurred. One of the cardinal features of rings is that of instability (Figure 6.10), because a breakage – fusion – bridge cycle occurs in some divisions, particularly if

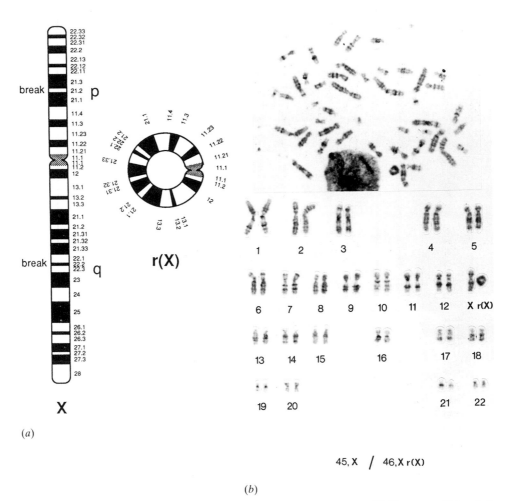

(a)

45, X / 46, X r(X)

(b)

Figure 6.10 (a) Idiogram of ring X with loss of both distal parts of both arms. (b) Karyotype (G banded) of a female with the phenotype of Turner's syndrome due to instability of the ring leading to a cell line with 45X as a result of absence (loss) of the ring

there are dicentric derivatives. The instability is related both to the breakpoints and the basic chromosomal structure of the segments involved.

The principal risks of phenotypic abnormality associated with ring chromosomes are those for small deletions or duplications of the chromosomal regions involved. These in general are for mental handicap which may be moderate to severe, often with only minor dysmorphic features. For example, for ring chromosome 13, the phenotype tends to be similar to that for 13q-deletions (Figure 6.11). In attempting to assess the risks when a ring chromosome is detected prenatally, the first and major priority is to determine the origin of the ring, i.e. whether it is inherited from

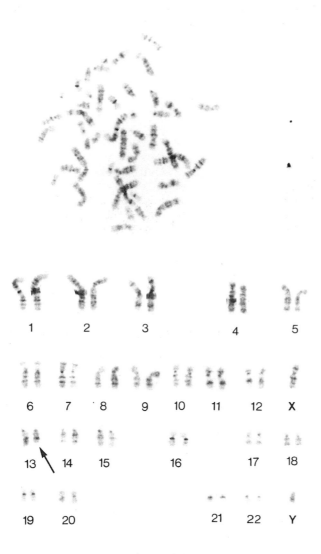

Figure 6.11 13q – G banded chromosome preparation of male fetus with deletion of distal part of terminal q. Child had microcephaly and radial aplasia

a parent or has occurred as a new mutation and whether it is present in pure or mosaic form. For the rare cases in which there is a familial ring chromosome, it is essential to check whether the parent carrying the ring has it in every cell or is a mosaic. A parent with a mosaic ring who has only minimal or no phenotypic abnormalities, may have a child who has the ring in every cell and is severely mentally handicapped. To complicate matters, there may be differences in the stability of the ring (and therefore in apparent mosaicism) in different tissues, so that comparisons of the frequency of mosaicism in parental blood samples and that in amniotic fluid cells or CVS samples may differ.

For *de novo* rings discovered prenatally, it is imperative to undertake detailed chromosome banding studies to determine the chromosomal breakpoints because this gives the basic information from which risks can be derived. For each different ring chromosome the risks of phenotypic abnormality can be assessed from the major atlases of cytogenetic abnormalities (Schinzel, 1984) and detailed literature searches.

Supernumerary marker chromosomes

The nomenclature of markers is complicated; they are variously described as extra chromosomes, structurally abnormal chromosomes, supernumerary markers, accessory chromosomes and fragments. Supernumerary marker chromosomes (SMC) represent a heterogeneous group of chromosomal abnormalities; they may have little in common except that they are extra chromosomes and they are structurally abnormal. They may arise *de novo*, as a new mutation, in other cases the marker may be familial.

Supernumerary marker chromosomes may be acrocentric, submetacentric or metacentric. They vary in size from those larger than a G group chromosome to minute chromosomes consisting of little more than a centromere. It is hardly surprising in the face of this tremendous variation in size and structure that the risks vary from those involving severe mental handicap or violence and behaviour disturbances to those without apparent phenotypic effect. Mosaicism, as expected in general leads to less severe effects. Much of the data for these 49 probands has been given in greater detail by Buckton *et al.* (1985).

Familial markers

Many supernumerary marker chromosomes are inherited from a parent who is normal but has 47 chromosomes and is a carrier of a marker chromosome. These are described as familial marker chromosomes. Inheritance is more often from the mother than from the father since marker chromosomes in the male may be associated with infertility. Usually the parent carries the supernumerary marker chromosome in all cells and is therefore non-mosaic, and a fetus with the marker would be expected to be like the parent. However, in a proportion of cases, the supernumerary chromosome may have arisen as a new mutation in the parent, in whom it occurs as an early mitotic error in the zygote, so that it is found in mosaic form. Prediction of the fetal phenotype in these circumstances causes problems. It may not be the same as that of the parent, since the proportion of abnormal cells may be greater and many markers are known to have a deleterious effect, particularly on neurological development. Parents who carry the marker in only a small proportion of cells may be of normal intelligence but they may have children who have a marker chromosome in every cell who may be severely mentally handicapped. Detailed studies of the parental karyotypes are mandatory in all cases where supernumerary markers are found because this will identify familial markers, reveal those markers which have arisen *de novo* and exclude mosaicism in a parent.

De novo *markers*

The frequency of supernumerary markers in prenatal samples depends upon the maternal age structure of the population as these show a very significant increase with advancing maternal age (*see* Table 6.1). *De novo* markers involving chromosome 15 have the strongest maternal age effect. The data from the New York Registry of 75 000 amniocenteses (Hook, 1983) show that the rate for all supernumerary markers is 0.8 per 1000 samples, of which 0.4–0.5 per 1000 are mutant and 0.3–0.4 per 1000 are inherited. The maternal age effect is thus quantitatively as strong as that for trisomy 21.

The risks for *de novo* supernumerary marker chromosomes depend upon the structure and the chromosomal segments from which they are derived. These include whether they are dicentric or monocentric. If they are dicentric then breaks must have occurred in the long arms of two different chromosomes increasing the risk of phenotypic abnormality or mental handicap. If they contain only highly repeated or ribosomal DNA, the risk for the fetus is less than if they involve crucial genetic sequences, particularly those which are derived from the proximal part of the long arm of chromosome 15, (15q). Abnormalities involving proximal 15q are often associated with mental handicap or violent behaviour (*see* Table 6.8). Provided familial cases have been excluded, the prediction of the effect of the additional material in *de novo* cases is complex. In a large proportion of cases it may have no phenotypic effect and this is more likely if the marker is derived from the short arms and cytological satellite regions of acrocentric chromosomes. In general, the larger the chromosomal segments involved and the more euchromatin present, the worse the prognosis for the fetus. Markers which involve chromosomal regions carrying specific unique DNA sequences may be associated with malformation syndromes such as the cat eye syndrome with partial duplication 22q. Many other cases involve neurological problems, mental retardation or behavioural problems.

Risks for supernumerary markers

Attempting to derive risks for supernumerary marker chromosomes is difficult for two reasons. The first is that the extra chromosomal segments involved are small, and it may therefore be impossible to determine their origin. Furthermore, like *de novo* translocations, markers are relatively rare in the newborn surveys (except those which include more older mothers) and there are many more data from biassed sources of ascertainment than unbiassed ones.

Many markers are relatively benign and have virtually no phenotypic effect, some markers, in particular those derived from chromosome 15 (Tables 6.9 and 6.10) are associated with antisocial behaviour such as arson or violence against the person. Even for those markers where the chromosomal segments for which the marker was formed have been identified, there may be tremendous differences in structure and risks. For example, many *de novo* markers are derived from short

Table 6.9 Phenotypic/clinical effects of supernumerary markers

Probands with markers derived from chromosome 15

Ascertainment	15p15p ≥Ggp			15p15p ≤Ggp			del15q11 ≤Ggroup		
	NF	F	M	NF	F	M	NF	F	M
1. Severe mental retardation	6	–	2	–	–	–	3	–	–
2. Maximum security hospital	1	–	–	1	–	–	1	–	–
3. Prison survey	–	–	–	–	1	–	–	1	–
4. Subfertility clinic	–	–	–	1	–	1	–	–	–
5. Unbiassed surveys (newborn)	–	–	–	1	–	–	–	–	1
6. Other *normal intelligence	4	–	–	1	–	1	–	–	1

NF: non-familial
F: familial
M: mosaic
≥G: larger than a G group chromosome
≤G: less than a G group chromosome in size.

Table 6.10 Phenotypic effects of markers

Probands with markers not derived from chromosome 15

Ascertainment	≥Ggp			≤Ggp		
	NF	F	M	NF	F	M
1. Severe mental retardation	1	–	–	1	1	2
2. Maximum security hospital	–	–	–	1	–	–
3. Prison survey	–	–	–	–	–	–
4. Subfertility clinic	1	1	–	2	2	1
5. Unbiassed surveys (newborn)	–	1	–	2	–	1
6. Other *normal intelligence	–	–	–	–	–	2

NF: non-familial
F: familial
M: mosaic
≥G: larger than a G group chromosome
≤G: less than a G group chromosome in size.

arms, centromeres and proximal long arm of chromosome 15, or even sections of two different chromosomes 15. More rarely, two segments appear to be the same. These markers are the reciprocal of a Robertsonian translocation but these involve the short arms instead of the long arms of acrocentric chromosomes, and perhaps most significantly involve a break or breaks in a euchromatic region in the long arm of chromosome 15.

Partial deletions and duplications, contiguous gene or chromosomal deletion syndromes

The delineation of many of the new chromosomal deletion syndromes and contiguous gene disorders is providing information on the phenotype when the specific chromosomal segments can be identified. Prader-Willi syndrome involving obesity, hypogenitalism and mental handicap was found to be associated with abnormalities of proximal 15q usually involving small deletions of bands 15q11–13 (Ledbetter *et al.*, 1982). Most of these conditions involve *de novo* rearrangements but some occur secondary to a parental rearrangement. It is important to recognize that molecular genetic studies using gene probes to measure gene dosage and deletions for particular chromosomal regions may be of help in addition to the cytogenetic studies. For small autosomal deletions or duplications which lead to partial monosomy or trisomy there are often phenotypic consequences as a result of abnormal cell growth and tissue differentiation. The most major effect is most frequently upon both pre- and postnatal growth and neurological deficit (mental handicap) (Table 6.11). When the growth patterns are severely distorted *in utero*, this may lead to major abnormalities such as cardiac or renal anomalies. More minor disruptions of differentiation may lead to dysmorphic features some of which will be quite characteristic for the chromosomal segments involved (Table 6.12). The birth incidence of these anomalies is about 1 in 2000.

Table 6.11 Growth retardation and malformations in partial monosomies and trisomies

Chromosome anomaly	Growth retardation	Major malformations	Dysmorphic features	Mental handicap
4p-	IUGR	M	FLC	Severe
5p-	IUGR	MC	FLcry	Severe
9p-	Normal	SC	FL	Severe
13q-	IUGR	CNSC	FLG	Severe
18p-	IUGR	CVS	FLHair	Severe
18q-	IUGR	MC	FELG	Severe
Trisomy 4p	IUGR	M	F	Severe
Trisomy 9p	IUGR	SR	FL	Severe
Trisomy 10q	IUGR	CNSCR	FLG	Severe
Tetrasomy 12p	Normal	CNS	DF	Mild–moderate
Trisomy 20p	Normal	CR	FLG	Mild–moderate
Tetrasomy 22q	Normal	CR	FEyesE	Mild

IUGR: intrauterine growth retardation
Major: M = microcephaly, C = cardiac, R = renal, S = skeletal, CNS = central nervous system.
Dysmorphism: F = facies, E = ears, L = limbs, G = genitalia, C = clefting, D = diaphragmatic hernia.
Some of these occur frequently and have descriptive syndromes. These include:
4p- Wolf-Hirshhorn syndrome
5p- cri-du-chat
Tetrasomy 12p Pallister Killian syndrome
Tetrasomy 22q cat eye syndrome

Table 6.12 Microdeletion syndromes and their chromosomal loci

Microdeletion/contiguous gene syndromes	Chromosomal region
Retinoblastoma	13q14 del
Aniridia/Wilms' tumour (WAGR)	11p13 del
Prader-Willi	15q11 del
Langer Giedion	8p24.2 del
DiGeorge	22q11 del
Miller-Dieker lissencephaly	17p13 del
Beckwith-Wiedemann	11p15 trisomy

Where each of these specific chromosomal rearrangements or deletions is detected then it is important to recognize the possible phenotypic associations which might be found in these disorders. Detailed fetal imaging studies and other investigations to assess the associated fetal abnormalities are crucial in these cases.

A number of DNA gene probes are now available and these include those in the chromosomal regions involved in the partial deletion syndromes 5p-, 5q-, 18p-, 20q-, Yp. The use of recombinant DNA probes for the appropriate chromosomal region in microdeletions and partial aneuploidies, which include 11p probes for aniridia-Wilms' tumour, proximal 15q probes for Prader-Willi syndrome, and 22q probes for the cat eye syndrome, may help to provide more definitive diagnosis. The use of chromosome specific probes and a combination of the polymerase chain reaction (PCR) for dosage and rapid *in situ* hybridization using biothylated or fluorescent probes may help in cases of 47,XYY Klinefelter's syndrome, 45X, trisomy 21 and trisomy 13 and partial trisomies 21, 13, 15 and 18.

High frequency of chromosomal breakage in culture

The chromosomal breakage syndrome (CBS) is relatively rare. However, a high frequency of breaks or rearrangements is sometimes encountered in AFC/CVS specimens. This may include a possible CBS in the fetus or it may simply be due to a culture artefact in the cultured cells. Patterns of breakage in the cells should be examined and genetic history and parental samples obtained for heterozygotic testing. It is important to carry out more detailed testing of the cells under appropriate culture conditions as detailed above and a further sample, preferably including a fetal blood sample should always be obtained to confirm the abnormality.

Sex chromosome anomalies

Sex chromosome anomalies are relatively common in the newborn. The frequency of XXX (Figure 6.12), XXY and XYY among newborns is about 1 in 600 for each of these anomalies and for 45,X, approximately 1 in 5000. The problems of 45,X mosaicism were discussed above because of the complex interrelationship of the degrees of mosaicism, X chromosome loss and the phenotypic sex of the fetus.

For 47XXX and for 47XXY, there are increasing frequencies with advanced maternal age. 47XYY arises either as a result of a meiotic error in the father during the second meiotic division or as a post-zygotic error and as expected no maternal age effect has been observed for this condition. For 45X there is actually a strong inverse maternal age effect and many of these cases are due to post-zygotic error with loss of either an X or Y sex chromosome. The frequencies of these abnormalities at each maternal age at amniocentesis are given in Table 6.1. Initial studies on individuals with sex chromosome abnormalities suggested that many of the individuals with an XXY or XYY karyotype were to be found in hospitals for the mentally handicapped or prisons. This occurred because there were only limited data at that time on the frequency of these conditions in the general population and it emphasizes the dangers of drawing genetic conclusions when the source of ascertainment is biased.

In order to try to assess the risks and the prognoses for each of the different sex chromosome abnormalities it is important to derive the information from unbiased sources of data such as the follow-up of children with sex chromosome

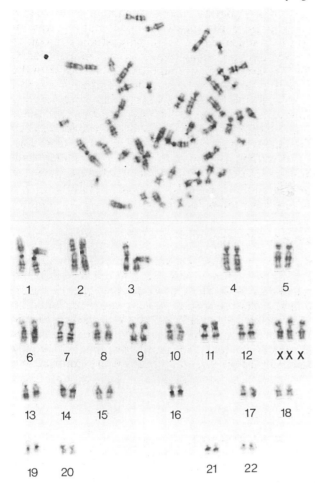

Figure 6.12 G banded preparation showing 3 X chromosomes 47, XXX

abnormalities found in newborn surveys, rather than using biassed sources of ascertainment such as data from institutions for the mentally handicapped, prisons and infertility clinics. Prospective longitudinal studies on children with sex chromosome abnormalities (SCA) began in the 1960s on 307 children with SCA identified in the large newborn cytogenetic studies carried out in Arhus, Boston, Denver, Edinburgh, New Haven, Toronto and Winnipeg. These studies are assessing physical and psychological development with siblings and case matched controls (Ratcliffe and Paul, 1986). These studies are helpful in assessing the prognosis when a sex chromosome abnormality in either non-mosaic or mosaic form is found prenatally because they are the major unbiassed source of information on physical, intellectual and behavioural problems and on the effects of therapy (such as testosterone therapy) for Klinefelter's syndrome (Ratcliffe and Paul, 1986; Stewart et al., 1986). The concerns of parents about sexuality and infertility in their sons with Klinefelter's syndrome are described by Robinson *et al.* (1986). There are a number of problems which occur in many children but may occur to a greater extent in children with SCA. These include childhood temper tantrums of 47XYY individuals, treatment of children with 45X or 47XXY karyotypes with hormonal supplementation, careful clinical management of the associated problems and the educational problems of 47XXX girls. There are alternatives to termination for sex chromosome abnormalities especially if the pregnancy is a much wanted one, e.g. in older mothers who have had infertility problems, but it is important to provide help and support for the management of specific childhood problems associated with each karyotype.

Non-mosaic triple X females have lower IQs on verbal performance and full scale tests than the controls and this obviously has a significant effect on their educational progress. Comparison of the results of the mosaics with the non-mosaics is interesting for two reasons. First they show the marked effect on IQ that the presence of normal cells has on an individual. The second is that 46,XX/47,XXX mosaics were indistinguishable from the controls on IQ testing and do not have significant increases in either behavioural or educational problems. These facts might well influence parental decisions about the prospect of further testing or termination in a pregnancy in which 47,XXX mosaicism was detected. A summary of the collaborative data from these follow-up studies is given for 47,XXY, 47,XXX, 47,XYY and 45,X mosaic karyotypes (Netley, 1986) in Tables 6.13, 6.14, 6.15 and 6.16.

When prenatal diagnosis reveals the presence of an SCA, the parents have to make difficult decisions about whether to seek a termination or to continue with the pregnancy. Most of the prospective studies have been conducted by paediatricians, psychologists and endocrinologists who have followed the children with SCA from infancy through adolescence. They usually feel most strongly that with information, help counselling and suitable resources, the vast majority of these children are

Table 6.13 Collaborative data from prospective studies on children (ascertained in newborn studies) on intelligence and behavioural problems in the sex chromosome abnormalities: 47,XXY Klinefelter's syndrome

	47,XXY			*Mosaics*		
	47,XXY *n=73*	*Controls* *n=60*	P	*46,XY/47,XXY* *n=6*	*Controls* *n=3*	P
Wechsler intelligence test results						
Verbal IQ mean	90.11	102.40	<0.01	97.33	107.67	NS
Verbal IQ s.d.	17.71	14.44		13.16	9.29	
Performance IQ mean	102.60	104.44	NS	109.33	116.00	NS
Performance IQ s.d.	13.11	12.22		12.99	13.11	
Full scale IQ mean	97.74	103.62	<0.01	102.67	113.00	NS
Full scale IQ s.d.	15.74	12.92		12.71	10.58	
Educational and behavioural development						
Educational problems	44/65 (67.6%)	14/63 (22%)	P<0.00001	3/5 (60%)	4/7 (57%)	NS
Behavioural problems	19/65 (29%)	13/62 (20.9%)	NS	1/5 (20%)	4/7 (57%)	NS

From Netley 1986 and Ratcliffe and Paul 1986.
For the non-mosaic Klinefelter's, verbal IQ but not performance IQ was significantly lower in probands than in controls so that intellectual limitations are confined to verbal areas.

Table 6.14 Collaborative data from prospectus studies on children (ascertained in newborn studies) on intelligence and behavioural problems in the sex chromosome abnormalities 47,XXX triple X syndrome

	47,XXX			*Mosaics*		
	47,XXX *n=32*	*Controls* *n=25*	P	*46,XX/47,XXX* *n=5*	*Controls* *n=7*	P
Wechsler intelligence test results						
Verbal IQ mean	86.63	105.64	<0.01	110.60	109.14	NS
Verbal IQ s.d.	16.70	13.71		11.13	16.47	
Performance IQ mean	95.19	109.60	<0.01	107.20	111.57	NS
Performance IQ s.d.	13.86	13.46		15.58	14.58	
Full scale IQ mean	90.06	108.40	<0.01	110.40	111.43	NS
Full scale IQ s.d.	14.84	13.39		14.29	15.63	
Educational and behavioural development						
Educational problems	25/35 (71%)	9/29 (32%)	P<0.001	1/5	3/9	NS
Behavioural problems	11/35 (31%)	11/29 (38%)	NS	2/5	4/9	NS

From Netley 1986

Table 6.15 Collaborative data from prospective studies on children (ascertained in newborn studies) on intelligence and behavioural problems in the sex chromosome abnormalities: 47,XYY

	47,XYY *n=28*	*Controls* *n=8*	P	*No mosaic in XYY series*
Wechsler intelligence test results				
Verbal IQ mean	100.75	104.50	NS	
Verbal IQ s.d.	14.28	14.48		
Performance IQ mean	107.20	111.57	NS	
Performance IQ s.d.	15.58	14.58		
Full scale IQ mean	110.40	111.43	NS	
Educational and behavioural development				
Educational problems	1/5	3/9	NS	
Behavioural problems	2/5	4/9	NS	

From Netley 1986.

developing within the normal range. The Danish study (Nielsen *et al.*, 1986) not only provided data on prospective studies on 58 children with SCA but also gave information about parental decisions about termination after prenatal diagnosis of an SCA in Denmark. From 1970 to 1982, 78% of the Danish parents chose to have an induced abortion for SCA. Oxford data on parental decisions about SCA have been given by Holmes-Siedle, Ryynanen and Lindenbaum, 1987) (Table 6.17).

Nielsen *et al.* (1986) felt that fewer parents would choose to have a termination of a fetus with an SCA if they received more comprehensive information about the developmental prospects for the children and offers of professional counselling, information and support for the child. Some of the authors produce cogent arguments against induced abortion for sex chromosome abnormalities discovered

Table 6.16 Collaborative data from prospective studies on children (ascertained in newborn studies) on intelligence and behavioural problems in the sex chromosome abnormalities: 45,X

	45,X/46,XX mosaics			*45,X partial X*		
	45,X/46,XX *n=11*	*Controls* *n=11*	P	*45,X partial X* *n=10*	*Controls* *n=11*	P
Wechsler intelligence test results						
Verbal IQ mean	104.09	104.36	NS	90.44	91.95	NS
Verbal IQ s.d.	14.27	12.07		21.72	19.72	
Performance IQ mean	104.64	106.18	NS	85.78	101.68	<0.05
Performance IQ s.d.	13.68	13.84		18.67	17.96	
Full scale IQ mean	104.82	105.82	NS	87.33	96.36	NS
Full scale s.d.	13.56	13.65		20.66	19.44	
Educational and behavioural development						
Educational problems	1/10 (10%)	4/11 (36%)	NS	6/9 (67%)	14/22 (63.6%)	NS
Behavioural problems	1/10 (10%)	5/11 (46%)	NS	3/9 (33%)	13/22 (59%)	NS

From Netley 1986

Table 6.17 Prenatal diagnosis of sex chromosome abnormalities and parental decisions to terminate affected pregnancies in Denmark 1970–1982

Karyotype	*No. of cases diagnosed*	*Induced abortion*	*Percentage of total*
47,XXY	19	15	79
XYY	13	11	85
47,XXX	24	18	75
45,X	21	16	76

From Nielsen *et al.*, 1986.

prenatally. However, there is a falling birthrate and parents are having fewer children. Parents expectations for their children, particularly for intellectual achievement, phenotypic normality and fertility are very high. For many couples problems such as gynaecomastia and infertility in 47,XXY or short stature, webbed neck and infertility in 45,X, or intellectual development and educational problems in 47,XXX are still major factors which influence their decision to terminate.

Normal chromosomal variants

Complex processing and banding studies must be carried out to detect small rearrangements. In a small proportion of cases, a number of clinical and significant anomalies may be revealed. However, such tests will also uncover a number of 'normal' chromosomal variants.

Chromosomal variants involve segments of varying size and staining properties, but principally the heterochromatic regions which contain highly repeated DNA sequences. Normal chromosomal variants are usually inherited in a Mendelian manner from a parent and most probably have no influence on phenotype or health.

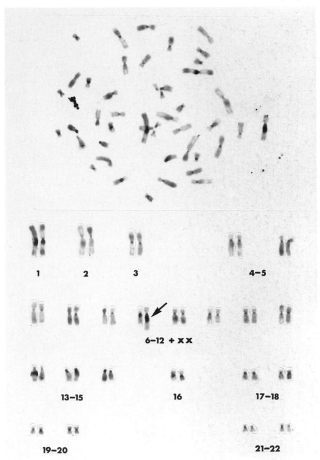

Figure 6.13 C banded karyotype of female with large C band region on chromosome 9 (9qh+)

These variant chromosomal regions include the large heterochromatic segments of chromosomes 1, 9, 16 and Y, and the differences involve both size and position. For example, variants of chromosome 9 are those most frequently encountered. Enlarged heterochromatic regions are described as 9qh+ (Figure 6.13), small heterochromatic blocks as 9qh− (Figure 6.14). A total pericentric inversion of the heterochromatic block leads to the presence of this region in the short arm of chromosome 9, instead of the long arm (Figure 6.15). This is described as inversion 9 and the breakpoints involved in this pericentric inversion occur at bands p11 in the short arm and q13 in the long arm so the cytogenetic nomenclature is inv(9)(p11q13). Sometimes not all the heterochromatic material is involved in the pericentric inversion, and remains in the long arm. This is described as a partial inversion. It is thus crucial to recognize that when a fetal karyotype is given as 46,XX or XY, inv(9)(p11q13) this means only that the fetus has a chromosomal variant, and essentially has a normal karyotype. Parental karyotyping will confirm whether this is a familial variant inherited from a parent. Obviously if a

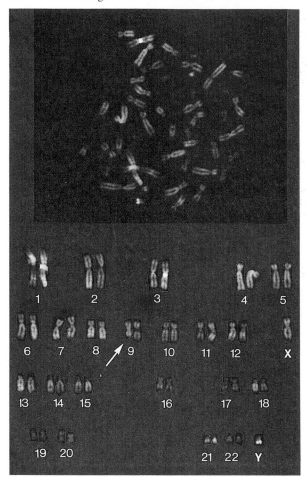

Figure 6.14 Q banded male karyotype lacking C band region on chromosome 9 (9qh–)

phenotypically normal parent is carrying the variant, the prognosis for the fetus is good.

Chromosomal variants occur in at least 3–4% of all prenatal diagnosis karyotypes and, as the frequency is high, it is important that there is clear reporting of these variants from the laboratory. There will frequently be requests for parental samples if necessary. An understanding of the significance of the laboratory results by obstetricians, antenatal clinic staff and genetic counsellors would ensure that these variants are not misinterpreted as signalling a significant abnormality in the fetus. In addition to the variable heterochromatic segments of 1,9,16 and Y, there are other variant regions which include the centromeres, short arms and cytological satellites of acrocentric chromosomes (13, 14, 15, 21 and 22), the variable fluorescent centromere reviews of chromosomes 3 and 4, the centromeric heterochromatin of other chromosomes such as variant satellited non-acrocentric

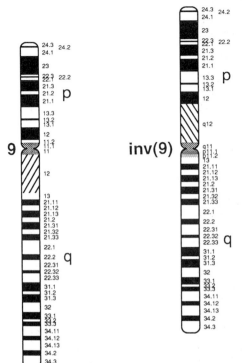

Figure 6.15 Idiogram showing pericentric inversion of C band region (heterochromatin) of chromosome 9

chromosomes (most usually observed in chromosome 17), and prominent secondary constrictions.

Pregnancies have been terminated because unusual chromosomal variants have been observed in the fetus, without investigating parental karyotypes. The subsequent discovery that a parent has a karyotype showing a variant identical to that of the fetus causes much anguish which could have been avoided by careful family studies for each variant.

Conclusions

The collaborative surveys of levels of mosaicism in amniotic fluid cells (Bui, Iselius and Lindsten, 1984; Hsu and Perlis, 1984; Worton and Stern, 1984) and preliminary reports of CVS studies have provided essential resources for the levels and types of mosaicism and confined placental anomalies (Mikkelsen and Ayme, 1986; Canadian Collaborative CVS-amniocentesis Clinical Trial Group, 1989). However, when faced with an individual case, the dilemma occurs of whether or not this is a true anomaly in the fetus and how the problem can be resolved with minimum risk to the fetus.

Even non-mosaic chromosome abnormalities such as some cases of autosomal trisomy, polyploidy and chromosome rearrangements may be associated with confined placental mosaicism. Rarer, more complex types of cell-specific

Table 6.18 Summary table: problem karyotypes

	Problems	*Methods of resolving problems*
Aneuploidy		
1 Recognized chromosomal abnormality syndromes (RCAS)		
A *Non-mosaic trisomies*		
Trisomy 18	False +ves frequent	Further sampling AFC or FBS
(1st and 2nd trimester CVS)	False −ves, i.e. normal result in true trisomy 18	Detailed USS, if this suggests 47,+18 then AFC or FBS
Trisomy 13	False +ves frequent	Further sampling AFC or FBS
(1st and 2nd trimester CVS)		
B *Mosaic trisomies for RCAS*		
46/47 + 7		Detailed scan of very limited use
46/47 + 8		because of dilution of phenotype.
46/47 + 9	90–95% are false +ves	Further sampling necessary; FBS
46/47 + 13	Do *not* assume these are real	most accurate
46/47 + 18		
46/47 + 21		
(CVS + AFC)		
C *Mosaic trisomies (not associated with CAS)*		
46/47 + 2		Check literature for risks monitor
46/47 + 3		pregnancy. Most do not require
46/47 + 16	Nearly all associated with confined placental mosaicism	further sampling
46/47 + 20		
46/47 + 22		
D *Polyploidy*		
69,XXX or XXY	Sometimes true mosaicism	Detailed scan for triploidy
46/69	but frequently confined	syndrome. Check markers for twins.
(CVS and AFC)	anomaly or twin pregnancy	Further sampling, FBS most
	with death of abnormal twin	accurate
46/92,XXXX or XXYY	Vast majority false +ves with	Detailed scan; further sampling but
92, XXXX or XXYY	endoreduplication	beware false + ves in fetal blood. Check using cell cycle studies to ensure cells in 1st division. Check nuclear size in non-dividing cells
E *Sex chromosome abnormalities*		
46,XX/46,XY	Most are maternal contamination or twin pregnancy. Few are true intersexes	Check maternal markers. Detailed USS of genitalia. Further sampling if necessary
45,X/46,XX	Most due to loss of X by anaphase lag, only 5–10% are real	Detailed scan only limited value because of dilution of phenotype. Further sampling, FBS if necessary
45,X/46,XY	Most due to loss of X in confined placental abnormality, 10% true karyotype. 3 possible phenotypes, male, intersex or Turner female	Detailed scan for genitalia. Further sampling, FBS. *See* literature for risks
45,X/46,XX/47,XXX	Many due to confined placental anomaly, some are true fetal mosaics	Further sampling, FBS if parents anxious
45,X/46,XY/47,XXY		
46,XY/47,XXY	Many due to confined placental anomaly, a few true fetal mosaics	Further sampling, FBS, only if parents would terminate pregnancy if true fetal karyotype. *See* text for phenotype of mosaics
46,XX/47,XXX		

	Problems	*Methods of resolving problems*
F *Supernumerary chromosomes* (Mosaic and non-mosaic)		
i. Derived from chromosome 15. ii. Derived from acrocentric short arms, 'cat eye' syndrome dup (22q)	50–60% of mosaics are real in the fetus	Test parents to see if *familial*. Further sampling, FBS to see if true mosaicism. Assess risks according to size and type of marker. *See* text for risks
Pallister Killian syndrome (isochromosome 12p tetrasomy for 12p)	Many cases represent true mosaicism in the fetus *but* the isochromosome is only present in fibroblastic cell lines	Detailed scan for associated fetal anomalies such as diaphragmatic hernia and polyhydramnios. NB Fetal blood karyotyping may not reveal abnormality as it is usually not present in lymphocytes, only in fibroblasts

2 *Other chromosome abnormalities*

A *Chromosomal rearrangements*

	Problems	*Methods of resolving problems*
Balanced translocations non-mosaic	30–40% are real May be false +ves (confined placental anomalies)	Check parental karyotypes to see if familial or *de novo*
Balanced translocations mosaic		Further sampling to see if real, FBS. Attempt to ascertain risks from literature
Unbalanced translocations Deletions		
i) RCDS	May be false +ves (confined placental anomalies)	Check parental karyotypes to see if translocation or other rearrangement present. FBS to test for confined placental mosaicism. Ascertain risks from literature
ii) non RCDS Inversions; pericentric Non-heterochromatic	May be false +ves (confined placental anomalies)	Check parental karyotypes to see if familial and balanced. FBS only if appears *de novo* or unbalanced. Ascertain risks
Inversions pericentric heterochromatic	Usually familial and *not* clinically significant	Check parental karyotypes (if necessary confirm paternity). Most familial
Inversions paracentric	Usually familial and not associated with abnormalities	Check parental karyotypes. Most familial
Rings mosaic Rings non-mosaic	May be false +ves (confined placental anomalies)	Check parental karyotypes to see if a parent has the ring even in mosaic form. FBS to confirm if it is real. Check literature for risks

B *Chromosomal breakage*

	Problems	*Methods of resolving problems*
i) Spontaneous in culture	May be false +ve effect. Test each culture flask separately	Check family history and test patients who should be heterozygotes in chromosome instability syndromes (CIS). Do detailed studies for CIS. If necessary, FBS and repeat AFC/ CVS
ii) In fetus at risk for chromosome breakage syndrome (CBS)	Beware false −ve tests	Test parents and affected sibling if possible. Fetal blood least risk of false −ve results

Table 6.18 continued

	Problems	Methods of resolving problems
C Fragile X		
i) Spontaneous in culture in a pregnancy not known to be at risk for fragile X	May be limited to a few cells, test several hundred cells	Take family history. Test mother and other family members. Further tests on cultures in stringent culture conditions. Ensure 5% of cells have Fra (X) (q27.3). Further sampling, FBS and testing if necessary
ii) In fetuses at risk for fragile X	Risk of false −ves, especially in AFC and CVS. Controls show that false +ve rate is very low	FBS most accurate. Check several hundred cells in stringent culture conditions with low folate or folate antagonists

CVS: chorionic villus sampling
AFC: amniotic fluid cells
FBS: fetal blood sampling
USS: ultrasound scan
RCDS: recognized chromosomal deletion (abnormality) syndrome

chromosomal anomalies also occur such as in the Pallister Killian syndrome in which only fibroblastic lines show the presence of the abnormal extra isochromosome 12p. Each of these abnormalities is individually rare but they cause cytogeneticists, obstetricians and parents much anxiety. The modes of resolving them depend upon the specific anomaly involved (Gosden, 1984; Gosden, Nicolaides and Rodeck, 1988; Nicolaides, Rodeck and Gosden, 1986) and have been covered in the preceding sections.

The danger of false-positive and false-negative diagnoses are also great when chromosomal breakage and fragile sites (particularly fragile X) are observed in either CVS, AFC or fetal blood samples. Rational modes of approach for breakage and fragile sites are essential if the problems are to be resolved before the gestation is too advanced. A summary of the major chromosomal problems in prenatal diagnosis is given in Table 6.18.

Many millions of amniotic fluid samples have now been successfully karyotyped worldwide and chromosome studies have been carried out on many thousands of CVS samples and fetal blood samples. In the vast majority of these cases an initial accurate prenatal diagnosis is achieved. In a very small proportion of cases, there is a risk of diagnostic inaccuracy. These problem cases must be identified rapidly. Initial assessments should be made on a combination of factors: the indication for karyotyping; a detailed ultrasound evaluation of the pregnancy; and the fetal karyotype. When difficulties occur then careful counselling and support for the parents is necessary to help them through a difficult and worrying time and to prevent precipitate termination if there are strong suspicions that the fetus may be normal. In cases of karyotypic abnormality the parents must be provided with the maximum amount of information and the possibilities of further evaluation and sampling with the associated risks and problems should be discussed. With care the accuracy of prenatal karyotyping might approach 100% and everyone, parents, obstetricians and geneticists, would feel that the first essential steps to the identification of major handicapping chromosome disorders were being taken. The overall goal, that of primary prevention of cytogenetic disorders, can only be achieved by understanding the aetiology of these conditions, but this has its roots in accurate diagnosis.

References

Anderson, W.F. (1984) Prospects for human gene therapy. *Science*, **226**, 401–409

Auerbach, A.D., Min, Z. and Ghosh, R. (1986) Clastogen induced chromosomal breakage as a marker for first trimester prenatal diagnosis of Fanconi anaemia. *Human Genetics*, **73**, 86–88

Auerbach, A.D., Sagi, M. and Adler, B. (1985) Fanconi anaemia: prenatal diagnosis in 30 fetuses at risk. *Pediatrics*, **76**, 794–800

Aurias, A., Prieur, M., Dutrillaux, B. and Leujeune, J. (1978) Systematic analysis of 95 reciprocal translocations of autosomes. *Human Genetics*, **45**, 259–264

Bardinger, S., Millard, C., Schmewing, D. and Bendel, R.P. (1987) Prenatal diagnosis of trisomy 20 mosaicism indicating an extra embryonic origin. *Prenatal Diagnosis*, **1**, 273–276

Benacerraf, B.R. and Frigoletto, F.D.J.R. (1987) Soft tissue nuchal fold in the second trimester fetus; standards for normal measurements compared with those in Down's syndrome. *American Journal of Obstetrics and Gynecology*, **157**, 1146–1149

Benn, P.A. and Hsu, L.Y.F. (1984) Incidence and significance of supernumerary marker chromosomes in prenatal diagnosis. *American Journal of Human Genetics*, **36**, 1092–1102

Blakemore, K.J., Samuleson, J., Breg, W.R. and Mahoney, M.J. (1985) Maternal metaphases on direct chromosome preparation of first trimester decidua. *Human Genetics*, **69**, 380

Bloom, S.E. and Goodpasture, C. (1976) An improved technique for selective silver staining of nucleolar organiser regions of human chromosomes. *Human Genetics*, **34**, 199–205

Borgaonkar, D.S. (1989) *Chromosomal Variation in Man*, 4th edn. New York: Alan R. Liss

Boué, J., Boué, A. and Lazar, P. (1975) Retrospective and prospective epidemiological studies of 1500 karyotyped spontaneous human abortions. *Teratology*, **12**, 11–26

Boué, J., Girard, S., Thépot, F.F., Choiset, A. and Boué, A. (1982) Unexpected structural rearrangements in prenatal diagnosis. *Prenatal Diagnosis*, **2**, 163–168

Brambati, B., Lanzani, A. and Oldrini, A. (1988) Transabdominal chorionic villus sampling. Clinical experience of 1159 cases. *Prenatal Diagnosis*, **8**, 609–617

Buckton, K.F., Spowart, G., Newton, M.S. and Evans, H.J. (1985) Forty four probands with an additional marker chromosome. *Human Genetics*, **69**, 353–370

Bui, T.-H., Iselius, L. and Lindsten, J. (1984) European collaborative study on prenatal diagnosis: mosaicism, pseudomosaicism and single abnormal cells in amniotic fluid cell cultures. *Prenatal Diagnosis*, **4**, 145–162

Callen, D.F., Korban, G., Dawson, G. *et al.* (1988) Extraembryonic/fetal karyotypic discordance during diagnostic chorionic villus sampling. *Prenatal Diagnosis*, **8**, 453–460

Canadian Collaborative CVS-Amniocentesis Clinical Trial Group (1989) Multicentre randomised clinical trial of chorionic villus sampling and amniocentesis. *Lancet*, **i**, 1–6

Cleaver, J.E. (1986) Xeroderma pigmentosum: biochemical and genetic characteristics. *Annual Review of Genetics*, **9**, 19–38

Crane, J.P. and Cheung, S.N. (1988) An embryogenic model to explain cytogenetic inconsistencies observed in chorionic villus versus fetal tissue. *Prenatal Diagnosis*, **8**, 119–129

Daniel, A., Hook, E.B. and Wulf, G. (1988) *Collaborative USA Data on Prenatal Diagnosis for Parental Carriers of Chromosome Rearrangements: Risks of Unbalanced Progeny. The Cytogenetics of Mammalian Autosomal Rearrangements*, (ed. A. Daniel) New York: Alan R. Liss, pp. 73–162

Daniel, A. and Lam-Po-Tang, P.R.L.C. (1976) Structure and inheritance of some heterozygous Robertsonian translocations in man. *Journal of Medical Genetics*, **13**, 381–392

Daniel, A., Williams, K. and Lam-Po-Tang, P.R.L.C. (1980) Higher risk to D:G translocation carriers of t dic (13:21) as compared to t dic (14:21) *Journal of Medical Genetics*, **17**, 491–496

Davies, K.E., Mattei, M.G., Mattei, J.F. *et al.* (1985) Linkage studies of X-linked mental retardation: high frequency of recombination in the telomeric region of the human X chromosome. *Human Genetics*, **70**, 249–255

Delozier-Blanchet, C.D., Engel, E., Extermann, P. and Pastori, B. (1988) Trisomy 7 in chorionic villi: follow up studies in pregnancy normal child and placental clonal anomalies. *Prenatal Diagnosis*, **8**, 281–286

Eichenbaum, S.Z., Krumins, E.J., Fortune, D.W. and Duke, J. (1986) False negative finding on chorionic villus sampling. *Lancet*, **ii**, 391

Ferguson-Smith, M.A. (1965) Karyotype-phenotype correlations in gonadal dysgenesis and their bearing on the pathogenesis of malformations. *Journal of Medical Genetics*, **2**, 142–155

Ferguson-Smith, M.A. and Yates, J.R.W. (1984) Maternal age specific rates for chromosome aberrations and factors influencing them; report of a collaborative European study on 52 965 amniocenteses. *Prenatal Diagnosis*, **4**, 5–44

Fraccaro, M., Lindsten, J., Ford, C.E. and Iselius, L. (1980) The 11q;22q translocation: a European collaborative analysis of 43 cases. *Human Genetics*, **56**, 21–35

Freiberg, A.S., Blumberg, B., Lance, H. and Mann, J. (1988) XX/XY chimerism encountered during prenatal diagnosis. *Prenatal Diagnosis*, **8**, 423–426

Fryns, J.-P. and Van den Berghe, H. (1982) Transmission of fragile (X)(q27) from normal male(s). *Human Genetics*, **61**, 262–263

Funderburk, S.J., Spence, M.A. and Sparkles, R.S. (1977) Mental retardation associated with 'balanced' chromosome rearrangements. *American Journal of Human Genetics*, **29**, 136–141

Galt, J., Boyd, E., Connor, J.H.M. and Ferguson-Smith, M.A. (1989) Isolation of chromosome 21-specific DNA probes and their use in the analysis of non-disjunction in Down's syndrome. *Human Genetics*, **81**, 113–119

Glover, T.W. (1981) FUdR induction of the X-chromosome fragile site: evidence for the mechanism of folic acid and thymidine inhibition. *American Journal of Human Genetics*, **33**, 234–242

Gosden, C.M. (1983) Amniotic fluid cell types and culture. *British Medical Bulletin*, **39**, 348–354

Gosden, C.M. (1984) The recognition of clinically significant chromosome abnormality in prenatal diagnosis. In *Prenatal Diagnosis*, (eds C.H. Rodeck and K.H. Nicolaides) London: Royal College of Obstetricians and Gynaecologists

Gosden, C.M. and Brock, D.J.H. (1978) Combined use of alphafetoprotein and amniotic fluid cell morphology in early prenatal diagnosis of fetal abnormalities. *Journal of Medical Genetics*, **15**, 262–270

Gosden, J.R., Lawrie, S.S. and Gosden, C.M. (1981) Satellite DNA sequences in the human acrocentric chromosomes: information from translocations and heteromorphisms. *American Journal of Human Genetics*, **33**, 243–251

Gosden, C.M., Nicolaides, K.H. and Rodeck, C.H. (1988) Fetal blood sampling in investigation of chromosome moscaicism in amniotic fluid cell culture. *Lancet*, **i**, 613–617

Gosden, C.M., Rodeck, C.H., Nicolaides, K.H., Campbell, S., Eason, P. and Sharp, J.C. (1985) Fetal blood chromosome analysis: some new indications for karyotyping. *British Journal of Obstetrics and Gynaecology*, **92**, 915–920

Group de Cytogeneticiens Français (1987) Paracentric inversions in man: a French collaborative study. *Annals of Genetics*, **29**, 169–176

Hall, J.G. (1988) Somatic mosaicism: observations related to clinical genetics. *American Journal of Human Genetics*, **43**, 355–363

Hoehn, H., Rodriquez, M.L., Norwood, T.H. and Maxwell, C.L. (1978) Mosaicism in amniotic fluid cell cultures: classification and significance. *American Journal of Medical Genetics*, **2**, 253–266

Hogge, W.A., Schonberg, S.A. and Golbus, M.S. (1986) Chorionic villus sampling. Experience of the first 1000 cases. *American Journal of Obstetrics and Gynecology*, **154**, 1249–1252

Holmes-Siedle, M., Ryynanen, M. and Lindenbaum, R.H. (1987) Parental decisions regarding termination of pregnancy following prenatal detection of sex chromosome abnormality. *Prenatal Diagnosis*, **7**, 239–244

Hook, E.B. (1977) Exclusion of chromosome mosaicism: tables of 90%, 95% and 99% confidence limits and comments on use. *American Journal of Human Genetics*, **29**, 94–97

Hook, E.B. (1983) Chromosome abnormalities and spontaneous fetal death following amniocentesis: further data and associations with maternal age. *American Journal of Human Genetics*, **35**, 110–116

Hook, E.B., Cross, P.K., Jackson, L., Pergament, E. and Brambati, B. (1988) Maternal age-specific rates of 47, +21 and other cytogenetic abnormalities diagnosed in the first trimester of pregnancy in chorionic villus biopsy specimens: comparison with rates expected from observations at amniocentesis. *American Journal of Human Genetics*, **427**, 97–807

Hook, E.B. and Hamerton, J.L. (1977) The frequency of chromosomal abnormalities detected in consecutive newborn studies – differences between studies – results by sex and by severity of phenotypic involvements. In *Population Cytogenetics, Studies in Humans* (eds E.B. Hook and I.H. Porter) New York: Academic Press, pp. 63–79

Hook, E.B., Schreinmachers, D.M., Willey, A.M. and Cross, P.K. (1983) Rates of mutant structural chromosome rearrangements in human fetuses: data from prenatal cytogenetic studies and associations with maternal age and mutagen exposures. *American Journal of Human Genetics*, **35**, 96–109

Hook, E.B. and Warburton, D. (1983) The distribution of chromosomal genotypes associated with Turner's syndrome: livebirth prevalence rates and evidence of diminished fetal mortality and severity in genotypes associated with structural X abnormalities or mosaicism. *Human Genetics*, **64**, 24–27

Hsu, L.Y.F. (1989) Prenatal diagnosis of 45,X/46,XY mosaicism – a review and update. *Prenatal Diagnosis*, **9**, 31–48

Hsu, L.Y.F., Kaffe, S. and Perlis, T.E. (1987) Trisomy 20 mosaicism in prenatal diagnosis – a review and update. *Prenatal Diagnosis*, **7**, 581–596

Hsu, L.Y.F. and Perlis, T.E. (1984) United States survey on chromosome mosaicism and pseudomosaicism in prenatal diagnosis. *Prenatal Diagnosis*, **4**, 97–130

ISCN (1981) An international system for human cytogenetic nomenclature-high resolution banding. *Cytogenetics and Cell Genetics*, **31**, 1–84

Jacobs, P.A. (1981) Mutation rates for structural chromosome rearrangements in man. *American Journal of Human Genetics*, **33**, 44–54

Jacobs, P.A., Szulman, A.E., Funkhauser, J., Matsuura, J.S. and Wilson, C.C. (1982) Human triploidy: relationship between the parental origin of the additional haploid complement and development of partial hydatidiform mole. *Annals of Human Genetics*, **46**, 223–231

Jalbert, P., Sele, B. and Jalbert, H. (1980) Reciprocal translocations: a way to predict the mode of unbalanced segregation by pachytene-diagram drawing. A study of 151 human translocations. *Human Genetics*, **55**, 209–215

Jenkins, E.C., Brown, W.T., Krawczun, S. *et al.* (1988) Recent experience in prenatal fra(X) detection. *American Journal of Medical Genetics*, **30**, 329–336

Johnson, D.D., Dobyns, W.B., Gordon, H. and Dewald, G.W. (1988) Familial pericentric and paracentric inversions of chromosome 1. *Human Genetics*, **79**, 315–320

Kaiser, P. (1988) Pericentric inversions: their problems and clinical significance. In *The Cytogenetics of Mammalian Autosomal Rearrangements*, (ed. A. Daniel) New York: Alan R Liss, pp. 163–247

Kalousek, D.K., Barret, I.J. and McGillivray, B.C. (1989) Placental mosaicism and intrauterine survival of trisomies 13 and 18. *American Journal of Human Genetics*, **44**, 338–343

Kalousek, D.K. and Dill, F.J. (1983) Chromosomal mosaicism confined to the placenta in human conceptions. *Science*, **221**, 665

Kalousek, D.K., Dill, F.J., Dantzar, T., McGillivray, B.C., Young, S.L. and Wilson, R.D. (1987) Confined chorionic mosaicism in prenatal diagnosis. *Human Genetics*, **77**, 163–167

Laird, C. (1987) Fragile sites in human chromosomes as regions of late-replicating DNA. *Trends in Genetics*, **31**, 274–279

Landy, H.L., Weiner, S., Corson, S.L., Batzer, F.R. and Bolognese, R.J. (1986) The 'vanishing twin'. Ultrasonographic assessment of disappearance in the first trimester. *American Journal of Obstetrics and Gynecology*, **155**, 14–19

Ledbetter, D.H., Mascarello, J.T., Riccardi, V.M., Harper, V.D., Airhart, S.D. and Strobel, R.J. (1982) Chromosome 15 abnormalities and the Prader-Willi syndrome: a follow up report of 40 cases. *American Journal of Human Genetics*, **34**, 278–286

Leschot, N.J., Wolf, H. and Weenink, G.H. (1988) False negative findings at third trimester chorionic villus sampling (CVS). *Clinical Genetics*, **34**, 204–205

Linton, G. and Lilford, R.J. (1986) False negative findings on chorionic villus sampling. *Lancet*, ii, 630

Llerena, J., Murer-Orlando, M., McGuire, M. *et al.* (1989) Spontaneous and induced chromosome breakage in chorionic villus samples: a cytogenetic approach to first trimester prenatal diagnosis of ataxia telangiectasia syndrome. *Journal of Medical Genetics*, **26**, 174–178

Luckett, W.P. (1978) Origin and differentiation of the yolk sac and extraembryonic mesoderm in presomite human and rhesus monkey embryos. *American Journal of Anatomy*, **152**, 59–98

McKinley, M.J., Kearney, L.U., Nicolaides, K.H., Gosden, C.M., Webb, T.P. and Fryns, J.P. (1988)

Prenatal diagnosis of fragile X syndrome by placental (chorionic villi) biopsy culture. *American Journal of Medical Genetics*, **30**, 355–368

McKusick, V.A. (1988) *Mendelian Inheritance in Man* 8th edn. Baltimore and London: Johns Hopkins University Press

Malin, J., Singer, N., Warburton, D., Kardon, N. and Kim, H.J. (1987) Pseudomosaicism for trisomy 13. Three case reports. *Prenatal Diagnosis*, **7**, 395–400

Manning, F.A., Harrison, M.R. and Rodeck, C. (1985) Catheter shunts for fetal hydronephrosis and hydrocephalus. Report of the international fetal surgery report. *New England Journal of Medicine*, **315**, 336

Martin, A.O., Elias, S., Rosinsky, A.B., Bombard, A.T. and Simpson, J. (1986) False negative findings on chorionic villus sampling. *Lancet*, **ii**, 391–392

Mattei, M.G. and Mattei, J.F. (1988) Use of recombinant DNA probes in determining the origin of chromosome rearrangements. *The Cytogenetics of Mammalian Autosomal Rearrangements*, New York, London: Alan R Liss, pp. 601–613

Mikkelsen, M. and Aymé, S. (1986) Chromosomal findings in Chorionic villi: a collaborative study. In *Human Genetics* (eds. F. Vogel and K. Sperling). Proceedings of 7th International Congress Berlin. Berlin, Heidelberg, New York: Springer-Verlag.

Mikkelsen, M., Hanne, P., Jorgen, G. and Aksel, L. (1980) Non-disjunction in trisomy 21: a study of chromosomal heteromorphisms in 110 families. *Annals of Human Genetics*, **44**, 17–28

Netley, C.T. (1986) Summary overview of behavioural development in individuals with neonatally identified X and Y aneuploidy. *Birth Defects Original Article Series*, **22**, 293–306

Nicolaides, K.H., Rodeck, C.H. and Gosden, C.M. (1986) Rapid karyotyping in non-lethal malformations. *Lancet*, i, 283–287

Nicolaides, K.H., Soothill, P.W., Rodeck, C.H. and Campbell, S. (1986) Ultrasound guided sampling of umbilical cord and placental blood to asses fetal wellbeing. *Lancet*, i, 1065–1067

Nicolaides, K.H., Soothill, P.W., Rodeck, C.H., Warren, R.C. and Gosden, C.M. (1986) Why confine chorionic villus (placental) biopsy to the first trimester? *Lancet*, i, 543–544

Niebuhr, E. (1978) The cri du chat syndrome: epidemiology, cytogenetics and clinical features. *Human Genetics*, **44**, 227–234

Nielsen, J., Wohlert, M., Faaborg-Andersen, J. *et al.* (1986) Chromosome examination of 20 222 newborn children. Results from a 7.5 year study in Aarhus, Denmark. In *Prospective Studies on Children with Sex Chromosome Aneuploidy* (eds. S.G. Ratcliffe and N. Paul). March of Dimes Birth Defects Original Article Series 22 no 3: New York: Alan R. Liss, pp. 209–219

Purvis-Smith, S.G., Laing, S., Sutherland, G.R. and Baker, E. (1988) Prenatal diagnosis of the fragile X – the Australasian experience. *American Journal of Medical Genetics*, **30**, 337–345

Ratcliffe, S.G. and Paul, N. (1986) *Prospective Studies in Children with Sex Chromosome Aneuploidy*. March of Dimes Birth Defects Foundation Original Article Series 22 no 3. New York: Alan R. Liss

Roberts, E., Duckett, D.P. and Lang, G.D. (1988) Maternal cell contamination in chorionic villus samples assessed by direct preparations and three different culture methods. *Prenatal Diagnosis*, **8**, 635–640

Robinson, A., Bender, B.G., Borelli, J.B., Puck, M.H., Salderblatt, J.A. and Winter, J.S.D. (1986) Sex chromosome aneuploidy, prospective and longitudinal study. In *Prospective Studies on Children with Sex Chromosome Aneuploidy* (eds S. Ratcliffe and N. Paul) Birth defects original article series 22 no 3. New York, Alan R. Liss, pp. 23–71

Rosenberg, C., Frota-Pessoa, O., Vianna-Morgante, Am. and Ottu, T.H. (1987) Phenotypic spectrum of 45,X/46,XY individuals. *American Journal of Medical Genetics*, **27**, 553–559

Sabbagha, R.E., Sheikh, Z., Tamura, R.K. *et al.* (1985) Predictive value, sensitivity and specificity of ultrasonic targeted imaging for fetal anomalies in gravid women at high risk for birth defects. *American Journal of Obstetrics and Gynecology*, **152**, 822–827

Sachs, E.S., Van Hemel, J.O., Den Hollander, J.C. and Jahoda, M.G.J. (1987) Marker chromsomes in a series of 10000 prental diagnoses: cytogenetics and follow-up studies. *Prenatal Diagnosis*, **7**, 81–89

Sarkar, R. (1983) Association between the degree of mosaicism and the severity of syndrome in Turner mosaics and Klinefelter mosaics. *Clinical Genetics*, **24**, 420–428

Schinzel, A. (1984) *Catalogue of Unbalanced Chromosome Aberrations in Man*. Berlin, New York: Walter de Gruyter

Schweitzer, D., Ambros, P. and Andrle, M. (1978) Modification of DAPI banding on human chromosomes by prestaining with a DNA binding oligopeptide antibiotic Distamycin A. *Experimental Cell Research*, **111**, 327–334

Shapiro, L.R., Wilmot, P.L., Murphy, P.D. and Breg, W.R. (1988) Experience with multiple approaches to the prenatal diagnosis of the fragile X syndrome: amniotic fluid, chorionic villi, fetal blood and molecular methods. *American Journal of Medical Genetics*, **30**, 347–354

Sherman, S., Iselius, L. and Galliano, P. (1986) Segregation analysis of balanced pericentric inversions in pedigree data. *Clinical Genetics*, **30**, 87–95

Simoni, G., Brambati, B., Danesino, C. *et al.* (1983) Efficient direct chromosome analyses and enzyme determinations from chorion villi samples in the first trimester of pregnancy. *Human Genetics*, **63**, 349–357

Simoni, G., Fraccaro, M., Terzoli, G. *et al.* (1984) Discordance between prenatal cytogenetic diagnosis after chorionic villi sampling and chromosomal constitution of the fetus. In *First Trimester Fetal Diagnosis*, (eds M. Fraccaro, G. Simoni and B. Brambati). New York: Springer-Verlag, pp. 99–108

Simoni, G., Fraccaro, M., Terzoli, G. *et al.* (1985) Cytogenetics of chorionic villi sampling: technical developments and diagnostic applications. In *First Trimester Diagnosis*, (ed. M. Fraccaro *et al.*) Berlin, Heidelberg: Springer-Verlag

Simpson, J.L. (1982) Abnormal sexual differentiation in humans. *American Review of Genetics*, **16**, 193–224

Stene, J., Stene, E. and Mikkelsen, M. (1984) Risk for chromosome abnormality at amniocentesis following a child with non-inherited chromosome aberration. *Prenatal Diagnosis*, **4**, 81–95

Stene, J. and Stengel-Rutkowski, S. (1988) Genetic risks of familial reciprocal and Robertsonian translocation carriers. In *The Cytogenetics of Mammalian Autosomal Rearrangements* (ed. A. Daniel). New York: Alan R Liss, pp. 3–72

Stewart, D.A., Bailey, J.D., Netley, C.T., Rovet, J. and Park, E. (1986) Growth and development from early to midadolescence of children with X and Y chromosome aneuploidy: the Toronto study. In *Prospective Studies on Children with Sex Chromosome Aneuploidy* (eds S. Ratcliffe and N. Paul) Birth defects original article series 22 no 3. New York, Alan R. Liss, pp. 119–182

Sumner, A.T. (1972) A simple technique for demonstrating heterochromatin. *Experimental Cell Research*, **75**, 304–307

Sutherland, G.R. (1979) Fragile sites on human chromosomes. III Distribution, phenotypic effects and cytogenetics. *American Journal of Human Genetics*, **32**, 136–148

Therkelsen, A.J., Jensen, P.K.A., Hansen, J.T., Smidt-Jensen, S. and Hahnemann, N. (1985) Choice of medium for cultivation and 24 hour incubation of chorionic villi: Selective effects *in vitro*. In *First Trimester Fetal Diagnosis*, (ed. M. Fraccaro *et al.*) Berlin, Heidelberg: Springer-Verlag.

Therkelsen, A.J., Jensen, P.K.A., Hertz, J.M., Smidt-Jensen, S. and Hahneman, N. (1988) Prenatal cytogenetic diagnosis after transabdominal chorionic villus sampling in the first trimester. *Prenatal Diagnosis*, **8**, 19–31

Turner, G. and Jacobs, P. (1986) Marker (X)-linked mental retardation. *Advances in Human Genetics*, **13**, 83–112

Van De Sande, H.J., Lin, C.C. and Deugau, K.V. (1979) Clearly differentiated and stable chromosome bands produced by spermidine bisacridine, a bifunctional intercalating analogue of quinacrine. *Experimental Cell Research*, **120**, 439–452

Van Dyke, D.L., Weiss, L., Roberson, J.R. and Babu, V.R. (1983) The frequency and mutation rate of balanced autosomal rearrangements in man estimated from prenatal genetic studies for advanced maternal age. *American Journal of Genetics*, **35**, 301–308

Verma, R.S. and Lubs, H.A. (1975) A simple R-banding technique. *American Journal of Human Genetics*, **27**, 110–113

Warburton, D., Kline, J., Stein, Z. and Susser, M. (1980) Monosomy X, a chromosomal anomaly associated with young maternal age. *Lancet*, **i**, 167–169

Warburton, D. (1984) Outcome of cases of *de novo* structural rearrangements diagnosed at amniocentesis. *Prenatal Diagnosis*, **4**, 69–80

Watanabe, M., Ito, T., Yamamoto, M. and Watanabe, G. (1978) Origin of mitotic cells of the chorionic villi in direct chromosome analysis. *Human Genetics*, **44**, 191–193

Webb, T.P., Rodeck, C.H., Nicolaides, K.H. and Gosden, C.M. (1987) Prenatal diagnosis of the fragile X syndrome using fetal blood and amniotic fluid. *Prenatal Diagnosis*, **7**, 203–214

Wheeler, M., Peakman, D., Robinson, A. and Henry, G. (1988) 45,X/46,XY mosaicism: contrast of prenatal and post natal diagnosis. *American Journal of Medical Genetics*, **29**, 565–571

Williams, J., Medearis, A.L., Chu, W.H., Kovacs, G.D. and Kaback, M. (1987) Maternal cell contamination in cultured chorionic villi: comparison of chromosome Q-polymorphisms derived from villi, fetal skin and maternal lymphocytes. *Prenatal Diagnosis*, **7**, 315–322

Wolstenholme, J., Crocker, M. and Jonasson, J. (1988) A study of chromosomal aberrations in amniotic fluid cell cultures. *Prenatal Diagnosis*, **8**, 339–353

Worton, R.G. and Stern, R. (1984) A Canadian collaborative study of mosaicism in amniotic fluid cell cultures. *Prenatal Diagnosis*, **4**, 131–144

Wyandt, H.E. (1988) Ring autosomes: identification, familial transmission, causes of phenotypic effects and *in vitro* mosaicism. In *The Cytogenetics of Mammalian Autosomal Rearrangements*, (ed. A. Daniel). New York: Alan R Liss, pp. 667–696

Chapter 7

An introduction to modern genetics

M. Super

Introduction

Parents may come to realize that they have a genetic risk following the birth of an affected child. Sometimes a couple is realized to be at significant risk of a serious genetic disorder in their offspring, before they themselves have had children – this may occur during investigation of siblings when the disorder has occurred in a family member; it could also occur during population screening for disorders known to be prevalent in particular population groups. Such couples are in an especially difficult position, having been denied the natural optimism which fuels the procreative drive. Couples seem more influenced by the possibility of severe mental handicap or physical deformity than by morbidity imposed by a genetic disorder. The more a condition can be treated, the less interested are couples in prenatal diagnosis. For example, a couple at 1:4 risk of having a further child with cystic fibrosis (CF), underwent chorionic biopsy because of a fear of Down's syndrome, with the mother aged 42. When tests showed that the fetus had CF but was chromosomally normal, the couple proceeded with the pregnancy. They already had four daughters. The fact that the chromosome analysis revealed female once more, caused them to consider termination on this score but they rejected the idea. An ethical point arose in the counselling – was it right for me to remind them that girls with CF often do worse than boys and die earlier?

In genetic counselling, couples are given information which they may use to help them in their procreative decisions. Though counselling seeks to be non-directive, the counsellor, simply by outlining details of the disorder and the options open to couples may introduce ideas which were not present before. Discussions need, of necessity, to be detailed and to cover aspects such as variability of a condition, its treatability or otherwise and the risk the couple run of having an affected child. Discussions need to include prenatal diagnosis, whether it exists for the condition, its timing and the exact techniques used to obtain material representative of the fetus. Couples are strongly influenced in their decision by the gestational age at which testing is carried out.

Most prenatal diagnosis in the first or second trimester is orientated today towards offering the option of termination of pregnancy. Second trimester tests involve ultrasound, blood tests on the mother, e.g. alpha-fetoprotein, amniocentesis or fetoscopy, often with fetal blood sampling. First trimester tests are becoming much more prevalent. Mostly they include chorionic villus sampling, either transabdominally or transvaginally. Society is about to be offered a further option –

the fertilization of the egg *in vitro*, followed by the testing of single cells from the developing zygote, after amplifying the DNA, with the option of replacing into the uterus only those zygotes found to be free of specific disease. The first people to make use of these advances will be those for whom *in vitro* fertilization is a necessity in its own right.

The options open to families are disease specific and depend on the state of our scientific knowledge in each one. Nevertheless, there are certain principles which may be applicable in many diseases. In particular this applies to the use of linked probes in the tracking of genes within families. In the process of discovering specific disease genes, an earlier stage which may last for many years is the discovery of the approximate location of the disease locus on a specific chromosome. Related genes or random DNA markers from this section of the chromosome can then be tracked within families. These markers must be situated very close to the gene in question and polymorphic (i.e. occurring in more than one normal form). These polymorphisms are detected by digestion of the DNA with specific enzymes – restriction fragment length polymorphisms (RFLP) (*see* Chapter 8). The closer the marker, the less likely a meiotic cross-over which, if it has occurred, would give misleading information about whether the disease gene has been coinherited. This could result in a false prenatal prediction and this possibility must be built into counselling.

Linked markers may be used predictively, either prenatally, (with the object of offering termination) or preclinically after birth, where they may allow specific health surveillance in those predicted to be affected (and release from surveillance in the unaffected), or they may be used for diagnosis thereby improving the accuracy and effectiveness of genetic counselling. Some other interesting factors must be taken into account. For example, the prognosis for myotonic dystrophy is different according to whether the mother or father is the carrier of this autosomal dominant condition. Only in the former case is there a risk of the lethal neonatal form.

Autosomal dominant conditions

The risk of new mutations in some of these conditions is associated with advanced *paternal* age, e.g. achondroplasia. Other than ultrasound scanning there are no prenatal tests performed simply because of advanced paternal age.

The condition, myotonic dystrophy, is chosen as an example of an autosomal dominant condition to describe in detail. Once symptomatic, the condition becomes debilitating fairly quickly, with death about 15 years after the onset of the symptoms of weakness, wasting and myotonia. The onset of the adult form is generally between 20 and 40 years. Affected females are at risk of having offspring with the congenital form. This is associated with significant perinatal problems for mother and child such as hydramnios and prolonged labour. The baby presents with hypotonia and feeding difficulties as well as talipes (hydramnios + talipes = myotonic dystrophy until proved otherwise).

The mother is quite often still in the preclinical state of her condition when the affected child is delivered and it is easy to blame the infant's problems on perinatal asphyxia, without realizing the underlying genetic diagnosis. A woman who has had such a child has a 1:4 risk that further *affected* offspring would present in the newborn period. This 1:4 is not a Mendelian risk figure but an empiric figure based on the frequency of affected neonates in women with myotonic dystrophy. Unaffected offspring, or those destined to present years later, are in some danger of intrapartum intracerebral haemorrhage, associated with difficult birth.

Pregnancy itself may cause a deterioration in muscle strength in the affected woman. She may have great difficulty caring for the infant and will require help. The above facts tempt one towards being directive in counselling an affected woman and her spouse – by advising against pregnancy or further pregnancy. One woman, realizing her poor prognosis, wanted to leave her husband with a healthy child – she undertook a pregnancy and proceeded with it when prenatal tests of secretor status of the amniotic fluid allowed a prediction with 92% accuracy of an unaffected fetus. Antenatal and postpartum care were carefully monitored and labour did not prove too difficult – the baby proved unaffected but the woman died before he reached the age of 2 years.

How did we arrive at a 92% figure of an unaffected fetus (or an 8% chance that it would be affected)? This was based on tests for secretor status – 80% of the population are secretors, i.e. their blood groups antigens can be determined from their secretions – tears, saliva etc.; 20% are non-secretors. The genetics of this system is exactly like the Rhesus (Rh) factor, i.e. the 20% are homozygotes for the recessive, non-secretor form; the other 80% comprise homozygotes for secretor status and heterozygotes who contain one gene for secretor, with the other being non-secretor.

It was established that the gene for myotonic dystrophy and that of secretor status are linked – many families with two or more affected and at least one unaffected first degree relative were tested. Families informative for secretor status in an index affected person, i.e. with one gene for secretor and one not, were analysed. They showed that a particular status, either for secretor or non-secretor, tracked with the disease in the majority of instances. Analysis of many families allowed the odds of the two genes being linked to be calculated – this is expressed as the logarithm of the odds (LOD) score. As we shall see in the next two chapters a LOD score of more than 3 indicates that the odds of this being a chance association are less than 1:1000, i.e. $<10^3$.

The error rate of prenatal prediction when linked genes are used depends on the chance of meiotic recombination between the two tested loci – in this case 5%. Again this is an empiric observation derived in many tested families. With a prior probability of 50:50 of an affected fetus, the error rate using this test is estimated from the most likely recombination rate at specific genetic distances. (In practice many geneticists prefer to lower the chance of giving false reassurance and therefore use a correction to take into account the possibility that the real genetic distance might be greater than that calculated from the number of recombinations observed in a limited number of families, i.e. they use the upper 95th confidence limit of the mean estimate of genetic distance based on family studies.) The recombination rate which gives the highest LOD score linking myotonic dystrophy and the secretor allele is 5% (also known as theta = 0.5). This distance is expressed in centiMorgans – so secretor and myotonic dystrophy are 5 centiMorgans apart. Some geneticists downgrade this figure to 8% to take account of possible higher order recombination fraction possibilities as mentioned above. This knowledge of the chance of cross-over (5 or 8%), the secretor status of normal and affected family members and the fetus and the prior risk (50%) is then used to calculate the probability (or odds) that the child will be affected – in this example 8%. The basis of these calculations will be explained in the next two chapters.

The observed distances, described above, based on cross-over frequency, do not imply an absolutely accurate specific distance in terms of base pairs because some parts of the chromosome form more cross-overs. Strictly speaking there ought to be separate recombination fractions for males vs females – for many paired loci throughout the genome there is increased crossing over in females compared with males. Where two probes linked to the disease in question are known to *flank* it on either side, then the error rate of using both becomes the one recombination rate multiplied by the other, or a much smaller number. In myotonic dystrophy, flanking markers are not known. Relevant individuals need to be informative for both markers (i.e. to have different markers) and this limits the usefulness of flanking gene probes in disorders where they have been discovered.

Since the time of the case presented above, it has become known that the genes for myotonic dystrophy and secretor status are on chromosome 19. We now have DNA probes which are closer to the myotonic locus, being about 3 cM away. Testing with such probes depends on exactly the same principles and are described in detail in the next two chapters. A polymorphism (i.e. more than one normally occurring allele at the marker site) is required in order to tell the chromosomes 19 apart at the site of the particular polymorphism. So tests today would be more accurate but would still include an error rate based on the chance of meiotic cross-over between the tested marker and the disease site. Tests using markers in myotonic dystrophy can be used in a predictive way, in a child or adult with two affected first degree relatives. Combined with DNA markers would be physical examination, electromyogram (EMG) and examination of the eyes for cataracts. We detected two young daughters of an affected man by secretor status tracting in the family – both were predicted to have a 92% chance of being affected and, although asymptomatic, both had myotonia on EMG. On the other hand, a 25-year-old man sharing the same DNA genotype as his affected sister and mother has a 95% chance of having the gene. However, if he is asymptomatic and has normal EMG and eye examination then his chances of having myotonic dystrophy are much less than the 95% predicted by DNA studies alone; in his case it is likely that cross-over between gene and marker *has* occurred.

Other dominant conditions for which genetic markers exist are Huntington's chorea and adult type polycystic kidney disease. Application of probes in preclinical detection, especially of the former disorder, requires careful thought.

Recessive disorders

As we shall see in the next two chapters, for linked probes to be applicable in a recessive disorder, both parents need to be informative, either with one probe or a combination of two probes, enabling the counsellor to determine which markers are linked to normal and abnormal genes *in a particular family*. If only one parent is informative then only half the time can one predict an unaffected fetus, in the other half a 50:50 chance of the disease remains. Error rates depend on the likelihood of cross-over between the marker locus and the gene locus. When the disease state is forecast, the error is theta; when carrier is predicted, theta, and when no disease genes (non-carrier), theta^2; the error rate for a partially informative family is theta.

Theta, the chance of cross-over in meiosis was discussed above and the logic behind this arithmetic will be explained in Chapter 9. Once again much smaller error rates are achievable if flanking probes prove informative in a family. Of course, once the genes themselves are discovered, the error rates depend only on the accuracy of tests in the laboratory and accurate DNA tests can be used in disease diagnosis or in identifying specific subclasses of disease. Screening for the disease or carrier state in the general population also becomes feasible once the specific genetic abnormalities are determined. Testing for feasibility of prenatal diagnosis should occur ideally *before* a pregnancy is undertaken. It is possible to detect carriers among the siblings of affected subjects in informative families and sometimes in the sibs of the parents.

The example chosen is cystic fibrosis (CF), since there has been widespread use of DNA probes since the discovery of the locus for CF on the long arm of chromosome 7 in 1985 by Tsui. Very close linkages were discovered by studying families with two or more affected subjects.

Before the discovery of accurate prenatal tests for CF, most couples decided to have no further children once a diagnosis of CF was made. In 1983, Brock established that microvillar enzymes in amniotic fluid taken at 17–18 weeks were reduced in *most* instances where the fetus had CF and the couple were at a 1:4 risk of having an affected child. *Most* fluids with a normal result were associated with an unaffected fetus. The lateness of the test and the error rates were serious limitations. The error rates associated with this test are 8% false-positive and 5% false-negative, for couples with a 1:4 prior risk.

The CF locus has been intensively studied and the generosity of laboratories like that of Professor Bob Williamson of St Mary's Hospital in London have ensured wide availability of probes extremely closely linked to the CF locus – so close that error rates of <1% are quoted when CF is diagnosed in the fetus, with even lower error rates for carrier or 'no CF genes' predictions. There is an important caveat however: diagnosis of the CF must be accurate (use of linked probes for all genetic disorders relies on the accuracy of the diagnosis and the lack of heterogeneity of the disease). Two particular pitfalls in CF are described. In the first a couple who have lost a child with CF have prenatal testing using a microvillar enzyme (e.g. in 1985), a diagnosis of CF is predicted with 92% certainty and the pregnancy terminated. DNA is extracted from the fetal tissue. The reliability of using the genotypes from this tissue in any subsequent pregnancy depends on the accuracy of the microvillar tests, i.e. one would start out with an 8% inbuilt error rate. However, newer probe testing with probes which show linkage disequilibrium with CF may come to our rescue and reduce the chances of error. This linkage disequilibrium means that some markers *tend* to go with the gene. The marker was probably present on the chromosome when the original mutation occurred and has tended to stay with it ever since because it is very close to the gene – cross-over between the marker and gene occurs infrequently and they are said to be in linkage disequilibrium. If DNA from the aborted fetus gives the classical CF pattern, then of these newer probes the likelihood of false prediction in a future pregnancy is reduced. The probes in present use which are in marked linkage disequilibrium are XV2c and Km19, both from Professor Williamson's laboratory. Most CF chromosomes of northern Europeans contain the larger allele of XV2c and the smaller allele of Km19 (weaker linkage disequilibrium is present in Spain and Italy). We return to the phenomenon of linkage disequilibrium, in more detail, in Chapter 9.

A second pitfall is based on diagnosis of CF on the basis of meconium ileus found at post-mortem following spontaneous abortion; meconium ileus often implies CF in these circumstances but this is not always the case. Again the new tightly linked probes in linkage disequilibrium can increase the likelihood that the child did in fact have CF.

Linked probes can also be used on the spouse who marries into a family where CF has occurred, e.g. the risk of a person from the North-West of England of being a carrier can be increased to 1:7 or reduced to 1:250 instead of the average population risk of 1:22. Parents of a person with CF have one CF and one non-CF allele and the genetic risk after remarriage can be recalculated on the basis of linked probes. This is explained in more detail in Chapter 9.

*Once the CF gene is discovered and cloned these calculations will become obsolete provided that it turns out that one molecular DNA abnormality is responsible for all cases of CF (i.e. like sickle cell disease but unlike beta thalassaemia).

Other autosomal recessive disorders in which linked probes are applicable are the thalassaemias and other haemoglobinopathies. Some of these are bedevilled by the lack of informative polymorphisms (e.g. thalassaemics from island communities like Cyprus where one allele of each polymorphism is likely to predominate). In sickle cell disease, one of the restriction enzymes cuts at the point mutation site and this allows definitive testing. However, the severity of the clinical phenotype depends on the characteristics of the rest of the globin genes. In Britain thalassaemia and haemoglobinopathy testing is centred at Professor Weatherall's department in Oxford. Clear clinical details need to accompany requests for test. In these diseases, analysis and prediction of prenatal feasibility can all occur before the onset of pregnancies. It is usually medical oversight that results in 'panic' testing during pregnancies. In the case of thalassaemias the molecular position may be too complex to allow emergency testing. Where DNA analyses are informative, first trimester prenatal diagnosis is feasible. Otherwise there is still the option of fetal blood sampling at 18 weeks for these blood diseases.

Not all genetic testing is DNA based, though this could be the case in the future. In certain inborn errors of metabolism the disease and carrier state can be identified by enzyme analysis. An example is Tay-Sachs disease, a condition with increased prevalence in Ashkenazi Jews. It is possible to screen for carriers among those with no family history and to offer prenatal diagnosis on chorionic material or amniotic fluid, as the enzyme (hexosaminidase A) is expressed in both.

Sex-linked disorders

Carrier detection in females is feasible because of Lyon's law that only one X chromosome per cell is active: carriers may show normal levels of testing products, simply because their cells happen to contain a higher than average proportion of active X chromosomes with the normal allele. As a result it is possible to say with relative confidence that a female *is* a carrier when tests are abnormal; when they are normal she may still be a carrier. To complicate matters further, germ cell mosaicism has been shown for some of these conditions, i.e. more than one egg with the genetic abnormality, though the woman does not carry the trait in her somatic cells. Prenatal diagnosis where feasible is always offered to women who already have an affected son, even when somatic cell testing suggests that she might not be a carrier.

Linked probes are also of less use on the X chromosome than is the case with many autosomal conditions – meiotic cross-over seems especially active in certain parts of the X, e.g. the site of Duchenne muscular dystrophy and the site of fragile

*The major mutation of the CF gene, delta F_{508} has now been discovered. It accounts for 80% of CF genes in Britain.

X, factor VIII and factor IX. The frequency of new mutation at some of these sites may be related to the amount of meiotic cross-over activity.

Duchenne muscular dystrophy (DMD) is chosen as the example. There is often no family story when this disorder of poor prognosis is diagnosed. Creatine kinase testing of the mother may indicate that she is a carrier, but 30% of definite carriers have normal levels. Female relatives on the maternal side might be carriers and need to be offered counselling and testing. Linked probe analysis combined with creatine kinase can allow one to reduce the chances of carrier status for some of the female relatives. Discovery of the actual DMD gene has allowed more clear-cut testing and advice for the boy's parents. Seventy per cent of boys will show a deletion with one of the probes developed from within the dystrophin site. The mother, even if she is deleted at that site, will have a normal dystrophin gene on her other X chromosome; therefore, a signal will be obtained with every dystrophin probe used. Thus it is technically difficult at present to tell whether the mother is deleted on one chromosome or whether the signal on the autoradiograph is from two normal (superimposed) dystrophin genes. If we could prove the latter case, we would be dealing either with a true new mutation or with germinal mosaicism; the woman's sisters would be at no greater risk of being carriers than someone from the general population; her daughters could still be carriers if germinal mosaicism is found. Gene dosage tests or tests based on the gene product, dystrophin, ought to enable differentiation of women with a deleted dystrophin locus from those without in the fairly near future, but tests for families at risk are not available at present. Sometimes a deletion results in a so-called junctional fragment, i.e. a restriction site happens to have been involved in the deletion and the part of the dystrophin gene tested gives a signal at a different place on the autoradiograph. In such a case it is possible to tell the mother's two X chromosomes apart and whether her daughter is a carrier or not. If the affected boy alone shows a junctional fragment then again new mutation or germinal mosaicism are proved and the mother's sisters would not share their nephew's Duchenne gene.

Advances in our knowledge are increasing options for families at risk of many genetic disorders. Earlier prenatal diagnostic tests are becoming feasible. There are many ethical issues on which society needs consulting and much public education is required. As treatment options become possible, either at a somatic or early embryonic level (which would involve germ cells and be passed on), a new set of ethical and practical guidelines will emerge.

References

Brock, D.J.H. (1983) Amniotic fluid alkaline phosphatase isoenzymes in early prenatal diagnosis of cystic fibrosis. *Lancet*, **ii**, 941–943

Tsui, L.-C., Buchwald, M., Barker, D. *et al.* (1985) Cystic fibrosis locus defined by a genetically linked polymorphic DNA marker. *Science*, **230**, 1054–1057

Chapter 8

Technology for DNA diagnosis

R. Mueller

Introduction

Prenatal diagnosis is one of the areas in clinical medicine which has been and will continue to be profoundly influenced by the recent advances in recombinant DNA technology.

There are in excess of 3000 known single gene disorders in man (McKusick, 1988) and it is estimated that approximately 1% of the population is or will be affected by a disorder inherited in a Mendelian fashion. Until the availability of recombinant DNA technology, prenatal diagnosis by conventional means was only possible in a very limited number of these disorders in which an abnormal or deficient gene product (protein or enzyme) had been identified and was known to be expressed in a tissue which could be obtained from the fetus without undue risk to the mother or fetus.

The use of recombinant DNA technology to find the mutation responsible or a polymorphic DNA marker linked to a disease locus will allow prenatal diagnosis of any single gene Mendelian disorder provided the families are available for study and funding and manpower are provided.

The molecular basis of inheritance, the principles of recombinant DNA technology and examples of its application will be illustrated in this chapter.

The molecular basis of inheritance

DNA: the hereditary material

The chromosomes contain a single Watson-Crick DNA (deoxyribonucleic acid) double helix (Watson and Crick, 1953). This consists of two complementary polynucleotide chains with opposite (anti-parallel) orientations composed of the four nucleotides, the two purines adenine and guanine and the two pyrimidines, cytosine and thymine. The pairing in the double helix is specific: guanine in one chain always pairs with cytosine in the other chain and adenine always pairs with thymine (Figure 8.1).

The genetic code

Genetic information in the DNA double helix is stored in the form of triplet codes, three nucleotides (a codon) determining a single amino acid. The code is, however,

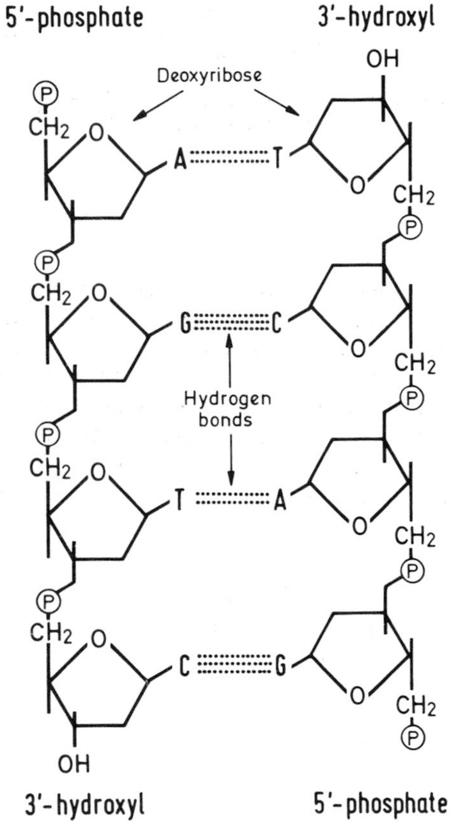

5'-phosphate   **3'-hydroxyl**

Figure 8.1 Diagrammatic representation of the DNA double helix. Phosphate (P) and deoxyribose sugar (D) form the backbone, the bases adenine (A), thymine (T), guanine (G) and cytosine (C) pair to form sidearms of the ladder-like structure. (From Emery and Mueller, 1988)

'degenerate', the 20 different amino acids of proteins being coded for by the 4^3 or 64 possible triplet codons and two 'stop' and one 'start' codons.

Gene structure

The human genome is approximately 3×10^9 base pairs in size. If the entirety of the nucleotide sequence in man were to code for proteins the size of the haemoglobin genes, then there would be as many as 3 million genes in man. Even allowing for a proportion of the genome to be involved in the control of gene expression, there is far in excess of the amount of DNA necessary for the 50–100 000 functional genes predicted to be present in man. Therefore, the majority of DNA in the human genome consists of 'intergenic' or 'spacer' DNA. A significant proportion of this DNA consists of repeated sequences of varying lengths, the function of which is not apparent.

The nucleotide sequence of the genes themselves is not translated in its entirety into messenger RNA (mRNA) for transcription into protein. The coding sequences or 'exons' are separated by intervening sequences or 'introns' which are removed or 'spliced out' before the mature mRNA is transported to the ribosomes for transcription into protein (Figure 8.2).

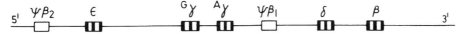

Figure 8.2 Representation of the coding sequences (—■—) and non-coding sequences (—□—) of the human beta globin gene and adjoining region (ψ represents the position of pseudogenes). (From Emery and Mueller, 1988)

Gene mutation

An understanding of the nature and types of mutations which can occur is vital to appreciate how DNA techniques are used in prenatal diagnosis. Changes in genetic material are called mutations, which can occur either spontaneously or be induced by a variety of mutagenic agents. There are two main types: macroscopic chromosomal alterations and submicroscopic or molecular changes which involve individual nucleotide(s). There are a number of different types of mutation, common ones which include deletions, insertions, inversions or substitution of one or more bases (Figure 8.3). Functionally, the various types of mutations can result

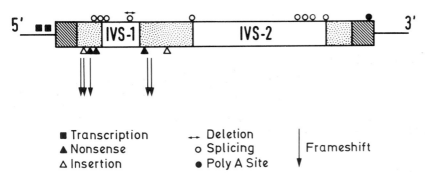

Figure 8.3 Examples of the location and types of mutations which occur in the beta globin gene and flanking region which result in beta thalassaemia (IVS-intervening sequence or intron). (From Emery and Mueller, 1988)

either in lack of or reduced production of the normal gene product, decrease of biological activity of an altered protein product or a 'silent' mutation with no biological effect.

Principles of recombinant DNA technology

There are four main steps in recombinant DNA technology:

1. generation of DNA fragments by restriction enzyme cutting
2. incorporation or recombination of these fragments into a suitable carrier or vector
3. transformation of a bacterial host organism with the recombinant vector to produce multiple copies of the DNA fragment of interest, the procedure of cloning

4. selection of clones, individual recombinant vectors, which contain specific DNA sequences or genes of interest.

Generation of DNA fragments: restriction fragments

DNA fragments can be generated by mechanical shearing techniques, but this produces a haphazard, indiscriminate collection of DNA fragments. The isolation of greater than 200 different enzymes from bacteria, restriction enzymes, which cleave double-stranded DNA at sequence specific sites (Smith and Wilcox, 1970) allows the generation of DNA fragments such that particular DNA sequences or genes can be isolated in a DNA fragment(s) in a reproducible consistent manner from a single individual (Table 8.1).

Table 8.1 Some examples of commonly used restriction enzymes, the bacteria from which obtained and their cleavage sites (+) (adapted from Emery and Mueller, 1988)

Enzyme	Organism	Cleavage site	
		5'	3'
Bam H1	*Bacillus amyloliquefaciens* H	G + G A T C	C
Eco R1	*Escherichia coli* RY 13	G + A A T T	C
Hae III	*Haemophilus aegyptius*	G G + C C	
Hind III	*Haemophilus influenzae* Rd	A ÷ A G C T	T
Hpa I	*Haemophilus parainfluenzae*	G T T + A A	C
Pst I	*Providencia stuartii*	C T G C A +	G
Sma I	*Serratia marcescens*	C C C + G G	G

Incorporation of DNA fragments into vectors

DNA fragments generated by restriction enzyme cleavage have either 'blunt' or 'staggered' termini of varying lengths. Under appropriate conditions the enzyme DNA ligase can make complementary termini of DNA fragments generated in this way unite to produce recombinant DNA molecules.

Incorporation of 'foreign' DNA into a carrier vector such as plasmids, bacteriophages or cosmids allows production of large amounts of the recombined DNA fragments by replication in a bacterial host organism (Figure 8.4).

Transformation of host organisms

After the production of recombinant vectors, they are introduced into host bacteria by the process known as transformation. The host-vector is then grown in culture medium to produce large amounts of the individual recombinants, known as clones.

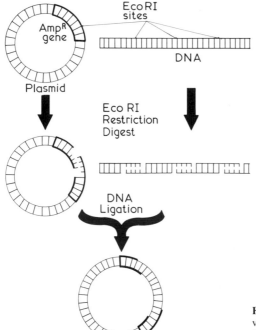

EcoRI
sites

DNA

Amp^R
gene

Plasmid

Eco RI
Restriction
Digest

DNA
Ligation

Figure 8.4 Generation of recombinant vector with DNA insert. (From Emery, 1984)

Screening of vectors with DNA inserts

Use of vectors with restriction sites within antibiotic resistance genes means that a recombinant vector with a DNA insert can be screened for by loss of resistance to that particular drug in selective culture media as opposed to a vector which has merely religated to itself.

The collection of DNA clones produced in this way is called a DNA library. When the DNA source is nucleated cells the library is called a total or genomic library, while a DNA library made from DNA produced by the action of the enzyme reverse transcriptase on mRNA is called complementary or cDNA.

Selection of clones with specific DNA sequences

The problem is to select the vector containing the particular DNA insert relevant to the disease we are interested in. There are a number of different techniques to detect clones with specific DNA inserts. If the DNA insert in the vector is expressed then the recombinant protein might be detected for example, by immunological methods (Broome and Gilbert, 1978; Korman et al., 1982). More frequently, however, nucleic acid hybridization techniques are employed. If the DNA sequence of the gene is known or can be inferred from the amino acid sequence of the protein, then a radioactively labelled chemically synthesized oligonucleotide DNA sequence can act as a probe (Grunstein and Hogness, 1975; Benton and Davis, 1977; Suggs et al., 1981; Singer-Sam et al., 1983). Alternatively, one can use mRNA from a cell source in which a particular mRNA species is

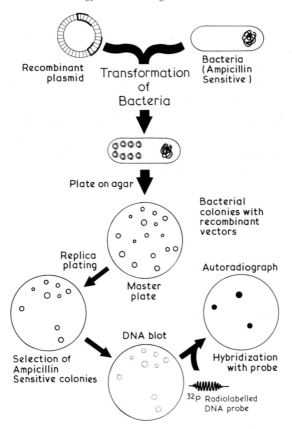

Figure 8.5 Identification of recombinant DNA clones with specific DNA inserts by loss of antibiotic resistance, nucleic acid hybridization and autoradiography. (Adapted from Emery, 1984)

predominant, e.g. the alpha and beta globin genes from immature red blood cells, reticulocytes (Paterson, Roberts and Kuff, 1977; Hastie and Held, 1978). Frequently neither of these methods is possible and we must rely on linkage (family) studies to relate a particular DNA fragment to a particular gene (*see below*).

DNA from the bacterial colonies containing the recombinant vectors are bound onto a nitrocellulose filter. The replica colonies are then allowed to hybridize with the radioactively labelled DNA or RNA probe and monitored by exposure to an X-ray film – autoradiography. In this way, a colony containing a DNA sequence complementary to the probe will be detected and from its position on the replica plate can be identified on the master plate and then cultured separately to produce large amounts of that particular DNA sequence (Figure 8.5).

Applications of recombinant DNA technology

The main application of recombinant DNA technology in prenatal diagnosis has, until recently, been restriction mapping using the method of Southern blotting.

Restriction mapping

This procedure consists of subjecting DNA fragments generated by a restriction enzyme to electrophoresis on an agarose gel to which an electric current is applied which results in an ordered separation of DNA fragments by size, the smaller fragments migrating more rapidly than the larger. The DNA fragments in the gel are then denatured with alkali which makes them single stranded. A permanent copy of these single-stranded fragments is made by transferring them on to a nitrocellulose filter, the so-called Southern blot (Southern, 1975). A particular DNA fragment can be localized by incubating the blot under appropriate conditions with a ^{32}P radioactively labelled DNA probe which has been made single stranded. Any complementary DNA sequences will hybridize and can be visualized by autoradiography (Figure 8.6).

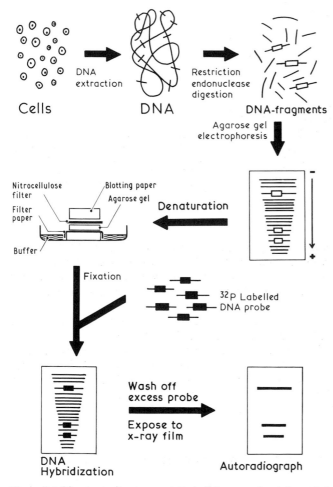

Figure 8.6 Diagrammatic representation of the procedure of restriction mapping. (Adapted from Emery, 1984)

A DNA probe can be specific for a gene, e.g. the human beta globin gene by making cDNA from mRNA derived from immature red blood cells, reticulocytes, where the majority of the mRNA codes for the two globin gene products, alpha and beta globin (Lawn *et al.*, 1978). Alternatively, a probe to a specific gene can be chemically synthesized, its sequence being inferred from the amino acid sequence of the protein (Wallace *et al.*, 1981; Connor *et al.*, 1983). Many unique sequence DNA probes are derived from DNA libraries and their location is unknown until assigned to the human genome by somatic cell genetics, linkage (*see* Chapter 9) or other techniques.

Restriction mapping techniques have been instrumental in our understanding of the mutational basis of certain single gene disorders and has had immediate application in the prenatal diagnosis of inherited disorders.

Defined/recognized molecular pathology

Deletion detection

In some of the haemoglobinopathies, such as alphathalassaemia or delta-beta thalassaemia where anaemia results due to an underproduction of one or more of the alpha globin chains (alpha or the delta and beta globin chains respectively), restriction mapping has shown that loss of one or more of the globin chain genes is the cause (Orkin *et al.*, 1978) (Figure 8.7). More recently, restriction mapping of DNA from males with Duchenne muscular dystrophy, has shown the majority to have a deletion of part of the dystrophin gene (Kunkel *et al.*, 1986).

Conventional agarose gel electrophoresis can only resolve DNA fragments up to approximately 20 000 base pairs in size. More recently, use of the technique of pulse field gel electrophoresis in which DNA fragments are subjected to two

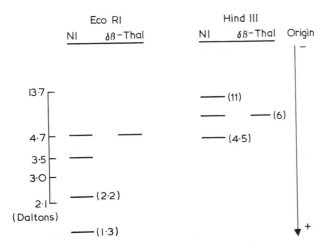

Figure 8.7 Representation of the EcoRI and HindIII restriction maps from normal (N1) subjects and persons homozygous for delta-beta thalassaemia (δβ-thal) with a beta globin cDNA radiolabelled probe showing loss of restriction fragments as evidence of a deletion as the mutational basis of delta-beta thalassaemia. (From Macleod and Sikora, 1984)

approximately perpendicular electrical fields alternately enables the separation of larger DNA fragments up to 2 million base pairs in size (Brown and Bird, 1986). Modifications of this technique along with use of infrequently cutting restriction enzymes for the DNA digests allows resolution of DNA fragments up to 5–10 million base pairs in size (Anand, 1986). This approach should facilitate the detection of deletions, if responsible, for single gene disorders when linked markers are found. Conventional restriction mapping would then subsequently allow more detailed resolution enabling definitive qualitative prenatal diagnosis.

Mutations within restriction sites

Some 200 different restriction enzymes are known with a consequent multiplicity and variety of recognition sites. If the mutation responsible for a single gene disorder were to occur within the DNA sequence of the recognition site of the restriction enzyme then the restriction map of DNA from a person with that disorder will be different from the remainder of the population. One of the first applications of this approach was in the prenatal diagnosis of sickle cell disease (Chang and Kan, 1982) (Figure 8.8).

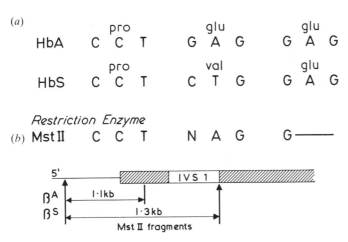

Figure 8.8 (a) Nucleotide sequence of the 5th, 6th and 7th codons of the normal beta (HbA) and sickle (HbS) globin genes. (b) Nucleotide recognition sequence of the restriction enzyme MstII and the restriction fragments of MstII digests of DNA from normal persons and persons with sickle-cell disease when hybridized with a 1.1 kb MstII genomic 5′ beta globin DNA sequence (N, any nucleotide). (Adapted from Emery and Rimoin, 1990)

Although identification of such a qualitative mutation allows unequivocal prenatal diagnosis in families at risk for other certain single gene disorders, such as alpha-1-antitrypsin deficiency (Kidd *et al.*, 1983), unfortunately in the majority of single gene disorders either the mutation responsible has not been identified, is not due to a deletion, or does not occur within a restriction site, so that alternative approaches will need to be utilized.

Restriction fragment length polymorphisms (RFLP)

It is for this reason that the observation of normal polymorphic DNA sequence variation is so important. In a significant proportion of the population, natural variation in the nucleotide sequence occurs – a polymorphism – approximately every 200 base pairs (Jeffreys, 1979). These DNA sequence differences are usually of no functional significance as they occur mainly in the intervening or intergenic DNA sequences. These differences in DNA sequence mean that the restriction fragments visualized with a specific DNA probe and a particular restriction enzyme will be of different lengths in different people. These alterations can be recognized in the restriction map by the altered mobility of the restriction fragments on gel electrophoresis due to the difference in fragment size.

By studying the pattern of the segregation of a particular single gene disorder in families with a battery of RFLP throughout the human genome, if the variation at a particular site can be shown to be linked to that disorder (*see* Chapter 9), then this polymorphism can be utilized for prenatal diagnosis using DNA either directly from chorionic villus sampling or cultured amniotic fluid cells. It is important to emphasize that this approach does not require any knowledge of the biochemical defect in the inherited disorder or the nature of the alteration in the DNA responsible for the disorder.

Allele-linked RFLP

In a limited number of single gene disorders, a particular RFLP has been found to be in linkage disequilibrium with the disease locus. This is when a particular polymorphic variant occurs together more commonly with a specific mutation than would occur by their individual frequencies in the population concerned. One of the early examples was the demonstration that the sickle cell mutation in persons of West African origin was usually within a 13 kb fragment when DNA digested with the restriction fragment HpaI was probed with a beta globin cDNA probe, whereas the normal beta globin gene was mainly found in a 7.0 or 7.6 kb fragment (Kan and Dozy, 1978) (Figure 8.9).

More recently, an RFLP has been found to be in linkage disequilibrium with the mutation for cystic fibrosis (Estivill *et al.*, 1987). As we saw in Chapter 7, this finding allows modification of the prior 1 in 20 carrier risk for the general population, often useful when counselling couples where one of the partners has/had a sibling with cystic fibrosis (*see* Chapter 9). A similar closely linked RFLP has been found to be in linkage disequilibrium with the mutation in phenylketonuria (DiLella *et al.*, 1986).

Observation of this type of RFLP is relatively rare and for most single gene disorders family studies of locus-linked RFLP is the approach of choice.

Locus-linked RFLP

This approach involves following the pattern of inheritance of a disorder and a battery of RFLP in families and looking for cosegregation. Once a particular RFLP has been linked to a disease locus (Murray *et al.*, 1982; Gusella *et al.*, 1983; Wainwright *et al.*, 1985; White *et al.*, 1985), then analysis of the pattern of segregation of the variants at that RFLP site must be established in each individual family.

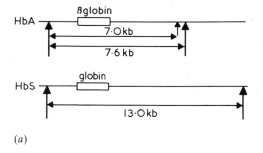

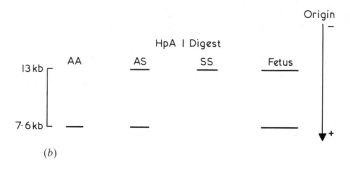

(b)

Figure 8.9 (a) Representation of the three types of HpaI restriction fragments observed containing the beta (HbA) and sickle (HbS) globin genes. (b) Diagrammatic representation of the restriction fragment pattern of the autoradiograph of the Southern blots of the HpaI digests of DNA from normal persons (AA) and persons with sickle-cell trait (AS), sickle-cell disease (SS) and a heterozygous fetus probed with a radiolabelled beta globin cDNA sequence. (From Macleod and Sikora, 1984)

An example of the use of a linked RFLP for an X-linked disorder is shown in Figure 8.10. Locus-linked RFLP will continue to be demonstrated in an ever increasing wide variety of single gene disorders.

Recent developments

Hypervariable DNA length polymorphisms

This form of polymorphism has been shown to be inherited in a Mendelian fashion and is due to the presence of variable numbers of tandem repeats of a short DNA sequence and are thought to have arisen by unequal exchanges either during recombination in meiosis, sister chromatid exchange in mitosis, or by means of slippage during DNA replication. These length variations are very highly polymorphic when compared to conventional RFLP and have the advantage that they can be demonstrated using any restriction enzyme provided it does not cleave within the DNA sequence of the repeat unit.

Such highly variable regions have been identified near the human insulin gene (Bell, Selby and Rutter, 1982) and the alpha globin gene on the short arm of

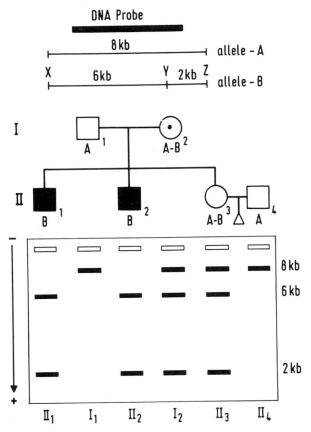

Figure 8.10 Hypothetical family with an X-linked disorder showing segregation of a linked RFLP at site Y which show individual II₃ to be a carrier for the disorder as she has inherited allele B from her mother, the one in common with her two affected brothers. (From Emery and Mueller, 1988)

chromosome 16 (Higgs *et al.*, 1981). The latter has been linked to the gene for adult onset polycystic kidney disease allowing presymptomatic gene detection in persons at risk for this late onset autosomal dominant disorder (Reeders *et al.*, 1986).

Jeffreys, Wilson and Thien (1985a) have identified a common short 10–15 base pair 'core' sequence which shares some nucleotide sequence similarity with other hypervariable sequences which simultaneously identifies many highly variable loci throughout the human genome, the so-called 'minisatellites' which are the basis of 'DNA fingerprinting' (Jeffreys, Wilson and Thien, 1985b).

Oligonucleotide probes

If the mutational basis of a single gene disorder is due to a point mutation, the single base pair mismatch can be shown by differential hybridization with allele-specific oligonucleotide probes (Connor *et al.*, 1983). It was suggested that this approach might find widespread application for particular populations at risk for the inherited disorders of haemoglobin but has not done so for technical reasons. It also is unlikely to be of use in most single gene disorders as it requires both the recognition of the mutation of the disease and for it to be due to a point mutation.

Non-radiolabelled probes

The established laboratory techniques depend on the use of radiolabelled DNA probes. While there are practical problems with the sensitivity of non-autoradiographic techniques such as fluorescent-labelled probes (Langer, Waldrop and Ward, 1981), use of DNA sequence amplification techniques may allow more widespread use of this latter type of probe.

DNA sequence amplification

A promising development in prenatal diagnosis using these techniques involves a novel application of oligonucleotide probes. Use of conventional oligonucleotide probes in prenatal diagnosis such as that reported in sickle cell disease (Connor *et al.*, 1983) requires restriction digestion of the DNA, gel electrophoresis to separate the DNA fragments containing the DNA sequence/gene of interest, and hybridization of the allele-specific oligonucleotides to these fragments. Prenatal diagnosis of disorders such as beta-thalassaemia (Pirastu *et al.*, 1983) or alpha-1-antitrypsin deficiency (Kidd *et al.*, 1983) using these techniques requires high activity probes which have been gel-purified, 5–10 µg of DNA for analysis and several days exposure of the resulting autoradiograph.

A modification of this approach offers significant practical advantages (Saiki *et al.*, 1985, 1986; Scharf, Horn and Erlich, 1986). Two oligonucleotide primers complementary to opposite DNA strands flanking a DNA sequence of interest are used to amplify a target sequence by means of repeated cycles of denaturation, primer annealing and primer extension (Figure 8.11). This polymerase chain reaction (PCR) consists of successive cycles of DNA synthesis resulting in an amplification of the DNA target sequence which can result in an increase up to 10^5-fold. This process enables analysis of quantities of DNA as small as 1 ng using the standard allele-specific oligonucleotides. The use of the heat-stable DNA polymerase from *Thermus aquaticus* which increases the specificity of the amplification process compared to that with the Klenow fragment of DNA polymerase I allows direct visualization of the PCR amplified sequence in an agarose gel by ultraviolet fluorescence after staining with ethidium bromide without previous DNA extraction and purification reactions. Restriction digests of the target DNA sequence looking for mutation specific or linked polymorphisms is carried out as described previously, but all the subsequent steps of DNA denaturation, Southern blotting, hybridization with radioactive probes and autoradiography are eliminated. DNA sequence amplification with oligonucleotide restriction analysis has been used in the prenatal diagnosis of sickle cell disease (Embury *et al.*, 1987) and haemophilia A (Kogan, Doherty and Gitschier, 1987). It can be used to sex blastomeres from the pre-implantation embryo (Handyside *et al.*, 1989; Holding and Monk, 1989).

While the PCR is fairly labour intensive if carried out manually, results can still be available within 24 h and, with automation of the PCR, results can be available within the same day as the prenatal diagnostic procedure!

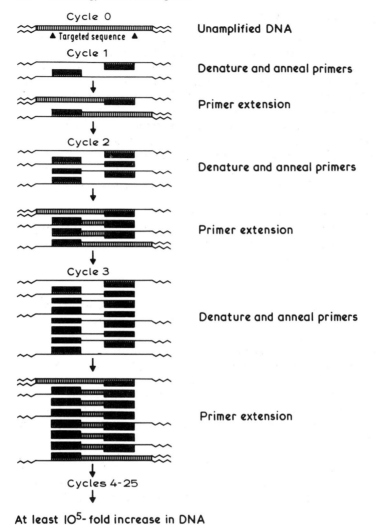

Figure 8.11 Representation of the polymerase chain method of DNA sequence amplification

The availability of a non-invasive means of prenatal diagnosis using fetal cells obtained from the maternal circulation is a logical concurrent obstetric development (Lo *et al.*, 1989). While there are likely to be practical developmental problems, the increased acceptability of prenatal diagnosis this might allow is obvious.

Problems and pitfalls in the application of DNA technology

There is, however, a number of theoretical and practical problems and/or pitfalls in the use of these approaches which must always be kept in mind.

Availability of appropriate DNA samples

Simple practical problems may limit the usefulness of these techniques. It must be stressed that the use of locus-linked RFLP for the prenatal diagnosis of most single gene disorders often requires a DNA sample from an affected individual within the family concerned. With potentially lethal disorders such as cystic fibrosis or Duchenne muscular dystrophy, it is vital to store DNA at the earliest available chance so that the opportunity is not missed. This situation will also commonly arise with late-onset autosomal dominant disorders in which the persons at risk seeking advice are below the usual age of onset and affected persons in the previous generation are no longer alive, e.g. as commonly occurs in Huntington's chorea. Sometimes it is possible to infer the RFLP allele(s) of such a person by looking at the rest of the family, e.g. the normal male sibs of a male with Duchenne muscular dystrophy.

Use of more recently developed techniques such as polymerase chain reaction may mean, however, that this problem can be overcome if pathological/histological material from such an individual is still available for analysis (Mueller *et al.*, 1990).

Informativeness

A proportion of families at risk for any single gene disorder may not be informative at a particular RFLP site, i.e. show the necessary polymorphic variation at that site to be of use. Although DNA sequence variation due to restriction site polymorphisms is estimated to be present every 100 base pairs in the human genome (Jeffreys, 1979), even if a family is screened with a large panel of restriction enzymes and a variety of probes, there is often a significant proportion of families in which the DNA sequence variation necessary to be informative for clinical use may not be demonstrated. The greater the number of RFLP linked to a particular disease locus, the greater the chance a family will be informative for one or more linked RFLP.

If a DNA probe is available which detects hypervariable DNA sequences this problem can be overcome. One example, as mentioned, is the hypervariable region near the alpha globin gene on chromosome 16 (Higgs *et al.*, 1981) which has been linked to the locus for adult onset polycystic kidney disease (Reeders *et al.*, 1986).

Genetic heterogeneity

The clinical geneticist is fully familiar with the potential pitfall of genetic heterogeneity. It is not uncommon to find with time that what was thought to be a single entity turns out to be genetically heterogeneous, i.e. due to more than one cause. This possibility needs to be particularly kept in mind when using linked RFLP in prenatal diagnosis. A number of disorders have been shown to be genetically heterogeneous being inherited in more than one way or due to genes at more than one loci. A pertinent example is the existence of an autosomal recessive pseudohypertrophic muscular dystrophy in which affected individuals have clinical features similar to males with Duchenne muscular dystrophy (McKusick, 1988).

It is vital to remember that demonstration of linkage of a disease locus with a polymorphic marker does not necessarily prove that in an individual family the disease is due to a mutation at the same locus no matter how large the LOD score. An example of this is the recent report of a second locus for adult onset polycystic kidney disease (Romeo *et al.*, 1988), i.e. defects of two quite separate genes may produce the same disease.

Phase

It may not be possible to determine on which of a chromosome pair the mutant allele is in relation to the linked RFLP – phase – unless one carries out extended families studies (Emery, 1986). When using linked RFLP in prenatal diagnosis one must allow for the possibility of a cross-over event having occurred in the parental meiosis(es) for the first affected child as well as in the fetus in the prenatal diagnostic procedure itself (*see* Chapter 9). With a partially informative pedigree for an autosomal recessive disorder it may not be possible to differentiate between the homozygous normal, heterozygotes and affected individuals in prenatal diagnosis. It is vital that the clinician counselling the families using these techniques has discussed the results of the family studies with the laboratory to ensure which situation pertains.

Recombination

Family studies of disease loci and RFLP provide a measure of the likelihood of linkage at a variety of cross-over (recombination) frequencies. The measure of the likelihood of linkage of a disease locus to an RFLP is known as the LOD (or Z) score which is calculated as the log (to the base 10) of the chance of the two being linked as opposed to being unlinked. A score of 3 (10^3 or 1000 to 1) is taken as proof of linkage (Emery, 1986). Once an RFLP has been shown to be linked to a disease locus, it can be used for prenatal diagnosis. The recombination frequency is known as theta (θ). It is a measure of the chance of a cross-over occurring between an RFLP and the disease locus in any single meiosis (Emery, 1986). The value of theta must be taken into account when using these techniques in prenatal diagnosis and will be the basis for an expected false-positive/false-negative rate. Demonstration of closely linked RFLP with smaller values of theta will minimize this chance. The use of RFLP on either side or 'flanking' the disease locus will further reduce this possibility as two cross-over events would need to have occurred to result in an outcome at odds with that predicted (*see* Chapter 9).

With a number of single gene disorders, the structural gene itself has been cloned. In this case intragenic (within introns) or closely flanking RFLP can be used and one might expect to be able to ignore the possibility of crossing-over. However, several loci, such as the Duchenne muscular dystrophy locus, appear to be a recombination 'hot-spot' with the consequence that this is always a possibility.

It is important to keep in mind the confidence limits of recombination fractions with linked markers (Renwick, 1986; Krawczak, 1987). A vital part of prenatal diagnosis is assiduous follow-up for confirmation of predicted outcomes. In couples at risk for cystic fibrosis this means testing all children born predicted to be carriers or unaffected homozygotes by means of immune reactive trypsin (IRT) levels in the newborn period with a subsequent sweat test, as well as examining all fetuses aborted predicted to be affected. Similarly, males born to couples at risk for Duchenne muscular dystrophy predicted as being unlikely to be affected should have creatine phosphokinase estimations carried out as soon as is reliable. The nature of linked markers and the assigned probability of a cross-over event means that in a predictable proportion of instances prenatal diagnosis will result in affected offspring (Darras, Harper and Francke, 1987).

As well as advising couples of the obvious advantages of these new techniques it is vital to keep in mind that there is likely to be a minimum error rate due to human fallibility.

Normal polymorphic DNA variation

Not every DNA sequence alteration in a likely candidate gene for a single gene disorder necessarily represents the mutational basis of a genetic disorder. This is illustrated by the report of an apparent 300 base-pair deletion in an alpha 1(I)-like collagen gene in four children with Type II or the perinatal lethal form of osteogenesis imperfecta (Pope *et al.*, 1984). As this finding was uncommon in DNA from a normal control population and one parent in each instance was shown also to have this same deletion, it was proposed that affected children were genetic compounds having a second undetected mutation at this site. It has subsequently been shown that this apparent deletion probably represents a normal polymorphism common in persons of Asian Indian origin (of which three of the four affected children reported were) in what is now known to be a gene encoding the alpha-chain subunit of Type II collagen (Sykes and Ogilvie, 1984). The report of a normal individual from this population homozygous for this polymorphism supports this conclusion (Sykes, Ogilvie and Wordsworth, 1985). In genes consisting of a large number of coding and non-coding sequences the normally occurring polymorphic variation possible means that it will be important to keep this sort of finding in mind.

Non-paternity

The use of linked RFLP in prenatal diagnosis will not be able to exclude the possibility of non-paternity. In the majority of instances non-paternity will result in a false-positive diagnosis, but false-negative diagnoses due to this cause might occur in populations at high risk for certain recessive disorders, e.g. the haemoglobinopathies in persons of Afro-Carribean origin (Hutton *et al.*, 1985). Use of internal controls such as 'DNA fingerprinting' could help detect misdiagnoses due to this cause (Jeffreys, Wilson and Thien, 1985b).

References

Anand, R. (1986) Pulsed field gel electrophoresis: a technique for fractionating large DNA molecules. *Trends in Genetics*, **2**, 278–283

Bell, G.I., Selby, M.J. and Rutter, W.J. (1982) The highly polymorphic region near the human insulin gene is composed of simple tandemly repeating sequences. *Nature*, **295**, 31–35

Benton, W.D. and Davis, R.W. (1977) Screening λgt recombinant clones by hybridization to single plaques *in situ*. *Science*, **196**, 180–182

Broome, S. and Gilbert, W. (1978) Immunological screening method to detect specific translation products. *Proceedings of the National Academy of Sciences, USA*, **75**, 2746–2749

Brown, W.R.A. and Bird, A.P. (1986) Long-range restriction site mapping of mammalian genomic DNA. *Nature*, **322**, 477–481

Chang, J.C. and Kan, Y.W. (1982) A sensitive new prenatal test for sickle-cell anaemia. *New England Journal of Medicine*, **307**, 30–32

Connor, B.J., Reyes, A.A., Morin, C., Itakura, K., Teplitz, R.L. and Wallace, R.B. (1983) Detection of sickle cell β-globin allele by hybridization with synthetic oligonucleotides. *Proceedings of the National Academy of Sciences, USA*, **80**, 278–282

Darras, B.T., Harper, J.F. and Francke, U. (1987) Prenatal diagnosis and detection of carriers with DNA probes in Duchenne's muscular dystrophy. *New England Journal of Medicine*, **316**, 985–992

DiLella, A.G., Marvit, J., Lidsky, A.S., Guttler, F. and Woo, S.L.C. (1986) Tight linkage between a splicing mutation and a specific DNA haplotype in phenylketonuria. *Nature*, **322**, 799–803

Embury, S.H., Scharf, S.J., Saiki, R.K. *et al.* (1987) Rapid prenatal diagnosis of sickle cell anaemia by a new method of DNA analysis. *New England Journal of Medicine*, **316**, 656–661

Emery, A.E.H. (1986) *Methodology in Medical Genetics*, 2nd edn. Edinburgh: Churchill Livingstone

Estivill, X., Farrall, M., Scambler, P.J. *et al.* (1987) A candidate for the cystic fibrosis locus isolated by selection for methylation-free island. *Nature*, **326**, 840–845

Grunstein, M. and Hogness, D.S. (1975) Colony hybridization: a method for the isolation of cloned DNAs that contain a specific gene. *Proceedings of the National Academy of Sciences, USA*, **72**, 3961–3965

Gusella, J.F., Wexler, N.S., Conneally, P.M. *et al.* (1983) A polymorphic DNA marker genetically linked to Huntington's disease. *Nature*, **306**, 234–238

Handyside, A.H., Pattinson, J.K., Penketh, R.J.A., Delhanty, J.D.A., Winston, R.M.L. and Tuddenham, E.G.D. (1989) Biopsy of human reimplantation embryos and sexing by DNA amplification. *Lancet*, **i**, 347–349

Hastie, N.D. and Held, W.A. (1978) Analysis of mRNA populations by cDNA.mRNA hybrid-mediated inhibition of cell-free protein synthesis. *Proceedings of the National Academy of Sciences, USA*, **75**, 1217–1221

Higgs, D.R., Goodbourn, S.E.Y., Wainscoat, J.S., Clegg, J.B. and Weatherall, D.J. (1981) Highly variable regions of DNA flank the human α globin genes. *Nucleic Acids Research*, **9**, 4213–4224

Holding, C. and Monk, M. (1989) Diagnosis of beta-thalassaemia by DNA amplification in single blastomeres from mouse preimplantation embryos. *Lancet*, **ii**, 532–535.

Hutton, E.M., Shuman, C., Boehm, C. and Kazazian, H.H. (1985) False paternity as a problem in the use of restriction fragment length polymorphisms for prenatal diagnosis. *American Journal of Human Genetics*, **37**, A221

Jeffreys, A.J. (1979) DNA sequence variants in γ, α, δ and β globin genes of man. *Cell*, **18**, 1–10

Jeffreys, A.J., Wilson, V. and Thien, S.L. (1985a) Hypervariable 'minisatellite' regions in human DNA. *Nature*, **314**, 67–73

Jeffreys, A.J., Wilson, V. and Thein, S.L. (1985b) Individual-specific 'fingerprints' of human DNA. *Nature*, **316**, 76–79

Kan, Y.W. and Dozy, A.M. (1978) Polymorphism of DNA sequence adjacent to human beta-globin structural gene: relationship to sickle mutation. *Proceedings of the National Academy of Sciences, USA*, **75**, 5631–5635

Kidd, V.J., Wallace, R.B., Itakura, K. and Woo, S.L.C. (1983) α-1-antitrypsin deficiency detection by direct analysis of the mutation in the gene. *Nature*, **304**, 230–234

Kogan, S.C., Doherty, M. and Gitschier, J. (1987) An improved method for prenatal diagnosis of genetic diseases by analysis of amplified DNA sequences. *New England Journal of Medicine*, **317**, 985–990

Korman, A.J., Knudsen, P.J., Kaufman, J.F. and Strominger, J.L. (1982) cDNA clones for the heavy chain of HLA-DR antigens obtained after immunopurification of polysomes by monoclonal antibody. *Proceedings of the National Academy of Sciences, USA*, **79**, 1844–1848

Krawczak, M. (1987) Genetic risk and recombination fraction – an example of non-monotonic dependency. *Human Genetics*, **75**, 189–190

Kunkel, L.M. *et al.* (1986) Analysis of deletions in DNA from patients with Becker and Duchenne muscular dystrophy. *Nature*, **322**, 73–77

Langer, P.R., Waldrop, A.A. and Ward, D.C. (1981) Enzymatic synthesis of biotin-labelled polynucleotides: novel nucleic acid affinity probes. *Proceedings of the National Academy of Sciences, USA*, **78**, 6633–6637

Lawn, R.M., Fritsch, E.F., Parker, R.C., Blake, G. and Maniatis, T. (1978) The isolation and characterization of linked delta- and beta-globin genes from a cloned library of human DNA. *Cell,* **15**. 1157–1174

Lo, Y.-MD., Patel, P., Wainscoat, J.S., Sampietro, M., Gillmer, M.D.G. and Fleming, K.A. (1989) Prenatal sex determination by DNA amplification from maternal blood. *Lancet,* **ii**, 1363–1365

McKusick, V. (1988) *Mendelian Inheritance in Man,* 8th edn. London: Johns Hopkins University Press

Mueller, R.F., Taylor, G.R., Stewart, A.D., Noble, J.S., Quirke, P. and Ivinson, A. (1990) Polymerase chain reaction on fixed necroscopy material. *Journal of Medical Genetics,* **27**, 67–68

Murray, J.M., Davies, K.E., Harper, P.S., Meredith, L., Mueller, C.R. and Williamson, R. (1982) Linkage relationship of cloned DNA sequences in the short arm of the X chromosome to Duchenne muscular dystrophy. *Nature,* **300**, 64–71

Orkin, S.H., Alter, B.P., Altay, C. *et al.* (1978) Application of endonuclease mapping to the analysis and prenatal diagnosis of thalassaemias caused by globin gene deletions. *New England Journal of Medicine,* **229**, 166–172

Paterson, B.M., Roberts, B.E. and Kuff, E.L. (1977) Structural gene identification and mapping by DNA.mRNA hybrid arrested cell-free translation. *Proceedings of the National Academy of Sciences, USA,* **74**, 4370–4374

Pirastu, M., Kan, Y.W., Cao, A., Conner, B.J., Teplitz, R.L. and Wallace, R.B. (1983) Prenatal diagnosis of β-thalassaemia. Detection of a single nucleotide mutation in DNA. *New England Journal of Medicine,* **309**, 284–287

Pope, F.M., Cheah, K.S.E., Nicholls, A.C., Price, A.B. and Grosveld, F.G. (1984) Lethal osteogenesis imperfecta congenita and a 300 base pair deletion for an α1(I)-like collagen. *British Medical Journal,* **288**, 431–434

Reeders, S.T., Breuning, M.H., Corney, G. *et al.* (1986) Two genetic markers closely linked to adult polycystic kidney disease on chromosome 16. *British Medical Journal,* **292**, 851–853

Renwick, J.H. (1986) Letter: chance that individual in Duchenne family is recombinant. *Lancet* ii, 351

Romeo, G., Devoto, M., Roncuzzi, L. *et al.* (1988) A second genetic locus for autosomal dominant polycystic kidney disease. *Lancet,* ii, 8–11

Saiki, R.K., Bugawan, T.L., Horn, G.T., Mullis, K.B. and Erlich, H.A. (1986) Analysis of enzymatically amplified β-globin and HLA-DQα DNA with allele-specific oligonucleotide probes. *Nature,* **324**, 163–166

Saiki, R.K., Scharf, S., Faloona, F. *et al.* (1985) Enzymatic amplification of β-globin genomic sequences and restriction site analysis for diagnosis of sickle cell anemia. *Science,* **230**, 1350–1354

Scharf, S.J., Horn, G.T. and Erlich, H.A. (1986) Direct cloning and sequence analysis of enzymatically amplified genomic sequences. *Science,* **233**, 1076–1078

Singer-Sam, J., Simmer, R.L., Keith, D.H. *et al.* (1983) Isolation of a cDNA clone for human X-linked 3-phosphoglycerate kinase by use of a mixture of synthetic oligonucleotides as a detection probe. *Proceedings of the National Academy of Sciences, USA,* **80**, 802–806

Smith, H.O. and Wilcox, K.W. (1970) A restriction enzyme from *Haemophilus influenzae* I. Purification and general properties. *Journal of Molecular Biology,* **51**, 379–391

Southern, E.M. (1975) Detection of specific sequences among DNA fragments separated by gel electrophoresis. *Journal of Molecular Biology,* **98**, 503–517

Suggs, S.V., Wallace, R.B., Hirose, T., Kawashima, E.H. and Itakura, K. (1981) Use of synthetic oligonucleotides as hybridization probes: isolation of cloned cDNA sequences for human β-2-microglobulin. *Proceedings of the National Academy of Sciences, USA,* **78**, 6613–6617

Sykes, B. and Ogilvie, D. (1984) Lethal osteogenesis imperfecta and a gene deletion. *British Medical Journal,* **288**, 1380

Sykes, B.C., Ogilvie, D.J. and Wordsworth, B.P. (1985) Lethal osteogenesis imperfecta and a collagen gene deletion. Length polymorphism provides an alternative explanation. *Human Genetics,* **70**, 35–37

Wainwright, B.J., Scambler, P.J., Schmidtke, J. *et al.* (1985) Localization of cystic fibrosis locus to human chromosome 7 cen-q22. *Nature,* **318**, 384–385

Wallace, R.B., Johnson, M.J., Hirose, T., Miyake, T., Kawashima, E.H. and Itakura, K. (1981) The use of synthetic oligonucleotides as hybridization probes. II Hybridization of oligonucleotides of mixed sequences to rabbit β-globin DNA. *Nucleic Acids Research,* **9**, 879–894

Watson, J.D. and Crick, F.H.C. (1953) Molecular structure of nucleic acids – a structure for deoxyribose nucleic acid. *Nature*, **171**, 737–738

White, R., Woodword, S., Leppert, M. *et al.* (1985) A closely linked genetic marker for cystic fibrosis. *Nature*, **318**, 382–384

Further reading

Alberts, B., Dennis, B., Lewis, J. *et al.* (1983) *Molecular Biology of the Cell*. London: Garland

Caskey, C.T. (1987) Disease diagnosis by recombinant DNA methods. *Science*, **236**, 1223–1229

Emery, A.E.H. (1984) *An Introduction to Recombinant DNA*. Chichester: John Wiley

Emery, A.E.H. and Mueller, R.F. (1989) *Elements of Medical Genetics*, 7th edn. Edinburgh: Churchill Livingstone

Emery, A.E.H. and Rimoin, D.L. (eds) (1990) *Principles and Practice of Medical Genetics*, 2nd edn. Edinburgh: Churchill Livingstone

Macleod, A. and Sikora, K. (eds) (1984) *Molecular Biology and Human Disease*. Oxford: Blackwell

Maniatis, T., Fritsch, E.F. and Sambrook, J. (1990) *Molecular Cloning – a Laboratory Manual*, 2nd edn. New York; Cold Spring Harbour Laboratory Press

Old, R.W. and Primrose, S.B. (1985) *Principles of Gene Manipulation: an Introduction to Genetic Engineering*, 3rd edn. Oxford: Blackwell

Weatherall, D.J. (1985) *The New Genetics and Clinical Practice*, 2nd edn. Oxford: Oxford Medical Publications

Chapter 9

DNA diagnosis: calculation of genetic risk

I.D. Young

Introduction

During the last decade there has been an explosion in molecular biology which has revolutionized counselling and risk assessment for many of the common single gene disorders, particularly those in which the basic defect at the protein level is unknown. Ultimately it is hoped that this technology, which has been outlined at length in the previous chapter, will lead to isolation of the genes concerned thus paving the way for elucidation of their protein products through the approach known as reverse genetics. Perhaps the best example of this is the recent isolation of dystrophin (Hoffman, Brown and Kunkel, 1987), a protein involved in maintaining the integrity of the muscle fibre cytoskeleton. Defective production of dystrophin results in the severe sex-linked Becker and Duchenne forms of muscular dystrophy (Hoffman *et al.*, 1988).

For most of the more common Mendelian disorders which precipitate requests for prenatal diagnosis, isolation of the miscreant gene has not yet been achieved. In these situations recourse has to be made to the use of polymorphic DNA markers known to be genetically linked to the disorder in question. The use of linked markers can generate some very difficult calculations which, in many instances, are best solved by reference to specially designed computer programs (Lathrop and Lalouel, 1984). However, some of the less complex situations can be handled perfectly adequately without calling upon the help of the microchip, as outlined in the following pages.

Linkage

Two gene loci are said to show linkage if they are so close together on the same chromosome that they are unlikely to be separated by a cross-over (recombination) during meiosis. Linked genes on the same chromosome are said to be in coupling; those on opposite homologous chromosomes are described as being in repulsion. This is known as the linkage phase. The recombination fraction (θ) is a measure of the distance separating two loci, or more precisely an estimate of the likelihood of recombination occurring between them. Thus if $\theta=0.05$, there is a probability of 1 in 20, i.e. 5%, that a cross-over will occur between two linked genes during meiosis.

It is now apparent that the human genome contains numerous base pairs at which 'silent' mutations of no clinical significance have occurred during evolution. The discovery of restriction enzymes which may by chance cleave DNA at one of these polymorphic sites of silent mutation, along with the development of Southern blotting (*see* Figures 8.6 and 8.9), has enabled the study of the cosegregation of these silent mutations with specific diseases. These polymorphic cutting sites constitute the DNA markers, which, if known to be closely linked to a specific disease locus, can be used as an aid in carrier detection and prenatal diagnosis. Exactly how these linked markers can be utilized is illustrated in the examples which follow.

Reference should also be made to a phenomenon known as linkage disequilibrium. This is best understood by considering a disease locus (D = good gene, d = bad gene) and a closely linked polymorphic DNA cutting site (A = presence of cutting site, B = absence of cutting site). If the gene frequency of A and B are equal (i.e. A = B = 0.5), then it could be anticipated that 50% of patients with the disease (D) would have marker A, whereas the other 50% would have marker B. In this instance the loci are said to be in equilibrium. If there is a statistically significant deviation from this 1:1 ratio, then the loci are said to show linkage disequilibrium. The demonstration of very strong linkage disequilibrium can be utilized for indirect carrier detection or prenatal diagnosis since in this situation the linkage phase can be deduced from knowledge of the disequilibrium rather than by study of the extended family. In general, linkage disequilibrium is of very limited value in counselling with the possible exception of general population carrier detection for conditions such as cystic fibrosis (*see* example 6).

Bayes' theorem

In order to understand the approach used in the examples which follow, it is necessary to be familiar with a particularly useful means of calculating probabilities, known as Bayes' theorem. This enables an overall risk to be calculated taking into account the initial (prior) probability of an event plus factors which influence (condition) this initial probability. This is best illustrated by an example. Consider a female consultand who had two brothers with a sex-linked recessive disorder. Their mother must have been a carrier so that the consultand must have commenced life with a 50% (= 0.5 = $\frac{1}{2}$ in terms of probability) risk of being a carrier. Intuitively it can be seen that if this woman has had five sons all of whom are healthy, then it becomes rather unlikely that she is in fact a carrier. Bayes' theorem provides a means for quantifying this intuition, by taking into account the prior and conditional probabilities if the patient is a carrier and comparing these with the probability obtained if she is not a carrier, i.e.

	Consultand is a carrier	Consultand is not a carrier
Probability		
Prior	$\frac{1}{2}$	$\frac{1}{2}$
Conditional 5 healthy sons	$(\frac{1}{2})^5$	1
Joint	$(\frac{1}{2})^6 = 1/64$	$\frac{1}{2}$

Thus the overall or posterior probability that this woman is a carrier equals the joint probability of having five healthy sons if she is a carrier (1/64) divided by the sum of all the joint probabilities (1/64 + ½). This gives a final probability of 1/33, so that the risk that a future son would be affected would equal 1/33 × ½ = 1/66.

Autosomal dominant inheritance

Linked DNA markers are now available for several autosomal dominant disorders such as Huntington's chorea (Harper and Sarfarazi, 1985), neurofibromatosis (Upadhyaya *et al.*, 1989), and adult polycystic kidney disease (Reeders *et al.*, 1986). Several situations are illustrated to show their potential value in counselling and prenatal diagnosis.

Example 1. Phase known

In Figure 9.1, A and B are allelic marker genes at a locus closely linked to the disease locus. Analysis of the family indicates that in II2 the disease gene must be coupled with marker B since both have been inherited from her mother I2. It is important to note that this does not automatically imply that the disease gene is coupled with marker B in I2, since a cross-over could have occurred during meiosis in the gamete which went to form II2.

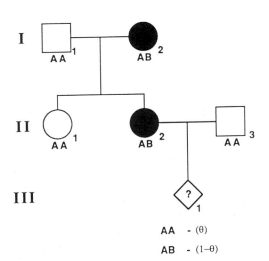

Figure 9.1 *See* example 1. Autosomal dominant inheritance. The disease gene in II2 must be coupled with marker B. The probability that III1 will be affected is indicated for each possible genotype

Knowledge of the linkage phase in II2 enables the probable disease status to be predicted in her unborn baby III1. If this child inherits the B marker from its mother, then there is a probability of $1-\theta$ that the baby will be affected. If, as is likely, θ equals 0.05 or less, this means that the baby is at high risk. If the baby inherits the A marker from its mother, then the baby will only be affected if a cross-over occurs, i.e. the risk will be equal to the value of θ.

Thus in this example prenatal diagnosis carries with it a predictive error equal to the value of θ.

Example 2. Phase unknown

In Figure 9.2 the linkage phase is known in II1 as indicated in the preceding example. In I2 the disease is probably coupled with marker B, but could be coupled with marker A in which case a cross-over occurred in the gamete which went to

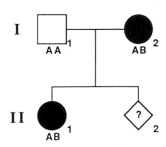

I

II

AA

AB

AB

AA - $(2\theta - 2\theta^2)$

AB - $(1 - 2\theta + 2\theta^2)$

Figure 9.2 *See* example 2. Autosomal dominant inheritance. The linkage phase in I2 is not known with certainty although information about it can be deduced from II1. The probability that II2 will be affected is indicated for each possible genotype

form II1. Thus, in assessing the risk to II2, the calculation has to take into account the possibilities that the disease in I2 is coupled with either A or B. This is most easily achieved using Bayes' theorem.

	Disease in I2 coupled with A	Disease in I2 coupled with B
Probability		
Prior	½	½
Conditional. II1 is affected and has inherited B	θ	$1 - \theta$
Joint	$\dfrac{\theta}{2}$	$\dfrac{1 - \theta}{2}$

Thus the posterior probability that the disease in I2 is coupled with A equals

$$\frac{\dfrac{\theta}{2}}{\dfrac{\theta}{2} + \dfrac{1 - \theta}{2}}$$

which reduces to θ.

Similarly the posterior probability that the disease in I2 is coupled with B equals

$$\frac{\dfrac{1 - \theta}{2}}{\dfrac{\theta}{2} + \dfrac{1 - \theta}{2}}$$

which reduces to $1 - \theta$.

For II2 in Figure 9.2 risks can be calculated as follows. If this baby inherits marker A from its mother then the probability that it will be affected equals the sum of:

1. the probability that the disease in I2 is coupled with A (θ) multiplied by $1 - \theta$ plus
2. the probability that the disease in I2 is coupled with B ($1 - \theta$) multiplied by θ.

This summates to $2\theta - 2\theta^2$.

If II2 inherits marker B from its mother then the probability that it will be affected equals the sum of:

1. the probability that the disease in I2 is coupled with B ($1 - \theta$) multiplied by ($1 - \theta$) plus
2. the probability that the disease in I2 is coupled with A (θ) multiplied by θ.

This summates to $1 - (2\theta - 2\theta^2)$.

Thus in this situation there will be a predictive error of $2\theta - 2\theta^2$, which is considerably greater than in example 1 when the linkage phase in the mother undergoing prenatal diagnosis was known with certainty.

An alternative approach to arriving at risks for II2 involves constructing a larger Bayesian tree which takes into account all possibilities. This is illustrated for the situation in which II2 inherits marker B from its mother.

	Disease in I2 coupled with A		Disease in I2 coupled with B	
Probability				
Prior	½		½	
Conditional. II1 is affected and has inherited B	θ		$1 - \theta$	
II2	Affected	Not affected	Affected	Not affected
Prior	½	½	½	½
Conditional. has inherited B	θ	$1 - \theta$	$1 - \theta$	θ
Joint	$\dfrac{\theta^2}{4}$	$\dfrac{\theta(1 - \theta)}{4}$	$\dfrac{(1 - \theta)^2}{4}$	$\dfrac{\theta(1 - \theta)}{4}$

From this tree it can be seen that the posterior probability that II2 will be affected if marker B is inherited from the mother equals:

$$\frac{\dfrac{\theta^2}{4} + \dfrac{(1 - \theta)^2}{4}}{\dfrac{\theta^2}{4} + \dfrac{\theta(1 - \theta)}{4} + \dfrac{(1 - \theta)^2}{4} + \dfrac{\theta(1 - \theta)}{4}} = 1 - (2\theta - 2\theta^2)$$

Once again it is apparent that there will be a predictive error of $2\theta - 2\theta^2$.

Example 3. Prenatal exclusion diagnosis

In Figure 9.3, II1 is a young man who has not yet shown any signs of the late onset disorder which affects his father. The linkage phase in the father is not known so

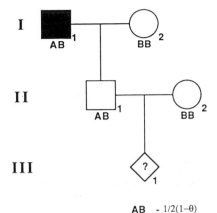

Figure 9.3 *See* example 3. Autosomal dominant inheritance. The linkage phase in I1 is not known. The probability that III1 will be affected is indicated for each possible genotype

AB - 1/2(1–θ)

BB - 1/2(θ)

that there is no means of predicting disease status for II1. However, it is clear from the pedigree that II1 must have inherited marker B from his mother and therefore marker A must have come from his father. Thus marker A conveys a risk of 50% for being coupled with the disease gene in II1.

This means that it would be possible to test any pregnancy conceived by II1 and II2 to determine if the fetus inherits marker A or B with a view to estimating risk for the unborn baby. Thus if the fetus inherits A there will be a probability of ½ (i.e. the probability that marker A is coupled with the disease in II1) × (1 – θ) (i.e. the probability that a cross-over between the disease gene and marker gene A will not occur) that the baby will also inherit the disease. If marker B is inherited then there will only be a very small probability (½ × θ) that the disease will also be inherited. Thus by this approach the disorder can be excluded with a predictive error of θ/2 if parents opt to terminate the 'high risk' pregnancy. Without the availability of linked markers any baby born to II1 would commence life with a 25% risk of being affected. Essentially the use of these markers means that the risk can be raised to almost 50% or lowered to almost zero.

Autosomal recessive inheritance

Linked markers have proven particularly valuable for the prenatal diagnosis of cystic fibrosis (Super *et al.*, 1987) and have largely superseded measurement of microvillar enzymes in amniotic fluid. Their application is considered in the following three examples.

Example 4. Information from one child

In Figure 9.4 the first child has an autosomal recessive disease, the locus for which is known to be closely linked to a polymorphic marker locus with alleles A and B. Calculation that the fetus (II2) will be affected, given different genotypes AA, AB and BB, has to take into account the posterior probabilities for the carrier

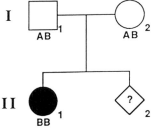

AA - $(4\theta^2)$

AB - (2θ) **Figure 9.4** *See* example 4. Autosomal recessive inheritance.
                        Approximate values for the probability that II2 will be
BB - $(1-4\theta)$ affected are indicated for each possible genotype

haplotypes in the parents based upon information provided by II1 who is affected
and has BB markers. These posterior probabilities are calculated as shown.

   Phase of disease gene in father (F) and mother (M)

	F(A) M(A)	F(A) M(B)	F(B) M(A)	F(B) M(B)
Probability				
Prior	¼	¼	¼	¼
Conditional. II1 has BB	θ^2	$\theta(1-\theta)$	$(1-\theta)\theta$	$(1-\theta)^2$

From this table it is apparent that the posterior probabilities for each of the four
different parental disease haplotypes are:

   Father A : Mother A – θ^2
   Father A : Mother B – $\theta(1-\theta)$
   Father B : Mother A – $(1-\theta)\theta$
   Father B : Mother B – $(1-\theta)^2$

1. Fetus (II2) has AA genotype

The total probability that the fetus will be affected if it inherits an AA genotype will
be the sum of:

a. the probability if the disease gene is coupled with A in the father and A in the
    mother i.e.

   $\theta^2 \times (1-\theta)^2$ plus

b. the probability if the disease gene is coupled with A in the father and B in the
    mother, i.e.

   $\theta(1-\theta) \times (1-\theta)\theta$ plus

c. the probability if the disease gene is coupled with B in the father and A in the
    mother, i.e.

   $(1-\theta)\theta \times \theta(1-\theta)$ plus

d. the probability if the disease gene is coupled with B in the father and B in the
    mother, i.e.

$$(1 - \theta)^2 \times \theta^2$$

This summates to $4\theta^2(1 - \theta)^2$ which equals

$$4\theta^2 - 8\theta^3 + 4\theta^4.$$

2. Fetus (II2) has BB genotype

The total probability that the fetus will be affected if it inherits a BB genotype will be the sum of:

a. the probability if the disease gene is coupled with A in the father and A in the mother, i.e.

$\theta^2 \times \theta^2$ plus

b. the probability if the disease gene is coupled with A in the father and B in the mother, i.e.

$\theta(1 - \theta) \times \theta(1 - \theta)$ plus

c. the probability if the disease gene is coupled with B in the father and A in the mother, i.e.

$(1 - \theta)\theta \times (1 - \theta)\theta$ plus

d. the probability if the disease gene is coupled with B in both parents, i.e.

$$(1 - \theta)^2 \times (1 - \theta)^2$$

This summates to $\theta^4 + 2\theta^2(1 - \theta)^2 + (1 - \theta)^4$ which equals

$$1 - 4\theta + 8\theta^2 - 8\theta^3 + 4\theta^4.$$

3. Fetus (II2) has AB genotype

In this situation the fetus could have inherited A from father and B from mother or vice-versa. If it is assumed that the A has come from the father and the B from the mother then the total probability that the fetus will be affected will be the sum of:

a. the probability if the disease gene is coupled with A in the father and A in the mother, i.e.

$\theta^2 \times (1 - \theta)\theta$ plus

b. the probability if the disease gene is coupled with A in the father and B in the mother, i.e.

$\theta(1 - \theta) \times (1 - \theta)^2$ plus

c. the probability if the disease gene is coupled with B in the father and A in the mother, i.e.

$(1 - \theta)\theta \times \theta^2$ plus

d. the probability if the disease gene is coupled with B in the father and B in the mother, i.e.

$$(1 - \theta)^2 \times \theta(1 - \theta)$$

This summates to $2\theta(1 - \theta)^3 + 2\theta^3(1 - \theta)$ which equals

$2\theta - 6\theta^2 + 8\theta^3 - 4\theta^4$.

An identical result will be obtained if the fetus has inherited A from the mother and B from the father. Thus whichever way the AB genotype has been derived, it conveys a probability of $2\theta - 6\theta^2 + 8\theta^3 - 4\theta^4$ for being affected. Note that this value should not be doubled since the fetus cannot have inherited both A from father with B from mother *plus* B from father and A from mother.

Since θ is likely to be a very small number (e.g. less than 0.01 for most of the linked markers used in the prenatal diagnosis of cystic fibrosis) reasonable approximations for the probability that the fetus will be affected are:

Genotype   AA – $4\theta^2$
             AB – 2θ
             BB – $1 - 4\theta$.

Example 5. Information from two children

In Figure 9.5 two children are affected and fortunately they show concordance for the linked marker genotypes. If they were totally discordant with, e.g. II1 having an AA genotype and II2 a BB genotype, then the family would not be 'informative' and prenatal diagnosis could not be offered. If they were partially discordant so that II1 had an AA genotype and II2 an AB genotype then the family would be partially informative in that a fetus inheriting a BB genotype would be at very low risk, but at relatively high risk for each of the other two genotypes.

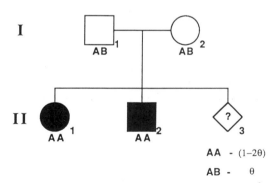

AA - $(1-2\theta)$

AB - θ

BB - θ^2

Figure 9.5 *See* example 5. Autosomal recessive inheritance. Approximate values for the probability that II3 will be affected are indicated for each possible genotype

In situations such as these the calculations become very lengthy. However, in the example shown in Figure 9.5 the fact that the linkage information is concordant in the two children means that the linkage phase in the parents can reasonably be assumed, i.e. the disease gene in both parents is in coupling with marker A. This enables risks for II3 given different genotypes to be calculated relatively easily. Thus if the fetus inherits an AA genotype then the likelihood that it will be affected equals $(1 - \theta)^2$ which equals $1 - 2\theta + \theta^2$ and approximates to $1 - 2\theta$. If the fetus inherits an AB genotype then the likelihood that it will be affected equals $(1 - \theta) \times$

θ which equals $\theta - \theta^2$ and approximates to θ. Finally, if the fetus inherits a BB genotype then the likelihood that it will be affected equals θ^2.

Example 6. Use of linkage disequilibrium

Recent studies have revealed that cystic fibrosis shows very strong linkage disequilibrium* with two very tightly linked markers identified by the probes CS.7 and XV-2c (Estivill *et al.*, 1987). These markers are so closely linked to the cystic fibrosis locus that, for practical purposes, it can be assumed that recombination never occurs between them. Furthermore, the disequilibrium is such that on 90% of chromosomes carrying the cystic fibrosis gene there will also be a CS.7 number 2 marker allele and an XV-2c number 1 marker allele. In contrast the CS.7(2)/XV-2c(1) haplotype is found on only 29% of normal chromosomes (Farrall, Estivill and Williamson, 1987).

This information can be used to modify risks for family members and their spouses as indicated in Figure 9.6. The top half of this figure shows the haplotypes for the CS.7 and XV-2c probes in the parents, their three children and their healthy daughter's spouse. A few moments study indicates that in both parents the cystic fibrosis gene must be coupled with a CS.7(2)/XV-2c(1) haplotype as indicated in the lower diagram. Remembering that a cross-over is extremely improbable

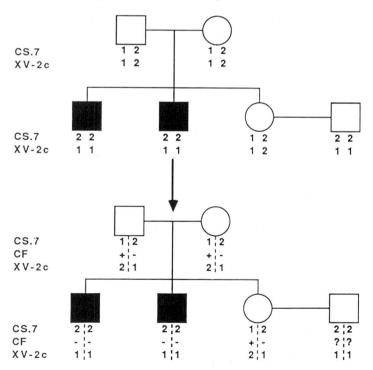

Figure 9.6 *See* example 6. The two affected boys have cystic fibrosis. Haplotypes obtained using the CS.7 and XV-2c probes are indicated. + equals the normal allele. − equals the cystic fibrosis allele. *See* text for full explanation

*The CF gene has now been identified and 70% of Caucasian defective genes carry a specific 3 base pair deletion. Diagnosis by RFLP is therefore now needed less often for this condition.

between these loci, it is apparent that the healthy sister has inherited one cystic fibrosis gene and is therefore a carrier.

It is also apparent that the healthy spouse of the sister has two 'high risk' cystic fibrosis haplotypes. What is the probability that this healthy spouse is also a carrier? This is calculated as follows remembering that the CS.7(2)/XV-2c(1) haplotype is found on 90% of cystic fibrosis chromosomes and on 29% of normal chromosomes, and that the gene frequency of cystic fibrosis equals 1 in 40 (everyone has two genes so that the incidence of carriers equals 1 in 20). Consider 1000 chromosomes in the general population: 25 of these carry the cystic fibrosis gene, of which $25 \times 0.9 = 22.5$ have the CS.7(2)/XV-2c(1) haplotype. The remaining 975 chromosomes do not carry the cystic fibrosis gene. Of these $975 \times 0.29 = 282.75$ have the CS.7(2)/XV-2c(1) haplotype. Thus for any chromosome with this haplotype there is a probability of

$$\frac{22.5}{22.5 + 282.75}$$

that it also carries the cystic fibrosis gene. This equals 0.0737 or approximately

$$\frac{1}{13.5}.$$

Thus for the healthy sister's spouse, who has two high risk haplotypes, there is a probability of $(0.0737)^2$ that he is homozygous affected, $2 \times 0.0737 \times 0.9263$ that he is heterozygous (i.e. a carrier) and $(0.9263)^2$ that he is homozygous normal, i.e.

homozygous affected – 0.0054
heterozygous   – 0.1365
homozygous normal – 0.8580

If the healthy sister's spouse is in good health then he clearly does not have cystic fibrosis so that the overall probability that he is a carrier equals

$$\frac{0.1365}{0.1365 + 0.8580}$$

which equals 0.137. or approximately 1 in 7.

Returning to Figure 9.6, it is now possible to inform the healthy sister and her spouse that there is a probability of approximately 1/28 (i.e. $1 \times 1/7 \times 1/4$) that their first baby would be affected with cystic fibrosis. This would rise to 1/14 if the fetus was found to have inherited its mother's cystic fibrosis chromosome. In a situation such as this some parents might feel that they would wish to avail themselves of microvillar enzyme assay in amniotic fluid even though this technique does carry a small risk of giving an incorrect result (Brock, 1988).

Sex-linked recessive inheritance

It is with sex-linked recessive disorders that linked markers have been of greatest value. This applies particularly to Duchenne muscular dystrophy in which, despite isolation of the gene and its protein product, carrier detection is still often very difficult. Other conditions susceptible to the linkage approach include Bruton's agammaglobulinaemia, Norrie's disease and the sex-linked form of retinitis pigmentosa.

Example 7. Phase unknown

In Figure 9.7, the mother II2 must be a carrier since she has had both an affected brother and an affected son. However, the phase in the mother is not known since all of the relatives needed to establish phase have died. Thus, as in example 2, account has to be taken of the possibility that the disease gene in II2 could be in coupling with either marker A or marker B.

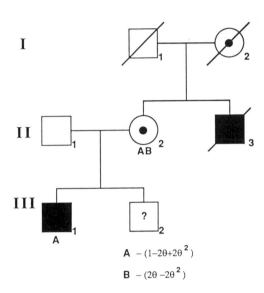

Figure 9.7 *See* example 7. Sex-linked recessive inheritance. The probability that III2 will be affected is indicated for each possible genotype

$$A - (1-2\theta+2\theta^2)$$

$$B - (2\theta - 2\theta^2)$$

Using the method outlined in example 2 it can be shown by taking into account information provided by III1 that there is a posterior probability of $1 - \theta$ that the disease is coupled with marker A in II2. Similarly it can be shown that there is a probability of θ that the disease is coupled with B in II2. Thus if III2 inherits marker A, there is a probability of $(1 - \theta)(1 - \theta)$ (if the disease is coupled with A) plus $\theta \times \theta$ (if the disease is coupled with B) that III2 will be affected. This summates to $1 - 2\theta + 2\theta^2$. In the same way it can be shown that there is a probability of $2\theta - 2\theta^2$ that III2 will be affected if he inherits marker B. Thus, as in example 2, there will be a predictive error of $2\theta - 2\theta^2$.

Example 8. Mother's carrier status unknown

In Figure 9.8, II1 represents an isolated case of a 'lethal' sex-linked recessive condition such as Duchenne muscular dystrophy. This is a relatively common situation in genetic counselling. To estimate risks for II3 it is necessary to take into account the likelihood that the mother I2 is a carrier as opposed to the likelihood that the disease has arisen in II1 as the result of a new mutation occurring in his mother's ovum. This involves some simple understanding of basic genetics.

It can be shown relatively easily that there is a probability of four times the mutation rate (μ) that any woman is a carrier of a particular sex-linked recessive

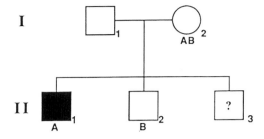

Figure 9.8 *See* example 8. Sex-linked recessive inheritance. When estimating risks for II3 the possibility that II1 represents a new mutation has to be taken into account. *See* text for full explanation

disorder. This value can thus be used as the prior probability that the mother I2 is a carrier.

	I2 is a carrier		I2 is not a carrier
Probability Prior	4μ		$1 - 4\mu = 1$
	Disease is coupled with A ½	Disease is coupled with B ½	
Conditional 1. Affected son has inherited A	$1 - \theta$	θ	μ
2. Healthy son has inherited B	$1 - \theta$	θ	1
Joint	$2\mu(1 - \theta)^2$	$2\mu\theta^2$	μ

Thus the posterior probability that the mother is a carrier and that the disease is coupled with A equals:

$$\frac{2\mu(1 - \theta)^2}{2\mu(1 - \theta)^2 + 2\mu\,\theta^2 + \mu} \quad \text{which reduces to} \quad \frac{2 - 4\theta + 2\theta^2}{3 - 4\theta + 4\theta^2} \quad (1)$$

Similarly the posterior probability that the mother is a carrier and that the disease is coupled with B equals:

$$\frac{2\mu\,\theta^2}{2\mu(1 - \theta)^2 + 2\mu\,\theta^2 + \mu} \quad \text{which reduces to} \quad \frac{2\theta^2}{3 - 4\theta + 4\theta^2} \quad (2)$$

The great value of this technology is illustrated by considering risks for II3 given different genotypes. If this baby inherits marker A the probability that he will be affected equals **(1)** × $(1 - \theta)$ plus **(2)** × θ. This will give a risk close to 2/3 if θ is small. However, if II3 inherits marker B, then the probability that he will be affected equals **(1)** × θ plus **(2)** × $(1 - \theta)$. This reduces to

$$\frac{2\theta - 2\theta^2}{3 - 4\theta + 4\theta^2}$$

If θ equals 0.05 this gives a risk of approximately 1 in 30 which is very much less than the risk of ¼ which would have been given if no information had been available using linked markers.

Discussion

There are a number of important points and potentially limiting factors which should be borne in mind when using linked markers for carrier detection and prenatal diagnosis.

1. First of all it is apparent that it is often necessary to study blood samples from members of the extended family so that linkage phase can be determined. Thus problems can arise if relatives who are critical for establishing phase refuse to give blood or have died. It is for this reason that vigorous efforts are now made to store blood and 'bank DNA' from relevant family members whenever possible.
2. If the family is not 'informative', in the sense that critical family members do not show heterozygosity for marker genes then obviously no predictive tests can be carried out. The only way to resolve this problem is to use different probe-enzyme combinations and hope that eventually an informative pattern is obtained.
3. Incorrect conclusions may be reached if the family contains instances of non-paternity. This can be tested for using the relatively new genetic fingerprinting probes. However, demonstration of non-paternity can clearly present major ethical problems which have to be handled with great care.
4. Using linked markers invariably means that there is a possibility of recombination so that every test carries with it a degree of predictive error, as illustrated by the examples in this chapter. Increasingly the use of more tightly linked probes is reducing the likelihood of recombination. The use of two flanking probes which bridge the disease locus reduces predictive error to almost negligible proportions. However, it has to be pointed out that the application of flanking probes can generate some very difficult calculations (Winter, 1985)!
5. Many apparently homogeneous genetic disorders show non-allelic heterogeneity. Thus the possibility of a second locus for a disease should always be kept in mind. Ideally every family should be tested to ensure that the disease cosegregates with the linked markers, but in practice this is rarely possible.

Despite these considerable limitations it is apparent that the use of linked markers can be of great value in predicting disease status and many families have benefited enormously from their introduction. Those who are totally confused by the complex mathematics can derive comfort from the fact that eventually this approach will become obsolete as disease specific mutations are identified. Meanwhile it is hoped that the contents of this chapter will help provide at least some insight into the intricacies of risk prediction using linked DNA markers.

References

Brock, D.J.H. (1988) Prenatal diagnosis of cystic fibrosis. *Archives of Disease in Childhood*, **63**, 701–704

Estivill, X., Scambler, P.J., Wainwright, B.J. *et al.* (1987) Patterns of polymorphism and linkage disequilibrium for cystic fibrosis. *Genomics*, **1**, 257–263

Farrall, M., Estivill, X. and Williamson, R. (1987) Indirect cystic fibrosis carrier detection. *Lancet*, ii, 156–157

Harper, P.S. and Sarfarazi, M. (1985) Genetic prediction and family structure in Huntington's chorea. *British Medical Journal*, **290**, 1929–1931

Hoffman, E.P., Brown, R.H. and Kunkel, L.M. (1987) Dystrophin: the protein product of the Duchenne muscular dystrophy locus. *Cell*, **51**, 919–928

Hoffman, E.P., Fischbeck, K.H., Brown, R.H. *et al.* (1988) Characterisation of dystrophin in muscle-biopsy specimens from patients with Duchenne's or Becker's muscular dystrophy. *New England Journal of Medicine*, **318**, 1363–1368

Lathrop, G.M. and Lalouel, J.M. (1984) Easy calculations of lod scores and genetic risks on small computers. *American Journal of Human Genetics*, **36**, 460–465

Reeders, S.T., Zerres, K., Gal, A. *et al.* (1986) Prenatal diagnosis of autosomal dominant polycystic kidney disease with a DNA probe. *Lancet,* **ii**, 6–8

Super, M., Ivinson, A., Schwarz, M. *et al.* (1987) Clinic experience of prenatal diagnosis of cystic fibrosis by use of linked DNA probes. *Lancet,* **ii**, 782–784

Upadhyaya, M., Sarfarazi, M., Huson, S.M., Broadhead, W., Fryer, A. and Harper, P.S. (1989) Close flanking markers for neurofibromatosis Type 1 (NF1). *American Journal of Human Genetics*, **44**, 41–47

Winter, R.M. (1985) The estimation of recurrence risks in monogenic disorders using flanking marker loci. *Journal of Medical Genetics*, **22**, 12–15

Chapter 10

Invasive diagnostic procedures

R.J. Lilford

Introduction

Prenatal diagnostic tests, like Gaul, can be divided into three groups: those involving measurement of chemicals in maternal blood; imaging the fetus; and invasive tests to remove tissues of fetal origin (including embryo biopsy). Maternal blood tests are essentially screening tests and these have been covered in Chapter 4. Fetal imaging, mostly by ultrasound at present, has characteristics of both a screening and a diagnostic test. Invasive tests, on the other hand, are by and large diagnostic tests which are carried out in people who are already known to be at increased risk. For the patient and her doctor the most important consideration is the risk to the fetus. The indications for invasive prenatal diagnostic tests have been discussed in the chapters dealing with chromosomal and single gene disorders. It should be said, however, that the final indication for an invasive test occurs when a patient perceives the expected utility of the test to be greater than that of no test. This in turn will depend on her perception of the probability of the disease in question and the probability of a harmful result from the invasive test, along with her valuation of these outcomes. The preceding chapters of this book have been concerned with the probabilities of congenital disease. The present chapter concerns the probability of harmful effects from invasive tests. Chapter 11 discusses the measurement and ascertainment of human values and how these can be combined with the probabilities to construct a decision tree.

Amniocentesis

Amniocentesis may be carried out at all gestational ages, between about 10 weeks and term. Traditionally this test is offered at about 16 weeks of gestational age, although we often carry out the procedure at 14 or 15 weeks. In most cases, culture of amniotic fluid cells is required for prenatal diagnosis and this takes a further 1–4 weeks, depending on the number of cells required and individual variations in the speed of cell growth. Depending on the length of time required for analysis, results of 16-week amniocentesis are therefore available somewhere between 18 and 22 weeks of gestational age. More recently, amniocentesis has been carried out at much earlier gestational ages, down to about 10 weeks of pregnancy. I will, therefore, discuss amniocentesis in two sections, one dealing with traditional amniocentesis and the other with early amniocentesis. For traditional amniocentesis I refer to those cases where the amniocentesis is carried out beyond 13 completed weeks of gestational age.

Traditional amniocentesis

Technique

The correct line for insertion of the needle is chosen by ultrasound. There is some difference of practice between those who select a point of entry and then carry out the technique with no further reference to ultrasound, and those who guide the needle into the correct position under continuous ultrasound control. The latter technique is greatly to be preferred, not because it is necessarily safer but because it is more reassuring for the patient. Patients are aware that the fetus is highly mobile within the amniotic sac and are therefore concerned about the possibility of a direct fetal hit if the operator cannot watch the needle tip at all times.

There are a number of measures which have been recommended to decrease the chance of miscarriage and although some of these have achieved universal acceptance, I recommend that they should all be followed where possible. A small needle should be used, and in practice this usually involves gauge 23. As little fluid as possible should be removed (15–20 ml). The placenta should be avoided and if the procedure is guided by ultrasound in real time, then it is almost always possible to thread the needle into the amniotic cavity, while avoiding both the placenta and the fetus. The fetal surface of the placenta contains a large number of thin walled veins, which do not have the retractile properties of the main umbilical vein and fatal haemorrhage following puncture of these chorial vessels has been documented. We also recommend full aseptic skin preparation since both acute and chronic infections are possible following amniocentesis.

Accuracy

The first problem that may occur is complete failure of culture and although the incidence of this complication is less than 1%, patients should be warned in advance of this possibility. The next problem is that of maternal cell contamination which could occasionally lead to false-negative diagnosis. Again the incidence of contamination is low (about 1 in 600 cases). Finally there is the problem of mosaicism and this topic has been dealt with in detail in Chapter 6.

Danger of amniocentesis

A small risk of relative pulmonary hypoplasia is reported and confirmed in both animal experiments and a randomized trial (Tabor et al., 1986). There is also a minute (less than 1 in 10000) risk of severe sepsis. The main danger is that of miscarriage. It is always difficult to generalize about the safety of any surgical procedure, since this is inevitably strongly influenced by personal skill. There are series of amniocenteses with miscarriage rates of the order of 0.5% (Katayama and Roesler, 1986). Most people believe, on the basis of large series, that the miscarriage rates following amniocentesis are of the order of 0.5–2% (Kappel et al., 1987). A recent randomized trial, in women under 35 (Tabor et al., 1986), has suggested that the overall excess risk of miscarriage due to this test is 1%. Although in their original paper they stated that the amniocenteses in this series were carried out with an 18-gauge needle, they have subsequently retracted this statement and indicated that a smaller needle was in fact used. I think it is reasonable for an expert in invasive diagnostic procedures to quote patients a procedure-related miscarriage rate of the order of 0.5%.

Early amniocentesis

The miscarriage rates of this procedure have not been published but animal experiments show that pulmonary hypoplasia occurs to a greater degree when the amniotic fluid is removed very early in pregnancy (Hislop, Howard and Fairweather, 1984). This technique also requires precise ultrasound directed biopsy similar to that necessary for transabdominal chorionic villus sampling (CVS) (*see below*) and there is therefore no advantage over CVS in terms of ease of sampling. First trimester amniocentesis will also not overcome the problem of placental mosaicism (*see* Chapter 6) because amniotic fluid contains a very high proportion of trophoblast derived cells in early pregnancy and culture is prone to failure before 12 weeks' gestational age (MacLachlan *et al.*, 1989). This technique, does, however, have a special place for the diagnosis of certain inborn errors of metabolism, where confirmatory backup amniocentesis is sometimes required after chorionic villus sampling has given a reassuring result (e.g. in the diagnosis of tyrosinaemia).

Chorionic villus sampling (biopsy)

The history of chorionic villus biopsy

The possibility of harvesting chorionic tissue has been known for over a decade, following attempts to obtain biopsies under direct vision through a hysteroscope. The methodology at this time was relatively crude and this technique was never introduced into clinical practice (Hahnemann, 1974). Subsequently, attempts were made to harvest exfoliated trophoblast cells from the internal os by means of a simple throat swab. Such cells were highly contaminated by maternal decidual tissue and this precluded the use of exfoliative cytology as a clinical method (Rhine, Palmer and Thompson, 1977). A simple technique of transcervical villus aspiration was developed in the Tietung hospital of an iron and steel company in Mainland China (Tietung Hospital of Ansham, 1975). This technique was not ultrasound-guided and the authors claimed a very high success rate and an abortion rate of only 5% of continuing pregnancies.

The next report of a transcervical villus aspiration technique came from the Soviet Union (Kazy, Rozovsky and Bakharev, 1982), where the technique was used in clinical practice for fetal sexing, in fetuses at risk of sex-linked disorders, and for a number of enzyme assays. Kazy has since returned to his native Hungary. The technique was first introduced to the West on an experimental basis prior to termination of pregnancy at St Mary's Hospital in London. This technique was initially carried out without ultrasound control but it was soon found that this was necessary for clinical use and all serious investigators throughout the world now use an ultrasound-directed technique (Horwell, Loeffler and Coleman, 1983). Over the last 8 years, since the first report in the West from St Mary's Hospital, the technique has been widely applied in Britain, Italy, Scandinavia, Denmark, the

Netherlands, France and the USA. A central registry has been formed in Philadelphia and over 100 000 cases have been reported to this source.

A more recent refinement of this technique has been the development of a transabdominal method for obtaining chorionic villus tissue. A blind transabdominal placental biopsy was carried out for the diagnosis of hydatidiform mole in 1965 (Alvarez, 1965). The theoretical and practical advantages of this technique are discussed later. However, the present method was developed independently by my team and a Danish group (Lilford and Maxwell, 1984; Smidt-Jensen and Hahnemann, 1984; Maxwell et al., 1986; Lilford et al., 1987). It is also possible to obtain chorionic villi at very early stages of gestation by aspiration through the vaginal fornices, guided by the vaginal probe.

The anatomy of the chorion in the first trimester of pregnancy

The chorion consists of an outer layer of trophoblast and an inner mesodermal layer containing blood vessels. At 5 weeks of pregnancy (3 weeks post-fertilization) the entire chorion participates equally in villus formation producing 200 tree-like colonies of villi which completely surround the embryo. Over the following weeks the villi facing towards the uterine cavity gradually degenerate to form the chorion laevae while those adjacent to the decidua basalis proliferate to form the placenta. Further growth takes place in this area due to fresh villus formation from the villus stems and progressive arborization of previously formed villi. At 6 weeks of pregnancy (4 weeks after fertilization) the chorionic vesicle begins to intrude into the cavity of the uterus. The decidua covering the vesicle is the decidua capsularis and that on the maternal aspect of the vesicle is the decidua basalis. The decidua parietalis lines the remainder of the body of the uterus. The cervical mucous membrane does not undergo decidual change but secretes a thick mucous plug which *seals* the cervical canal.

At 8 weeks of pregnancy (6 weeks of embryonic life) chorionic villus sampling becomes a possibility. The embryo is now 15 mm in length and the chorion frondosum is 3–6 mm thick while the decidua capsularis measures less than 2 mm. At 10 weeks (8 weeks of embryonic life), probably the optimal time for chorion villus biopsy, the embryo measures 25 mm and further thinning of the chorion laevae has taken place. The chorionic vesicle almost fills the uterine cavity but this will not be completely obliterated until the decidua capsularis fuses with the parietalis at 16–20 weeks of pregnancy (Hamilton and Boyd, 1970). By the end of the first trimester (10 weeks post-fertilization) the villi adjacent to the decidua capsularis are reduced to microscopical stumps and the extra-embryonic coelom has disappeared by fusion of the amnion with the chorion.

The timing of chorionic villus biopsy

Most workers feel that it is undesirable to perform a chorionic villus biopsy before 8 weeks of gestation because of the rapid embryonic development and organogenesis which takes place prior to this time. Nevertheless, this is entirely intuitive advice and, in the case of transabdominal or cervical aspiration, as opposed to transvaginal aspiration or hysteroscopic methods, there is a more important practical reason why the technique is normally deferred until 8 weeks, namely because the chorion frondosum is not clearly identifiable prior to this time. It is widely believed that the optimal time for transcervical chorionic villus biopsy is between 8 and 11 weeks of gestation. The transabdominal technique may, however, be carried out at any subsequent stage of pregnancy.

The technique of chorionic biopsy

Current techniques for *transcervical* chorionic biopsy may be grouped into those dependent on biopsy forceps (Gosden *et al.*, 1982; Rodeck and Morsman, 1983) and those where various forms of cannula are used (Maxwell *et al.*, 1985b). The latter are far more widely used but an adaption of the former demonstrates the technological refinement which may be applied to this technique. The method has been described by Gustavii (Gustavii, 1983; Gustavii *et al.*, 1984; Nordenskjold and Gustavii, 1984) in Sweden and is carried out as follows: a hysteroscope is passed through the interal os and the uterine cavity is filled with up to 150 ml of warmed saline. A tiny punch biopsy is taken at the point where the decidua capsularis reflects back onto the side wall of the uterus to form the decidua parietalis. A fibreoptic scope is introduced through this tiny hole affording direct visualization of the villus fronds (villoscopy or chorionoscopy). (This creates an appearance analogous to that seen by a scuba diver in a coral reef.) The first villi to be encountered on the edge of the chorion frondosum are short and white, and grow poorly in culture. The operator therefore directs the tip of the fibreoptic scope into the lush, more central area where highly sprouting and vascular villi are found and takes his biopsy from this area under direct vision.

This level of refinement is obviously not applicable to widespread use and is not associated with the lowest achievable fetal loss rates. The majority of operators use metal or plastic cannulae (Rodeck *et al.*, 1983a,b; Elias *et al.*, 1985; Maxwell *et al.*, 1985b; Perry *et al.*, 1985; Green *et al.*, 1988). The placental site is identified by ultrasound with the operator's fingers in the vagina so that the exact relationship to the cervix may be ascertained. The malleable cannula is then bent to the appropriate shape (Figure 10.1) and inserted through the cervix and guided into the

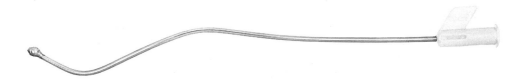

Figure 10.1 A malleable metal cannula with a smooth tip, suitable for atraumatic transcervical CVS

chorion frondosum. The aspiration is normally taken about half way between the edge of the forming placenta and the umbilical insertion. The aspirate is immediately examined in theatre. 'Bush-like' villi with many sprouts will contain more mitotic figures than smooth 'root-like' villi (Verlinsky *et al.*, 1985). Chorionic villi have a characteristic fluffy, white appearance and float to the surface of the culture medium (Figure 10.2). There are, however, many traps for the unwary operator with this deceptively simple technique.

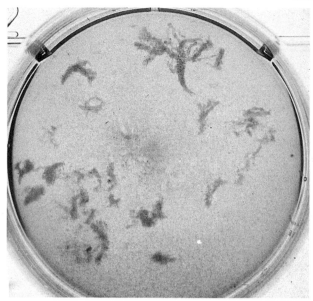

Figure 10.2 Magnified picture of bushy chorionic villi floating in culture medium after aspiration

The technique of transabdominal chorionic villus biopsy

The fundus of the pregnant uterus usually comes to lie against the abdominal wall after about 8 weeks of gestational age. The uterus can therefore be reached through the abdominal wall at this point without traversing the bladder or bowel (Figure 10.3). This route provides access to both the anterior and posterior walls of the uterus but, in order to reach the latter without penetrating the amniotic cavity, an empty bladder is required (Figure 10.4). In very rare cases, the uterus may still be acutely retroverted at this stage of pregnancy, but even this can be corrected by vaginal manipulation.

At St James's Hospital, Leeds, an 18-gauge stilette pointed needle is inserted through the abdominal and uterine walls to reach the placental edge. This is used as a conduit for a thinner 20-gauge needle which is inserted to a point midway between the placental edge and the umbilical cord insertion. It is from here that villi are aspirated and, if the first attempt is unsuccessful, the outer needle can again serve to guide the aspirating needle to the correct position. In this way, the need for multiple insertions through the uterine wall is obviated.

The technique may be carried out 'free-hand' (Brambati, Oldrini and Lanzani, 1987) or by means of a biopsy attachment on the transducer. The latter is easier for beginners and modern equipment allows the exact depth of required penetration to be measured.

Dangers of chorionic villus biopsy

The best figures available for fetal loss after chorionic biopsy come from the international register maintained by Laird Jackson in Philadelphia. A record is kept

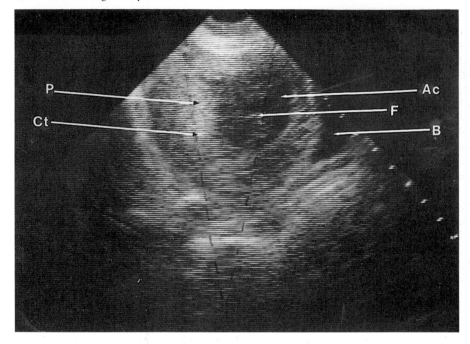

Figure 10.3 Ultrasound picture of a 9-week uterus showing: P – placenta; Ct – cannula tip; Ac – amniotic cavity; F – fetal parts; B – maternal bladder

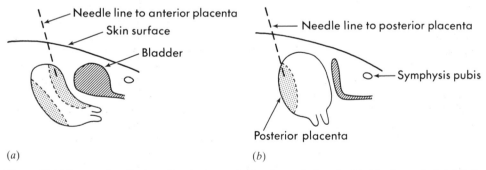

(a)   (b)

Figure 10.4 Diagram showing how the uterus usually tips forward when the bladder is emptied. (a) Full bladder; (b) empty bladder

of pregnancies, where the result of the chorionic biopsy was normal, and where abortion occurred. The most striking feature of this register is the wide variation in reported abortion rates for transcervical chorionic biopsy, with figures varying from 2% to 30%. The six European and American centres with the greatest experience report an abortion rate of approximately 3%. In order to calculate procedure-related fetal losses, the background abortion rate for similar cases must be subtracted from this overall figure. Overall abortion rates at various stages of pregnancy have been documented (Gustavii, 1984; Hobbins, 1984) but these are of little relevance to the risk of miscarriage where the fetus is seen to be intact on ultrasound.

A number of studies have now addressed specifically the probability of fetal loss in pregnancies shown by ultrasound to be intact and viable at around 10 weeks' gestation (e.g. Wilson *et al.*, 1984). Exclusion of patients with missed abortions shows that the background abortion rate for ultrasonically viable pregnancies at 10 weeks' gestation is no more than 2%. This is probably an overestimate as patients having ultrasound in the first trimester are a selected group. The procedure-related fetal loss rate in the best hands would therefore seem to be 2% and thus compares unfavourably to amniocentesis (0.3–1%) (National Institute of Child Health and Development, 1976; Tabor *et al.*, 1986). This argument, however, remains inconclusive; patients requiring chorionic biopsy are often older and may therefore have a higher risk of abortion. On the other hand, it can be argued that this higher rate is due to chromosomal abnormalities and, as affected fetuses are eliminated from the quoted abortion rates, this factor does not apply. CVS is undertaken, on average, at an earlier gestational age and this confounding variable might bias results in favour of amniocentesis. A prospective trial found no increased risk with CVS but selection bias may have been at work (Crane, Beaver and Cheung, 1988). The only way to resolve this issue is by randomized trials using amniocentesis patients as controls. The Canadian trial suggests an excess fetal loss of at least 1% with transcervical CVS, although the losses were extraordinarily high in both groups and the relatively small sample size (2600) of this trial makes measurement imprecise. Results of the large British trial are awaited with interest but transabdominal CVS appears to be safer (*see below*). Randomized trials of transabdominal versus transcervical CVs are underway but are unlikely to show large differences, since it is the learning curves of these techniques that seem to differ most.

Abortions after invasive tests follow two patterns. A proportion occur within the first week of chorionic villus sampling and manifest with bleeding followed by abortion. A second and equally common form of abortion occurs between 1 and 5 weeks after the procedure. The fetus grows initially but this is followed by severe oligohydramnios, loss of the fetal heart and then abortion. The first pattern can be ascribed to mechanical disruption and this is seldom seen in units with considerable experience. The second pattern of abortion, however, is presumed to be due to infection, possibly of a chronic form, with an organism such as *Listeria*, *Chlamydia* or *Mycoplasma* (Scialli, Neugebauer and Fabro, 1985). A number of factors are known to increase the risk of abortion following *transcervical* chorionic biopsy. These include the need for repeated aspiration, a gestational age of greater than 11 weeks and immediate bleeding or sac puncture. In addition, ultrasonic demonstration of a subchorial haematoma or tract after the procedure may be associated with a higher chance of subsequent abortion (Maxwell and Lilford, 1985). Unfortunately, it is not possible to predict which pregnancies are at greatest risk of spontaneous abortion; gestational age related human chorionic gonadotrophin or gestation sac volume measurements correlate very poorly with pregnancy outcome (Jouppila *et al.*, 1984).

Not all these infections are of a chronic and incipient form leading to late abortion. Predictably, since the cervix is a highly contaminated area, cases of septic shock following transcervical chorionic biopsy have been reported (Jackson and Wapner, 1987) and this provides a strong argument in favour of the transabdominal technique. Admittedly a proportion of fetal losses following amniocentesis are accompanied by some evidence of amnionitis but septic shock and disseminated coagulation are much rarer features of transcutaneous techniques, while every gynaecologist is aware of the danger of ascending infection when the cervical barrier is breached. Signs of septicaemia following transcervical chorionic villus biopsy may appear before the fetus dies or any other signs of abortion become apparent.

Fetal blood cell antigens are expressed in the first trimester giving rise to the possibility of Rhesus sensitization. A small fetomaternal haemorrhage after chorionic sampling can be inferred from the demonstrated rise in alpha-fetoprotein immediately after the procedure (Warren et al., 1985). However, this is not confirmed by Kleihauer testing (Maxwell et al., 1985b; Warren et al., 1985). Nevertheless, the likelihood that fortuitous sensitization will be ascribed to the procedure has persuaded many workers to recommend anti-D prophylaxis for unsensitized Rhesus negative mothers. In addition, 0.1 ml of fetal blood is required to cause sensitization and as this represents half the total blood volume of a 9-week fetus the possibility of sensitization must be remote.

Follow-up after chorionic villus biopsy to date has shown no increase in the incidence of obstetric complications in surviving fetuses (Williams et al., 1987).

Multiple pregnancy

Twin pregnancy (or greater order) always presents a special challenge in prenatal diagnosis (Lilford, 1985). Amniocentesis is feasible because ultrasound identification of the septum separating all dizygotic and many monozygotic fetuses allows liquor to be drawn from each sac independently (Rodeck and Ivan, 1981). Selective fetocide can then be carried out if one twin is found to be affected. Separate sampling from the relatively amorphous placental mass is more difficult to ensure. Again the transabdominal method is advantageous as it affords precise localization of the needle tip. Confirmation of the separate origin of each sample can be obtained if they are of separate sex or if they have different chromosomal banding patterns. If these differences do not exist identification must rely on HLA antigens which have been demonstrated on cultured mesenchymal cells (Niazi et al., 1979) or on genetic finger-printing. Following diagnosis it may be more difficult to ensure selective termination of the appropriate fetus although this has been accomplished in the first trimester for a haemophiliac fetus (Mulcahy, Roberman and Reid, 1984).

Advantages of transabdominal chorionic biopsy

A number of series of transabdominal chorionic biopsies have now been reported (e.g. Lilford, et al., 1987, Smidt-Jensen and Hahnemann, 1988). Early results from the registry reported fetal losses of 2.1% with transabdominal CVS compared with over 3.0% with all transcervical techniques (Jackson, 1987). We have lost five fetuses in 520 CVS procedures, of which 470 gave normal results. Transabdominal biopsy avoids the contaminated cervical area and this should greatly reduce the chances of infection. We know from experience with amniocentesis that life-threatening infection is hardly ever carried in from the skin. In addition, there is a theoretical possibility that viral infections may be inoculated into the fetus following transcervical instrumentation. Ten per cent of pregnant women secrete cytomegalovirus from the cervix during pregnancy and 0.2–7% are asymptomatic carriers of Herpes simplex (Marchese et al., 1984). In theory, both procedures may be capable of inoculating HIV virus into the fetus.

The technique which has been described allows multiple sampling to be carried out from a single needle insertion, whereas recannulation is required if the transcervical method fails. A randomized trial has confirmed that the procedure is at least as effective as transcervical sampling in producing an acceptable sample (Brambati *et al.*, 1988). Our laboratory reports that the chorionic villi are relatively less contaminated with cervical mucus and decidua than was previously the case. Samples obtained through the fine needles used for the transabdominal method are much more predictable in size, whereas disturbingly large flushes of villi are sometimes obtained by transcervical aspiration. Many patients prefer this technique to the vaginal manipulation and lithotomy position which are necessary for transcervical biopsy. The transabdominal route is mandatory for patients with known genital herpes or those with an existing Shirodkar suture. However, all metal contains traces of copper and transcervical aspiration with a plastic cannula is therefore recommended for prenatal diagnosis of Menke's disease.

Economic aspects

The cost of medical technology is increasing more rapidly than the economic growth of most countries. Thus, if chorionic villus biopsy is to surplant amniocentesis for cytogenetic indications it must be both medically and economically acceptable. This is particularly so in countries where resources are allocated centrally and the consumer is less able to purchase the service which she requires directly. Prenatal diagnosis in general has considerable cost–benefit advantages over other branches of medicine, but this does not greatly influence regional budget holders preoccupied with the rigors of cash-flow rather than long-term national savings. A detailed cost–benefit analysis (Sadovnick and Baird, 1982) of chorionic villus biopsy in comparison to amniocentesis has not been carried out. Nevertheless, the author's personal enquiries suggest that the resources required for cytogenetic analysis of each chorionic villus biopsy are, at present, considerably greater than those needed for each amniocentesis. Direct preparations are popular with patients and avoid the risk of culture overgrowth with maternal cells but they require special handling and this consumes a similar amount of a technician's time to conventional analysis of amniotic fluid. Most laboratories then culture the tissue in order to detect the most subtle chromosome rearrangements on fully banded preparations and to lower the risk of a false-negative result. Thus the resources required for analysis of each chorionic villus biopsy are approximately double those required for conventional analysis of amniocentesis specimens. Furthermore, the ambiguous results which can arise from mosaic formation in the trophoblast will necessitate subsequent amniocentesis in some patients. The British Association of Clinical Cytogeneticists scores a blood sample and amniotic fluid sample at 250 units of work, while direct CVS scores 450 and culture CVS 550. These increased costs are unlikely to be offset by savings resulting from earlier and much simpler termination of pregnancy.

The costs resulting from amniocentesis are already limiting factors in some centres. If chorionic villus biopsy is to be offered on a national scale in most countries a less expensive approach should be sought. This could be achieved by relying on the direct preparation in most cases and performing culture only when the quality and quantity of metaphases is inadequate for confident diagnosis. A recent rapid and easy technique for freezing chorionic villi, pending the outcome of the direct preparation, would assist the implementation of this scheme (Endres *et al.*, 1985). Some very rare and small inversions and *de novo* translocations might go undetected, but this disadvantage would be offset as many more patients at risk of the more common and unambiguously deleterious aneuploidies could be offered prenatal diagnosis. At present chorionic villus biopsy specimens are analysed by enthusiastic laboratory staff with a research interest; routine laboratories will require a rationalized approach. The incidence of *de novo* rearrangements is very small; 66 were found in 76 952 amniocenteses (Warburton, 1984). This is less than 0.1% and many of these would be detectable on direct preparation. I know anecdotally of only one false-negative result for Down's syndrome on direct preparation only arising in Germany. Where either parent is known to carry a balanced translocation, full culture should be carried out. In other cases however, little would be lost by performing direct preparations only, in the first instance, provided it was understood that this was a Down's exclusion test rather than a full chromosome analysis.

Analysis of chorionic villus tissue

The most frequent indication for chorionic villus sampling is for karyotyping, but gene probe analysis, for which chorionic tissue is particularly suitable, is a rapidly growing indication. Admittedly this technique can be applied to cultured amniotic fluid cells which provide enough DNA for the technique; however, the large number of cells in chorionic villi provide sufficient DNA for direct processing without the need for culture. Enzyme analysis for a number of inborn errors of metabolism may also be carried out on this tissue.

Cytogenetic analysis

Samples may be prepared for cytogenetic analysis in one of two ways. The first is conventional culture. For this, villi must be trypsinized or cut into very thin slices to expose the mesenchymal cores (Niazi, Coleman and Loeffler, 1981; Heaton *et al.*, 1984). Fibroblasts from this area proliferate in culture medium and under suitable conditions provide sufficient cells for chromosomal analysis within 8 days (Schwab, Muller and Schmid-Tannwald, 1984). In addition, culture of chorionic cells in the presence of methotrexate has been used to diagnose the fragile site on the long arm of the X chromosome (Martin-Bell syndrome) (Tommerup *et al.*, 1985). This is an important development as this is the second commonest known cause of mental retardation in males. Nevertheless, this method is not completely reliable on chorionic villi and a negative result in a male fetus should be backed up with a culture of fetal blood obtained at 20 weeks' gestation.

Experiments with monoclonal antibodies directed against cellular microfilaments have confirmed the morphological impression that most cultured chorionic cells are of mesenchymal origin (Koskull *et al.*, 1985) and the further finding that they contain HLA antigens, absent from the trophoblast surface, adds additional evidence for this. The cytotrophoblast divides more slowly and the proportion of these cells decreases with duration of culture.

The so-called direct preparation chromosome analysis relies on the fact that a large number of cells in the Langhan's layer of the chorion frondosum will be in the process of division at any one time. These cells are therefore amenable to analysis without culture (Simoni *et al.*, 1983; Lilford *et al.*, 1983). A common practice involves overnight incubation in the presence of colchicine, which allows more cells in prophase to enter metaphase; the point where further division is arrested

(Terzoli *et al.*, 1985). One advantage of direct preparation is that the result is available to the patient within hours. An even greater advantage is that this method effectively eliminates concern over the possibility of maternal contamination. Thus, although one or two metaphases may be found in a deliberate decidual biopsy (Blakemore *et al.*, 1985), the finding of five or more identical karyotypes in a thoroughly cleaned and dissected chorionic sample may be regarded as entirely fetal in origin (Simoni *et al.*, 1984). In the case of culture techniques, there is a risk that maternal decidual fibroblasts (which divide more rapidly in culture), will overgrow fetal cells and cause an erroneous result. Although parallel culture of fetal and trophoblast samples in our own large series suggests that this occurs less often than one case in a hundred (Maxwell *et al.*, 1985b), the even greater certainty provided by the direct method is very welcome. The main disadvantage of the direct method is that the chromosomes are usually not as elongated and clearly separated as those obtained from cultured cells. A prolonged period of exposure to hypotonic saline improves separation of the chromosomes and this, together with the use of special stains, has been used to diagnose unbalanced translocations in uncultured cells (Sachs *et al.*, 1983; MacKenzie *et al.*, 1983). Most laboratories, however, rely on a direct preparation to provide a rapid answer regarding fetal sex or aneuploidy and culture to provide information about minor deletions and rearrangements. An adequate number of mitotic cells for direct analysis may be obtained at all stages of gestation.

It is now known that the chromosomal constitution of the trophoblast may not reflect that of the fetus itself (Kalousek and Dill, 1983) and placental mosaicism may aid survival in cases of fetal trisomy (Kalousek, Barrett and McGillivray, 1989). The formation of a mosaic in the early embryo may result in a normal cell line in the embryonic disc with the cells containing the abnormal chromosome complement confined to the trophoblast. It is interesting to note, therefore, that a number of cases have now been described where trisomy of chromosome 16 was detected on chorionic biopsy (*see* Chapter 6). This is a lethal malformation if present in the embryo and subsequent amniocentesis in these cases has, not surprisingly, shown that the fetus itself was unaffected. The trophoblast can apparently function normally in the presence of this trisomy. Mosaicism in culture is more likely to be represented in the fetus, since the mesenchyme (obtained in culture) is embryologically closer to the fetus than trophoblast which is analysed in direct and short-term incubation preparations. Mosaicism may also arise in trophoblast cultures (Ridler and Greural, 1984), but complete false-positive results, where both direct preparations and culture gave misleading results are extremely rare. We have reported (Lilford *et al.*, 1987) one such case where short- and long-term cultures showed a marker chromosome. This was not present in the fetal tissue cultured, but the fetus had multiple congenital abnormalities and the marker contained euchromatin. Thus, the fetus may have been mosaic after all. No case of a complete false-positive or negative diagnosis of Down's syndrome has been reported to this date (*see* Chapter 6). Furthermore, complete (i.e. occurring as both direct (or short-term culture) preparations and long-term culture) false-negative results are very rare (Martin *et al.*, 1986). We have had no such cases in nearly 500 samples and Callen *et al.* (1988) had no such case in 1312 cases. They encountered four false-positive results, but three of these were of a type which could be identified as such (e.g. trisomy 16) and one was monosomy X. Furthermore, no totally misleading results were found on analysis of 500 cases by Sachs *et al.* (1988). Discrepancies are, of course, not unique to trophoblast sampling (Hsu and Perlis, 1984); e.g. trisomy 20 mosaicism may occur with amniotic fluid culture and the fetus in these cases is almost always normal. The abnormal amniotic fluid (AF) cells in these cases are presumed to derive from extra-embryonic mesenchyme (Pan et al., 1976). Another easily recognized artefact which is more common in trophoblast cultures is tetraploidy (duplication of the entire diploid chromosome set) due to fusion of the nuclei. The proportion of polyploidic cells increases as cultures age.

The incidence of chromosomal abnormalities following amniocentesis for advancing maternal age is nearly twice that in liveborn populations. By the same token, autosomal and sex chromosome trisomies are two to three times as common in chorionic villus biopsy specimens as they are in amniotic fluid at the same maternal age (Mikkelsen, 1985).

Gene probe analysis

About 15 or 20 mg of chorionic tissue is reported to extract sufficient DNA (approximately 20 µg) to perform gene probe diagnosis based on Southern blots (Maxwell, et al., 1985c), but much smaller amounts can be used for the polymerase chain reaction. Since few hospitals have immediate access to laboratories carrying out this work, it is necessary to send samples to the appropriate centres. These techniques are described in Chapters 7, 8 and 9.

Enzyme diagnosis

The activities of lysosomal enzymes and of various enzymes involved in inborn errors of amino acid, organic acid and nucleic acid metabolism can be measured. The analysis may be carried out on cultured cells (Gibbs et al., 1984) or directly from uncultured chorionic villi (Kleijer et al., 1984; Vimal et al., 1984; Maxwell et al., 1985a). In the former case, specific measures may be used to separate the epithelial (trophoblastic) from the mesenchymal components of the villi prior to culture. As the expression of enzymes differs in the trophoblast and mesenchyme (Tsvetkova et al., 1982; Vimal et al., 1984), it is necessary to work out normal ranges of the particular method which the laboratory plans to use, and a number of misdiagnoses (false-positive and negative) have already been encountered. To date no enzymes have been detected in chorionic tissue which could not be assayed in cultured amniotic fluid cells and the hope that trophoblast would express enzymes, such as phenylalanine dehydrogenase and ornithine carbamyl transferase, has not been realized.

Techniques other than enzyme assay have been used for diagnosis of inborn errors of metabolism on chorionic villi. Incorporation studies on intact chorionic villi have been used for prenatal diagnosis of methylmalonicacidaemia and citrullinaemia (Galjaard, 1985) and the total copper concentration is of use in the diagnosis of Menke's syndrome (Horn et al., 1985).

Other laboratory tests on chorionic tissue

A number of other techniques are likely to be developed for the analysis of chorion tissue. Thus linkage studies have been used in the prenatal diagnosis of 21-hydroxylase deficiency by means of HLA typing of amniotic fluid cells. This can also be carried out on chorionic mesenchymal cultures, although gene probe rather than HLA linkage is now used and 'fetal therapy' (by maternal steroid administration) is often attempted in the case of an affected female fetus. It is also possible to detect Rhesus antigens, which are expressed from a very early gestational age. A mixture of maternal and fetal cells is usually obtained but provided a few fetal cells are present agglutination can be demonstrated (Kanhai *et al.*, 1984) in this way. Selective termination of Rhesus positive fetuses may prove more acceptable than plasmaphoresis and intrauterine transfusion for some sensitized mothers with heterozygous husbands. We have carried out 'forensic' prenatal diagnosis for a patient who wished to confirm, by genetic finger-printing using the Jeffrie's probe, that her fetus had resulted from rape by her father, before she requested pregnancy termination.

Fetal blood sampling and tissue biopsy

Fetal blood is traditionally obtained antenatally by fetoscopy, but this procedure has been almost completely abandoned in favour of cordocentesis (obtaining fetal blood by direct puncture of the umbilical vein) or sometimes by direct aspiration from the fetal heart.

These techniques are quite easy to perform, either transplacentally, in the case of an anterior placenta, or across the amniotic cavity in the case of a posterior implantation. We have found that colour flow Doppler system of the Acuson ultrasound machine greatly facilitates fetal blood sampling, since it makes the identification of the insertion of the umbilical vein into the placenta very much easier.

The trouble with these techniques at present, is that nobody knows quite what fetal loss rate to quote to patients, because most series contain many high risk cases, such as immune and non-immune hydrops. While Dr Daffos in Paris, claims a fetal loss rate of 1.4% (quoted by Whittle, 1989), it is unlikely that these excellent figures can be widely reproduced and most centres would be prudent to quote fetal loss rates of around 2% for the time being. We have experienced one fetal loss in 14 cases but this fetus was grossly abnormal. Foley, Sonek and O'Shaughnessy (1989) found 25 attributable fetal deaths among 1283 cases reported to the American Percutaneous Umbilical Blood Sampling Registry (PUBS); a rate of 1.9% per procedure, but we cannot be sure that all cases are correctly attributed and reporting bias is possible. The genetic indications for this technique are discussed in greater detail in Chapter 6 but amount essentially to clarifying ambiguous amniocentesis and CVS chromosome results, and the search for fragile X. The possibility of a false-negative result (especially direct preparations) for chromosome 18 trisomy inclines some practitioners away from CVS and towards blood sampling when a rapid karyotype is required in the case of anomalies associated with this trisomy (e.g. diaphragmatic hernia, exomphalos, finger deformity). In families who are partially or completely non-informative for gene probe diagnosis by fragment length polymorphisms, this technique is also required for diagnosis of haemoglobinopathies. It may also be necessary occasionally for the diagnosis of rare immune deficiency syndromes.

Fetal tissue sampling is very seldom required. Fetal liver biopsy was necessary until recently for the diagnosis of phenylketonuria, but gene probe diagnosis is now available both for this and ornithine carbamyl transferase deficiency. Thus, there remain only a handful of conditions, such as cystinosis, for which fetal liver biopsy is still required.

The other form of fetal tissue biopsy that is sometimes carried out is fetal skin biopsy which is necessary for the diagnosis of certain lethal bullous skin conditions. This is usually done under fetoscopic control, although ultrasound directed biopsies have been performed.

Endo and transcervical swabs have been used in an attempt to harvest fetal cells as mentioned earlier, but failure to confirm fetal tissue by cytological means hampered these investigations. The availability of the polymerase chain reaction, which can amplify tiny amounts of fetal DNA, is now allowing my co-workers to re-investigate these secretions. Similarly, gene amplification techniques appear capable of identifying fetal cells in maternal blood.

References

Alvarez, H. (1965) Diagnosis of hydatidiform mole by transabdominal placental biopsy. *Fetus and Newborn*, **95**, 538–541

Blakemore, K.J., Samuelson, J., Breg, W.R. and Mahoney, M.J. (1985) Maternal metaphases on direct chromosome preparation of first trimester decidua. *Human Genetics*, **69**, 380

Brambati, B., Oldrini, A. and Lanzani, A. (1987) Transabdominal chorionic villus sampling: a freehand ultrasound-guided technique. *American Journal of Obstetrics and Gynecology*, **157**, 134–137

Brambati, B., Oldrini, A., Lanzani, A., Terzian, E. and Tognoni, G. (1988) Transabdominal versus transcervical chorionic villus sampling: a randomized trial. *Human Reproduction*, **3**, 6

Callen, D.F., Korban, G., Dawson, G. *et al.* (1988) Extra embryonic/fetal karyotypic discordance during diagnostic chorionic villus sampling. *Prenatal Diagnosis*, **8**, 453–460

Crane, J.P., Beaver, H.A. and Cheung, S.W. (1988) First trimester chorionic villus sampling versus mid-trimester genetic amniocentesis. Preliminary results of a controlled prospective trial. *Prenatal Diagnosis*, **8**, 355–366

Elias, S., Simpson, J.L., Martin, A.O., Sabbagha, R.E., Gerbie, A.B. and Keith, L.G. (1985) Chorionic villus sampling for first-trimester prenatal diagnosis: Northwestern University Program. *American Journal of Obstetrics and Gynecology*, **152**, 204–213

Endres, M., Dawson, G., Wirtz, A. and Haindl, E. (1985) Freezing of chorionic villi. In *First Trimester Fetal Diagnosis* (Eds M. Fraccaro, G. Simoni and B. Brambati). Berlin: Springer-Verlag. pp. 201–204

Foley, M.R., Sonek, J. and O'Shaughnessy, R., (1989) Cordocentesis. Cracking the diagnostic and therapeutic barrier between fetus and physician. *Obstetrics/Gynecology Report*, **1**, 152–166

Galjaard, H. (1985) Biochemical analysis of chorionic villi: a worldwide survey of first trimester fetal diagnosis of inborn errors of metabolism. In *First Trimester Fetal Diagnosis* (Eds M. Fraccaro, G. Simoni and B. Brambati). Berlin: Springer-Verlag. pp. 209–217

Gibbs, D.A., Crawfurd, M.D'A., Headhouse-Benson, C.M. *et al.* (1984) First-trimester diagnosis of Lesch-Nyhan syndrome. *Lancet*, **ii**, 1180–1183

Green, J.E., Dorfmann, A., Jones, S.L., Bender, S., Patton, L. and Schulman, J.D. (1988) Chorionic villus sampling: experience with an initial 940 cases. *Obstetrics and Gynecology*, **71**, 208–212

Gosden, J.R., Gosden, C.M., Mitchell, A.R., Rodeck, C.H. and Morsman, J.M. (1982) Direct vision chorion biopsy and chromosome-specific DNA probes for determination of fetal sex in first trimester prenatal diagnosis. *Lancet*, **ii**, 1416–1419

Gustavii, B. (1983) First-trimester chromosomal analysis of chorionic villi obtained by direct vision technique. *Lancet*, **ii**, 507–508

Gustavii, B. (1984) Chorionic biopsy and miscarriage in first trimester. *Lancet*, **i**, 562

Gustavii, B., Chester, M.A., Edvall, H. *et al.* (1984) First-trimester diagnosis on chorionic villi obtained by direct vision technique. *Human Genetics*, **65**, 373–376

Hahnemann, N. (1974) Early prenatal diagnosis; a study of biopsy techniques and cell culturing from extraembryonic membranes. *Clinical Genetics*, **6**, 294–306

Hamilton, W.J. and Boyd, J.D. (1970) Development of the human placenta. In *Scientific Foundations of Obstetrics and Gynaecology* (Eds E. Philipp, J. Barnes and M. Newton) London: W. Heinemann Medical Books, pp. 185–253

Heaton, D.E., Czepulkowski, B.H., Horwell, D.H. and Coleman, D.V. (1984) Chromosome analysis of first trimester chorionic villus biopsies prepared by a maceration technique. *Prenatal Diagnosis*, **4**, 279–287

Hislop, A., Howard, S. and Fairweather, D.V.I. (1984) Morphometric studies on the structural development of the lung in *Macaca fascicularis* during fetal and postnatal life. *Journal of Anatomy*, **138**, 95–112

Hobbins, J.C. (1984) Consequences of chorionic biopsy. *New England Journal of Medicine*, **310**, 1121

Horn, N., Sondergaard, F., Damsgaard, E. and Heydorn, K. (1985) Prenatal diagnosis of Menkes' syndrome by direct copper analysis of trophoblastic tissue. In *First Trimester Fetal Diagnosis* (eds M. Fraccaro, G. Simoni, and B. Brambati) Berlin, Springer-Verlag. pp. 251–255

Horwell, D.H., Loeffler, F.E. and Coleman, D.V. (1983) Assessment of a transcervical aspiration technique for chorionic villus biopsy in the first trimester of pregnancy. *British Journal of Obstetrics and Gynaecology*, **90**, 196–198

Hsu, L.Y.F. and Perlis, T.E. (1984) United States survey on chromosome mosaicism and pseudomosaicism in prenatal diagnosis. *Prenatal Diagnosis*, (special issue) **4**, 97–130

Jackson, L. (1985) *Jefferson Medical College Newsletter* (28 August)

Jackson, L.G. (1987) Jefferson Medical College C.V.S. Newsletter **20**, (13), March, 1987.

Jackson, L.G. and Wapner, R.J. (1987) Risks of chorion villus sampling. *Clinical Obstetrics and Gynaecology*, **1**, 513–531

Jouppila, P., Huhtaniemi, I., Herva, R. and Piiroinen, O. (1984) Correlation of human chorionic gonadotrophin secretion in early pregnancy failure with site of gestational sac and placental histology. *Obstetrics and Gynecology*, **63**, 537–542

Kalousek, D.K. and Dill, F.J. (1983) Chromosomal mosaicism confined to the placenta in human conceptions. *Science*, **221**, 665–667

Kalousek, D.D., Barrett, I.J. and McGillivray, B.C. (1989) Placental mosaicism and intrauterine survival of trisomies β and α. *American Journal of Human Genetics*, **44**, 338–343

Kanhai, H.H.H., Bennebroek Gravenhorst, J., van 'T Veer, M.B., Maas, C.J., Beverstock, G.C. and Bernini, L.F. (1984) Chorionic biopsy in management of severe rhesus isoimmunisation. *Lancet*, **ii**, 157–158

Kappel, B., Nielson, J., Brogaard, H., Mikkelsen, M. and Therkelsen, A. (1987) Spontaneous abortion following mid-trimester amniocentesis. Clinical significance of placental perforation and blood-stained amniotic fluid. *British Journal of Obstetrics and Gynaecology*, **94**, 50–54

Katayama, K. and Roesler, M.R. (1986) Five hundred cases of amniocentesis without bloody tap. *Obstetrics and Gynecology*, **68**, 70–73

Kazy, Z., Rozovsky, I.S. and Bakharev, V.A. (1982) Chorion biopsy in early pregnancy: a method of early prenatal diagnosis for inherited disorders. *Prenatal Diagnosis*, **2**, 39–45

Kleijer, W.J., van Diggelen, O.P., Janse, H.C., Galjaard, H., Dumez, Y. and Boue, J. (1984) First trimester diagnosis of Hunter syndrome on chorionic villi. *Lancet*, **ii**, 472

Koskull, H.V., Ammala, P., Aula, P. and Virtanen, I. (1985) Cytoskeletal and lectin markers for cells cultured from chorionic villi and decidua. In *First Trimester Fetal Diagnosis* (Eds M. Fraccaro, G. Simoni and B. Brambati). Berlin: Springer-Verlag pp. 164–177

Lilford, R.J. (1985) Antenatal diagnosis of genetic disease. *Practitioner*, **229**, 729–734

Lilford, R.J., Irving, H.C., Linton, G. and Mason, M.K. (1987) Transabdominal chorion villus biopsy: 100 consecutive cases. *Lancet*, **i**, 1415–1416

Lilford, R.J. and Maxwell, D. (1984) The development of a transcutaneous technique for chorion biopsy. *Proceedings of Prenatal Diagnosis Group Meeting Progress in first trimester diagnosis*, London: Queen Charlotte's Hospital

Lilford, R., Maxwell, D., Coleman, D., Czepulkowski, B. and Heaton, D. (1983) Diagnosis, four hours after chorion biopsy, of female fetus in pregnancy at risk of Duchenne muscular dystrophy. *Lancet*, **ii**, 1491

MacKenzie, I.Z., Lindenbaum, R.H., Patel, C., Clarke, G., Crocker, M. and Jonasson, J.A. (1983) Prenatal diagnosis of an unbalanced chromosome translocation identified by direct karyotyping of chorionic biopsy. *Lancet*, **ii**, 1426–1427

MacLachlan, N.A., Rooney, D.E., Coleman, D. and Rodeck, C.H. (1989) Prenatal diagnosis: early amniocentesis or chorionic villus sampling. *Contemporary Reviews in Obstetrics and Gynaecology*, **1**, 173–180

Marchese, C.A., Carbonara, A.O., Viora, E., La Prova, A. and Campogrande, M. (1984) Biopsy of chorionic villi for prenatal diagnosis. *Acta Obstetrica et Gynaecologica Scandinavica*, **63**, 737

Martin, A.O., Elias, S., Roskinsky, B., Bombard, A.T. and Simpson, J.L. (1986) False negative finding on chorionic villus sampling. *Lancet*, **ii**, 391–392

Maxwell, D.J., Blau, K., Baker, S.P., Johnson, R.D. and Lilford, R.J. (1985a) Activities of alkaline phosphatase in chorion tissue. *Prenatal Diagnosis*, **5**, 283–286

Maxwell, D., Czepulkowski, B.H., Heaton, D.E., Coleman, D.V. and Lilford, R. (1985b) A practical assessment of ultrasound-guided transcervical aspiration of chorionic villi and subsequent chromosomal analysis. *British Journal of Obstetrics and Gynaecology*, **92**, 660–665

Maxwell, D.J. and Lilford, R.J. (1985) An interesting ultrasonic observation following chorionic villus sampling. *Journal of Clinical Ultrasound*, **13**, 343–344

Maxwell, D.J., Lilford, R.J., Czepulkowski, B., Heaton, D. and Coleman, D. (1986) Transabdominal chorionic villus sampling. *Lancet*, **i**, 123–126

Maxwell, D., Lilford, R., Morsman, J., Rodeck, C., Old, J. and Thein, S. (1985c) Direct DNA analysis for diagnosing fetal sickle status in first trimester chorion tissue. *Journal of Obstetrics and Gynaecology*, **5**, 133–135

Medical Research Council (1985) Report of inquiry into human fertilisation and embryology: Medical Research Council's response. *Lancet*, **i**, 270

Mikkelsen, M. (1985) Cytogenetic findings in first trimester chorionic villi biopsies: a collaborative study. In *First Trimester Fetal Diagnosis* (Eds M. Fraccaro, G. Simoni and B. Brambati). Berlin: Springer-Verlag, pp. 109–120

Mulcahy, M.T., Roberman, B. and Reid, S.E. (1984) Chorion biopsy, cytogenetic diagnosis, and selective termination in a twin pregnancy at risk of haemophilia. *Lancet*, **ii**, 866–867

Niazi, M., Coleman, D.V. and Loeffler, F.E. (1981) Trophoblast sampling in early pregnancy. Culture of rapidly dividing cells from immature placental villi. *British Journal of Obstetrics and Gynaecology*, **88**, 1081–1085

Niazi, M., Coleman, D.V., Mowbray, J.F. and Blunt, S. (1979) Tissue typing amniotic fluid cells: potential use for detection of contaminating maternal cells. *Journal of Medical Genetics*, **16**, 21–23

National Institute of Child Health and Human Development (1976) Mid-trimester amniocentesis for prenatal diagnosis. Safety and accuracy. *Journal of the American Medical Association*, **236**, 1471–1476

Nordenskjold, F. and Gustavii, B. (1984) Direct-vision chorionic villi biopsy for prenatal diagnosis in the first trimester. *Journal of Reproductive Medicine*, **29**, 572–574

Pan, S., Fatora, R., Hass, J. and Steele, M. (1976) Trisomy of chromosome 20. *Clinical Genetics*, **9**, 449–453

Perry, T.B., Vekemans, M.J.J., Lippman, A., Hamilton, E.F. and Fournier, P.J.R. (1985) Chorionic villi sampling: clinical experience, immediate complications, and patient attitudes. *American Journal of Obstetrics and Gynecology*, **151**, 161–166

Rhine, S.A., Palmer, C.G. and Thompson, J.F. (1977) A simple alternative to amniocentesis for first trimester prenatal diagnosis. The National Foundation. *Birth Defects, Original Article Series*, **XII**:3D, 231–247

Ridler, M. and Greural, M. (1984) Possible source of error in prenatal diagnosis via chorionic villus biopsy. *Lancet*, **i**, 1081

Rodeck, C.H. and Ivan, D. (1981) Sampling pure fetal blood in twin pregnancies by fetoscopy using a single uterine puncture. *Prenatal Diagnosis*, **7**, 43–49

Rodeck, C.H. and Morsman, J.M. (1983) First-trimester chorion biopsy. *British Medical Bulletin*, **39**, 338–342

Rodeck, C.H., Morsman, J.M., Gosden, C.M. and Gosden, J.R. (1983a) Development of an improved technique for first-trimester microsampling of chorion. *British Journal of Obstetrics and Gynaecology*, **90**, 1113–1118

Rodeck, C.H., Morsman, J.M., Nicolaides, K.H., McKenzie, C., Gosden, C.M. and Gosden, J.R. (1983b) A single operator technique for first-trimester chorion biopsy. *Lancet*, **ii**, 1340–1341

Sachs, E.S., Jahoda, M.G., Kleijer, W.J., Pijpers, L. and Galjaard, H. (1988) Impact of first-trimester chromosome, DNA, and metabolic studies on pregnancies of high genetic risk: experience with 1000 cases. *American Journal of Medical Genetics*, **29**, 293–303

Sachs, E.S., Van Hemel, J.O., Galjaard, H., Miermeijer, M.F. and Jahoda, M.G.J. (1983) First trimester chromosomal analyses of complex structural rearrangements with RHA banding on chorionic villi. *Lancet,* **ii**, 1426

Sadovnick, A.D. and Baird, P.A. (1982) A cost–benefit analysis of prenatal diagnosis for neural tube defects selectively offered to relatives of index cases. *American Journal of Medical Genetics*, **12**, 63–73

Schwab, M.E., Muller, C. and Schmid-Tannwald, I. (1984) Fast and reliable culture method for cells from 8–10 week trophoblast tissue. *Lancet,* **ii**, 1082

Scialli, A.R., Neugebauer, D.L. and Fabro, S. (1985) Microbiology of the endocervix in patients undergoing chorionic villi sampling. In *First Trimester Fetal Diagnosis* (Eds M. Fraccaro, G. Simoni and B. Brambati). Berlin: Springer-Verlag, pp. 69–73

Simoni, G., Brambati, B., Danesino, C. *et al.* (1983) Efficient direct chromosome analysis and enzyme determination from chorionic villi samples in the first trimester of pregnancy. *Human Genetics*, **63**, 349–357

Simoni, G., Brambati, B., Danesino, C. *et al.* (1984) Diagnostic application of first trimester trophoblast sampling in 100 pregnancies. *Human Genetics*, **66**, 252–259

Smidt-Jensen, S. and Hahnemann, N. (1984) Transabdominal fine needle biopsy from chorionic villi in the first trimester. *Prenatal Diagnosis*, **4**, 163–169

Smidt-Jensen, S. and Hahnemann, N. (1988) Transabdominal chorionic villus sampling for fetal genetic diagnosis. Technical and obstetrical evaluation of 100 cases. *Prenatal Diagnosis*, **8**, 7–17

Tabor, A., Madsen, M., O'Bell, E.B. *et al.* (1986) Randomised controlled trials of genetic amniocentesis in 4606 low risk women. *Lancet,* **i**, 1287–1292

Terzoli, G.L., Romitti, L., Guerneri, S., Carrera, P. and Camurri, L. (1985) Effect of incubation time and serum concentration on the number of mitoses in aspirated villi samples. In *First Trimester Fetal Diagnosis* (Eds M. Fraccaro, G. Simoni and B. Brambati). Berlin: Springer-Verlag, pp. 197–200

Tietung Hospital of Ansham Iron and Steel Company (1975) Fetal sex prediction by sex chromatin of chorionic villi cells during early pregnancy. *Chinese Medical Journal*, **2**, 118–125

Tommerup, N., Sondergaard, F., Tonnesen, T., Kristensen, M., Arveiler, B. and Schinzel, A. (1985) First trimester prenatal diagnosis of a male fetus with fragile X. *Lancet,* **i**, 870

Tsvetkova, E.V., Maltseva, H.A., Zolotuchina, T.V., Bartseva, O.B. and Bachareu, V.A. (1982) Comparison of properties of neuraminidase in cultures of amniotic fluid cells and cultures of chorion cells. *Questions of Medical Chemistry (Moscow)*, **3**, 41–45

Verlinsky, Y., DeChristopher, P.J., Pergament, E. and Ginsberg, N.A. (1985) Histomorphological aspects of chorionic villi in first trimester fetal diagnosis. In *First Trimester Fetal Diagnosis*, (Eds M. Fraccaro, G. Simoni and B. Brambati). Berlin: Springer-Verlag, pp. 178–188

Vimal, C.M., Fensom, A.H., Heaton, D., Ward, R.H.T., Garrod, P. and Penketh, R.J.A. (1984) Prenatal diagnosis of argininosuccinicaciduria by analysis of cultured chorionic villi. *Lancet,* **ii**, 521–522

Warburton, D. (1984) Outcome of cases of *de novo* structural rearrangements diagnosed at amniocentesis. *Prenatal Diagnosis*, **4**, 69–70

Warren, R.C., Butler, J., Morsman, J.M., McKenzie, C. and Rodeck, C.H. (1985) Does chorionic villus sampling cause fetomaternal haemorrhage? *Lancet,* i, 691

Whittle, M.J. (1979) The safety of cordocentesis. *British Journal of Hospital Medicine*, **41**, 511

Williams, B., Medearis, A.L., Bear, M.B. and Kaback (1987) Chorionic villus sampling is associated with normal fetal growth. *American Journal of Obstetrics and Gynecology*, **157**, 708–712

Wilson, R.D., Kendrick, V., Wittman, B.K. and McGillivray, B.C. (1984) Risk of spontaneous abortion in ultrasonically normal pregnancies. *Lancet,* **ii**, 290

Chapter 11

Decision analysis in prenatal diagnosis: measuring patients' values

J.G. Thornton

> The spirit of decision analysis is divide and conquer. Decompose a complex problem into simpler problems, get your thinking clear on these simpler problems, paste these analyses together with logical glue, and come out with a program for action for the complex problem. Experts are not asked complicated fuzzy questions, but crystal clear, unambiguous, elemental, hypothetical questions.
>
> (Raiffa, 1968)

Introduction

Many patients find the choice whether to undergo prenatal diagnosis difficult and ask their doctor for help. To give sensible advice the doctor needs to know not only the risks of each possible outcome, which may vary between patients, but also the values that she attaches to the various outcomes. They both also need a rational system for combining the two to reach a decision. Decision analysis (Weinstein and Fineberg, 1980) is such a system, in which the doctor is the expert on probability and the patient the expert on values.

Much of the rest of this book is concerned with estimating risks. This chapter will consider how to elicit patients' values and how to incorporate them into the decision making process. Decision analysis will first be introduced with the simple and rather trivial example of a gambler playing a game of chance where the uncertainties and values are already known. Next the weaknesses of current intuitive decision making for prenatal diagnosis will be examined, before two new methods of decision analysis are described in some detail. Finally the advantages and disadvantages of this approach will be discussed.

The gambler's decision: an example

Like doctors, players of games of chance also work under conditions of uncertainty and, if they are skilled, do not gamble wildly, but rather play to maximize their winnings over many games. A gambler playing well is using the same logic as a doctor maximizing the expected utility of his actions. Imagine a player with a choice between throwing in his hand and losing no more money or drawing another card

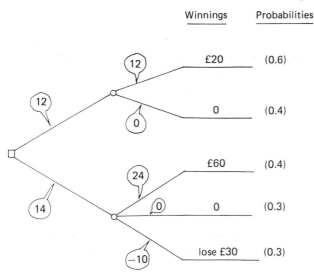

Figure 11.1 A hypothetical decision tree for a gambler deciding whether to gamble £30 in the hope of winning £60 (lower branch) or to make no further bet and accept his current 60% chance of winning £20 (upper branch). The outcomes have their own natural underlying scale, namely their value in pounds. The utilities of each outcome are calculated by multiplying probabilities and values and are marked in cartoon bubbles. At each chance node (○) the utilities are added to give an overall utility for each choice

which will cost him £30 and which gives him a 40% chance of winning £60, a 30% chance of breaking even, but a 30% chance of losing his £30 stake. The choice is displayed in Figure 11.1 using conventional decision theory symbols as follows. Decisions and chance outcomes are ordered from left to right across the page, points where choices can be made are represented by square nodes (□), and points where different outcomes can occur by chance are represented by round nodes (○). The probability of each outcome is represented in standard mathematical notation as a number between 0 (will never occur) and 1 (certain to occur). All possible outcomes are included so that the probabilities at each chance node always add up to 1. The values of each final outcome are represented here in monetary terms as winnings or losses. The utilities of each arm of a decision node are derived by multiplying the values and probabilities distal to it and adding them together. These computed utilities are represented in cartoon bubbles. This analysis reveals that the gambler should bet another £30 and draw another card. Expert gamblers would find this decision easy, but for the less numerate such a written down solution is a help and in more complex problems may be the only way to make the optimal decision.

Prenatal diagnosis: intuitive decision making

The usual method is that the counsellor simply describes the fetal abnormality being considered, tells the patient what the diagnostic test involves, and the risks of an affected child or test complication. The patient is then allowed to ask questions about risks and technical details but then encouraged to make up her own mind whether she wants the test. Most counsellors aim to avoid letting the patient know the counsellors values for fear that these might influence her. It is assumed that she is capable of incorporating her own values in the decision-making process but little guidance is usually given on how to combine probabilities and values.

Usually the patient succeeds in making a decision, although unless she is trained in risk revision and decision theory it may not be the choice that maximizes expected utility because people frequently make poor use of probabilistic information (Kahnemann, Slovic and Tversky, 1982). For example, patients may choose to avoid a risk of Down's syndrome more than they avoid a procedure-related abortion because they can easily recall seeing Down's children in the community and on television but have never met anyone who had had a procedure-related abortion. This is called 'the availability of recall' bias or simply 'availability' bias. In other patients the effect might be in the other direction if they equated all abortions and could easily recall a friend having had a miscarriage. Either way the availability bias can distort choices made by empirical methods. It is only one of many well documented similar effects (Kahnemann, Slovic and Tversky, 1982).

Many intelligent patients are aware, at least vaguely, of the potential biases affecting their decision. Others, faced with too much information to consider at once, become distressed that they cannot clearly make up their minds. They may compensate by latching on to an arbitrary element in the decision and ignoring the other issues. For example a 30-year-old patient who has had her Down's syndrome risk revised after a slightly reduced maternal serum alpha-fetoprotein (AFP) estimation (Cuckle, Wald and Thompson, 1987) and been told that her risk has changed from 1 in 1200 to 1 in 900 may not consider further the risks of amniocentesis but instead demand a test simply because her risk is 'increased'. The problem of information overload is severe even with intelligent patients who may have more than one possible and relevant fetal abnormality, and a number of different tests to consider, each of which may have different sensitivities, specificities and risks. Sometimes as fast as the counsellor tells the patient new information, she forgets the old.

There are a number of ways of improving patient understanding. The risks can be written down and the patient can be encouraged to take them away to think about at home. The method of framing of risks is important (Tversky and Kahnemann, 1974) and risks should be framed both ways. For example, procedure related risks of abortion should be expressed both as a 1 in n risk of abortion and as an n-1 in n chance of the test proceeding without complication. Understanding of low risks is improved if they are demonstrated pictorially. A simple method is to fill in n squares on 1000 squares of graph paper for an $n/1000$ risk.

None of these methods help the patient to combine probabilities and values in a way which will maximize expected utility. The only way to do this is by formal decision analysis.

Decision analysis for prenatal diagnosis

The method for prenatal diagnosis has been described by Richard and Susan Pauker of Massachusetts (Pauker and Pauker, 1977; 1987) who applied it to couples

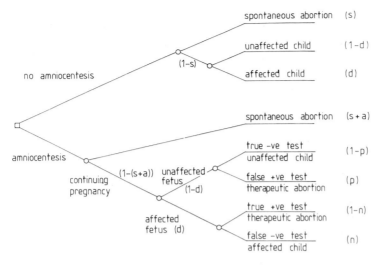

Figure 11.2 A decision tree for the amniocentesis decision (Pauker and Pauker, 1977). s the background abortion rate without amniocentesis; d the probability of having an affected child; a the increased risk of abortion after amniocentesis; p the rate of false-positive test results; n the rate of false-negative test results

having difficulty reaching a decision about amniocentesis for the diagnosis of Down's syndrome. The first phase of decision analysis is to structure the problem as a decision tree and the one the Paukers used is illustrated in Figure 11.2. The probabilities are shown enclosed in brackets using the following symbols:

s the background abortion rate without amniocentesis
d the probability of having an affected child
a the increased risk of abortion after amniocentesis
p the rate of false-positive test results
n the rate of false-negative test results
r (not shown on Figure 11.2) is the risk of amniocentesis causing the miscarriage of a pregnancy which would otherwise have continued and is the ratio a/1-s. r has been estimated to be between 0.005 and 0.01 (McNay and Whitfield, 1984; Tabor *et al.*, 1986).

The probabilities used will vary with the patient's age etc. and are obtained from the literature. Outcome utilities are measured using lotteries (*see below*). In practice the Paukers recommend that instead of the utilities of each outcome, the costs, which are the inverse of utilities, should be used and the course of minimum cost should be followed.

The next phase of the analysis is to discover the costs of the various intermediate outcomes between birth of a Down's syndrome affected child (cost 1) and the birth of a normal child (cost 0). (Note that some people might rank induced abortion as worse than live birth of a Down's syndrome affected child and would therefore cost induced abortion as 1 and rearrange the lotteries below.) Assuming the subject values the birth of an affected child as worse then termination of an unaffected child the scale of costs will be as follows:

Affected livebirth (C_A)   1
Cost of therapeutic abortion normal fetus (C_{TU})   intermediate
Cost of spontaneous abortion (C_S)   intermediate
Cost of therapeutic abortion affected fetus (C_{TA}) intermediate
Normal child   0

There are a number of ways of estimating the intermediate costs including representing them in monetary terms or marking them on linear scales. However the axiomatically correct method for decision analysis is to compare the cost of one outcome in terms of a gamble between two other relevant outcomes. The method is called the basic reference lottery.

The basic reference lottery

The precise cost of therapeutic abortion (C_T) is calculated by asking subjects to perform a gamble as in Figure 11.3. They are asked to imagine that they must choose between going through two doors. If they enter the left door, A, they will undergo a therapeutic abortion. If they enter door B, the pregnancy will continue with a 50% chance of the fetus being affected. For those who choose to enter door A (Figure 11.3a) the choice is repeated with the risk of an affected fetus through door B progressively *reduced* until they choose door B (Figure 11.3b). The risks through door B are adjusted until the patient cannot decide between the doors (Figure 11.3c). The subject is then said to be indifferent. For example the hypothetical subject above is indifferent between a 35% risk of Down's syndrome livebirth and a therapeutic abortion. For those patients who choose door B at a 50% Down's syndrome risk, the risks of Down's syndrome through door B are progressively *increased* until the point of indifference is reached. Put another way this gamble asks the patient the following question:

> Given no further diagnostic information, at what chance of a pregnancy resulting in a Down's syndrome affected child would you choose to have a therapeutic abortion?

Assuming, for example, that a woman is indifferent between a 35% risk of Down's syndrome and therapeutic abortion, we calculate that therapeutic abortion has a cost of 0.35.

A second similar lottery is performed to elicit the cost of spontaneous abortion (C_S). Again put into words the patient is asked this question:

> Given no further diagnostic information, at what chance of a pregnancy's resulting in the birth of a Down's syndrome affected child would you prefer that the pregnancy end in spontaneous abortion?

The Paukers suggest that extra lotteries are performed on those patients (the majority) who regard the therapeutic abortion of an affected fetus (C_{TA}) as of different cost to the therapeutic abortion of an unaffected fetus (C_{TU}). They do this by asking each patient to specify for various chances of having an affected child, a preference between that pregnancy and the therapeutic abortion of a different hypothetical pregnancy in which the fetus is found to be affected. The point of indifference determines the cost of therapeutic abortion of an affected fetus (C_{TA}). They then ask the patient to consider the choice between the 'no further information available' pregnancy and a different pregnancy in which the fetus is

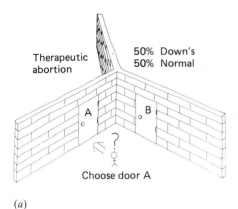

(a)

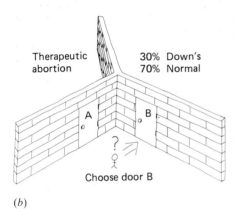

(b)

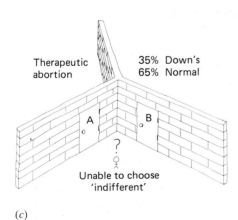

(c)

Figure 11.3 The basic reference lottery between therapeutic abortion and a gamble between a Down's syndrome child or a normal child. (a) The starting gamble. The example patient chooses therapeutic abortion. (b) The risks of a Down's syndrome affected child are reduced until the subject chooses to continue the pregnancy. (c) The risks are adjusted until the level of indifference is reached

found to be unaffected. The point of indifference in this lottery determines the cost of therapeutic abortion of an unaffected fetus (C_{TU}).

The costs obtained are used in the decision tree in Figure 11.2. At each terminal point on the tree the outcome cost is multiplied with the outcome probability to derive the expected cost of that outcome. The costs of outcomes arising from a single chance node are summated to provide a new cost for that chance node. This in turn is then multiplied with the relevant probability to derive the expected cost. Eventually the expected costs of amniocentesis and of no amniocentesis are derived. The course of minimum cost should be chosen.

In practice the whole decision process does not need to be worked out every time. Instead the utilities are used to calculate the threshold probability (T) for Down's syndrome above which amniocentesis would be the course of maximum utility and below which no test would be preferred. The formula below is used:

$$T = \frac{(1 - r)pC_{TU} + rC_S}{(1 - r)[pC_{TU} - (1 - n)C_{TA} - nC_A] + C_A}$$

This can be performed fairly easily for each patient with a programmable calculator.

The final part of decision analysis is to perform a sensitivity analysis. This involves varying the probabilities and costs in turn around typical values and re-analysing the decision using these new values to see if the course of maximum utility changes. If it does alter when a particular variable changes the decision is said to be sensitive to that variable and care must be taken to estimate that variable precisely. Sensitivity analysis has been carried out by the Paukers and reveals that the amniocentesis decision was most sensitive to the cost of therapeutic abortion, the additional chance of abortion after amniocentesis and the probability of the fetus being affected. In clinical practice therefore it may only be necessary to calculate the cost of therapeutic abortion. The Paukers found that most parents regarded C_{TA} to be approximately equal to C_{TU} and both approximately twice the cost of C_S. Making these assumptions, T can be plotted against C_{TA}. If the risks of Down's syndrome are assumed to vary only with maternal age (Mikkelsen and Stene, 1970) T can be replaced by maternal age. Such a graph is shown in Figure 11.4. Note also that a value of r (excess risk of miscarriage of a normal pregnancy after amniocentesis) of 0.005 and zero false-positive and false-negative test rates are assumed.

To use this graph in clinical practice one need only perform the lottery shown in Figure 11.3 to derive the cost of therapeutic abortion (C_T). If this, plotted against maternal age falls below and to the right of the line the patient should undergo amniocentesis and if it falls above and to the left she should not. One problem with this method is that it makes assumptions about the procedure-related abortion rate and age-related risks of Down's syndrome. If these are felt to be different then a new graph must be drawn.

An alternative method

The above method has disadvantages. First, it is complicated unless a number of possibly erroneous simplifying assumptions are made. For the prenatal diagnosis of Down's syndrome, consideration of false-positive and false-negative diagnoses only

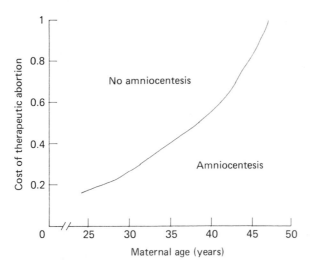

Figure 11.4 Graph of the threshold cost of therapeutic abortion plotted against maternal age for the decision whether to perform amniocentesis for the diagnosis of Down's syndrome (Pauker and Pauker, 1977). This graph assumes that C_{TA} is equal to C_{TU} and both are twice the cost of C_S, that r is 0.005 and there is a zero false-positive and false-negative test rate. The risks of Down's syndrome are assumed to vary only with maternal age (Mikkelsen and Stene, 1970)

add to the complexity and can justifiably be dropped. With other disorders such as Duchenne muscular dystrophy, where termination may be considered on the basis of fetal sex alone, false-positive diagnoses would be very important. Secondly, all spontaneous abortions are costed the same although some will be genuinely spontaneous while others may have resulted from the procedure. Finally, it provides no mechanism for considering the potential benefits of earlier diagnostic tests such as chorionic villus biopsy (CVB).

An alternative has been used by the author on a few selected patients. The relevant decision tree is simplified to that shown in Figure 11.5. Only those outcomes which could be affected by the prenatal diagnosis test and which might affect the decision are included. These are the risk of having a Down's syndrome child if amniocentesis is not chosen; and the risk of losing a normal child which would otherwise have survived if amniocentesis is chosen. It is assumed that there will be no false-positive or false-negative results from the amniocentesis procedure itself. The decision tree includes a third arm for CVB, but if this is not an option the lower arm should be omitted. Two lotteries are performed between accidental procedure-related abortion of a normal fetus and various risks of a Down's syndrome affected pregnancy (Figure 11.6a), and between 18-week termination of a Down's syndrome fetus and various risks of a Down's syndrome affected child (Figure 11.6b). If CVB is also being considered a third lottery is performed to measure the cost of suction termination of an affected child (Figure 11.6c).

As an example imagine a woman aged 33. The probabilities are as follows:

Down's (P_D) (1 in 588)   0.0017
Procedure-related abortion after amniocentesis ($P_{AMN\ PRA}$)   0.005
Procedure-related abortion after CVB ($P_{CVB\ PRA}$)   0.01

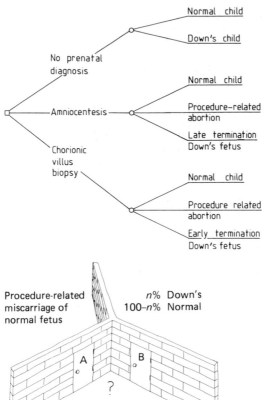

Normal child

Down's child

No prenatal
diagnosis

Normal child

Amniocentesis

Procedure-related
abortion

Late termination
Down's fetus

Chorionic
villus
biopsy

Normal child

Procedure related
abortion

Early termination
Down's fetus

Figure 11.5 An alternative decision tree including only the outcomes, Down's syndrome birth, procedure-related abortion, and termination of an affected fetus at varying gestation, for the choices, no test, amniocentesis, or CVB, for the prenatal diagnosis of Down's syndrome

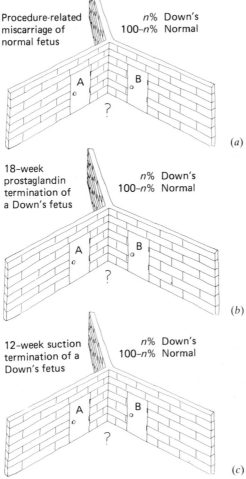

Procedure-related
miscarriage of
normal fetus

$n\%$ Down's
$100-n\%$ Normal

A
o

B
o

?

(a)

18-week
prostaglandin
termination of
a Down's fetus

$n\%$ Down's
$100-n\%$ Normal

A
o

B
o

?

(b)

12-week suction
termination of a
Down's fetus

$n\%$ Down's
$100-n\%$ Normal

A
o

B
o

?

(c)

Figure 11.6 (a) The basic reference lottery to measure the cost of procedure related abortion of a normal fetus (C_{PRA}). (b) The basic reference lottery to measure the cost of late termination of a Down's syndrome affected fetus (C_{LTD}). (c) The basic reference lottery to measure the cost of early termination of a Down's syndrome affected fetus (C_{ETD})

(The CVB procedure-related abortion rate is calculated from the Canadian collaborative trial data (1989) showing an excess fetal loss rate of 0.005 for CVB over amniocentesis.)

Imagine her costs have been derived from the three lotteries above (Figures 11.6a, b and c) as follows:

Livebirth of Down's syndrome affected child (C_D)	1.0
Procedure-related abortion of a normal fetus (C_{PRA})	0.5
Late termination of Down's syndrome affected fetus (C_{LTD})	0.2
Early termination of Down's syndrome affected fetus (C_{ETD})	0.05
Normal child	0.0

The cost of ño test ($C_D \times P_D$) = 0.0017
The cost of amniocentesis ($C_{LTD} \times P_D$) + ($C_{PRA} \times P_{AMN\ PRA}$)
$\quad$ =(0.2 × 0.0017) + (0.5 × 0.005) = 0.0028
The cost of CVB ($C_{ETD} \times P_D$) + ($C_{PRA} \times P_{CVB\ PRA}$)
$\quad$ = (0.05 × 0.0017) + (0.5 × 0.01) = 0.0051

This patient would therefore be advised not to undergo any prenatal diagnostic test.

Compare this with another patient of the same age with the same genetic risks who was more worried by the possibility of a Down's syndrome birth and relatively less averse to a procedure-related abortion or an early termination. However, she also felt that a late prostaglandin-induced termination after movements had been felt would be a severe burden. This second patient had the following costs derived from the three lotteries illustrated in Figures 11.6:

Livebirth of Down's syndrome affected child (C_D)	1.0
Procedure-related abortion of a normal fetus (C_{PRA})	0.1
Late termination of Down's syndrome affected fetus (C_{LTD})	0.5
Early termination of Down's syndrome affected fetus (C_{ETD})	0.05
Normal child	0.0

The cost of no test ($C_D \times P_D$) = 0.0017
The cost of amniocentesis ($C_{LTD} \times P_D$) + ($C_{PRA} \times P_{AMN\ PRA}$)
$\quad$ = (0.5 × 0.0017 + (0.1 × 0.005) = 0.0014
The cost of CVB ($C_{ETD} \times P_D$) + ($C_{PRA} \times P_{CVB\ PRA}$)
$\quad$ = (0.05 × 0.0017) + (0.1 × 0.01) = 0.0011

Despite her aversion to late termination this patient would be advised to choose amniocentesis in preference to no diagnostic test if that were the only test available. However, if CVB were also available it would be of even lower expected cost and should be chosen.

To perform an analysis like this is feasible in a clinic where time can be set aside for counselling and the calculations are not difficult. Most time is spent performing the lotteries and three of these are required if CVB is being considered. In practice, however, it is frequently unnecessary to complete all the calculations for every individual patient. For most the explanation in Figure 11.2 or Figure 11.5 will improve their understanding to such an extent that they will make a decision, and even those who need to perform the lotteries often quickly realize that one or other adverse outcome would have such a high cost for them that the correct course of action is obvious.

Discussion

Although the methods of decision analysis described above may appear complicated, I believe that they deserve a small but definite place in prenatal diagnosis counselling. The patient is under no obligation to accept the result but the process usually helps her decide, and not surprisingly most patients do finally choose the course of maximum expected utility (minimum cost). If a couple have differing opinions about amniocentesis and abortion, the lottery will help clarify their disagreement and may often indicate that although they have different values, their genetic risk is such that they should both choose the same course of action.

The consideration of decision analysis at all, even if it is never used in clinical practice, can have an important effect on our ways of thinking. For example, the facile analysis that amniocentesis should be recommended when the risk of Down's syndrome is greater than the risk of miscarriage from the procedure, should never be heard again.

An important area of debate is the issue of whose values should be used. Since it is the patient who must live with the result of a decision and we all have an ethical duty to respect autonomy, most people believe that the patient's values should be used. Patients usually want to be involved in decision making and appreciate decision analysis which incorporates their own values. The Paukers found that their technique increased the satisfaction of their patients with genetic counselling. On the other hand, some patients do not like to make decisions for themselves and prefer their doctor to decide. They may argue that the doctor who has seen other patients with the same disease is better able to value the outcomes than a patient who only knows about them from hearsay. They may not like to make decisions or there may be little time to consider all the issues in certain pressurized situations, and many patients will be confused and worried by non-directive counselling. A sensitive doctor, who has measured other similar patients' values may get a feel for a particular patient's value scale. If so, he or she can give such patients the directive counselling they desire, while still making a decision which broadly conforms with individual values.

The disutility ('cost') of abortion, measured by a basic reference gamble, between pregnancy termination and risk of mental handicap in the fetus, increases with gestational age (Thornton, Bryce and Bhabra, 1988). Similar lottery techniques might also be used to help decide whether resuscitation of very low birthweight infants should be continued or whether an intervention in labour such as Caesarean section should be performed when there was a severe risk of fetal handicap. The high emotions and drama surrounding such decisions would almost certainly preclude performing individual lotteries with the parents at the time, but experimental lotteries by parents who have been through such difficult decisions might provide a basis for rational debate and counselling.

A major criticism of decision analysis is the fear that the value measurements may simply be wrong. Possible reasons are that patients may have poor understanding of numbers, their values may change over time, the method of framing lotteries may influence the results, and value estimates obtained by a series of lotteries may be internally inconsistent (Llewellyn-Thomas et al., 1982; Thornton et al., 1989). These problems have not been completely resolved, although pictorial aids to display probabilities may help and measurement of the internal consistency of a series of lotteries may allow an objective measure of the accuracy of the resulting value estimates. To measure the internal consistency of patients' costs for early and late termination and for birth of a Down's syndrome affected infant a third lottery could be performed comparing early termination with a gamble between late termination and a live child. The cost of early termination obtained this way could be compared with the cost derived from the lottery illustrated in Figure 11.6c. If these were very similar we would say that the patient was internally consistent and place more weight on her values than if they were very different and she was inconsistent.

A particular attribute of value measurements which affects decision making is that decision analysis assumes that patients' values remain proportionally the same as the risk varies. For example, a patient who regards a Down's syndrome birth as twice as bad as the accidental loss of a normal fetus would be expected to regard a 1 in 200 risk of Down's syndrome birth as twice as bad as a 1 in 200 risk of the loss of a normal fetus. This is called the constant proportion risk attitude and unfortunately there is evidence that it does not strictly apply to human decision making (Kahnemann, Slovic and Tversky, 1982). This may be a weakness of decision analysis but it can also be argued that lack of a constant proportion risk attitude is irrational and a failure of human mental processes and that use of decision theory overcomes this 'problem'.

There are other ways in which real life decision making differs from the decision analysis approach. Patients may choose to decide on the basis of the advice of a respected figure, e.g. their doctor. Patients may request a test when their risk for a disease is above an arbitrary multiple of the population incidence rather than because of its absolute level – such patients are said to ignore the independence axiom and their reasoning is, by definition, faulty. Gamblers playing poker this way would undoubtedly lose in the long term! The principle of respect for autonomy would require a doctor to allow his patient to make suboptimal decisions this way if that was genuinely what she wanted. However, we believe that a doctor would also be justified in attempting to correct patients' faulty logic in the same way as he would be justified in correcting faulty probability estimates. It is axiomatic that decision analysis correctly applied will give the choice with the highest expected utility. Patients and doctors of course have the right to choose otherwise.

All the above methods and discussion have referred to decision making for individual parents. A similar concept can be used for policy makers who wish to decide whether to introduce a given prenatal screening programme. The author is not aware of any prenatal diagnosis test which has been accepted or rejected by health planners after decision analysis, but the way in which such an analysis could be performed has been described for both maternal serum alpha-fetoprotein testing (Tyrrell et al., 1988) and fetal anatomic ultrasonography (Pauker, Pauker and McNeil, 1981).

References

Canadian collaborative CVS-amniocentesis clinical trial group. (1989) Multicentre randomised clinical trial of chorion villus sampling and amniocentesis. *Lancet*, i, 1–6

Cuckle, H.S., Wald, N.J. and Thompson, S.G. (1987) Estimating a woman's risk of having a pregnancy associated with Down's syndrome using her age and serum alphafetoprotein level. *British Journal of Obstetrics and Gynaecology*, **94**, 387–402

Kahnemann, D., Slovic, P. and Tversky, A. (eds) (1982) *Judgement Under Uncertainty: Heuristics and Biases*. Cambridge: Cambridge University Press

Llewellyn-Thomas, H., Sutherland, H.J., Tibshirani, R., Ciampi, A., Till, J.E. and Boyd, N.F. (1982) The measurement of patients' values in medicine. *Medical Decision Making*, **2**, 449–462

McNay, M.B. and Whitfield, C.R. (1984) Amniocentesis. *British Journal of Hospital Medicine*, **31**, 406–416

Mikkelsen, M. and Stene, J. (1970) Genetic counselling in Down's syndrome. *Human Heredity*, **20**, 457–464

Pauker, S.P. and Pauker, S.G. (1977) Prenatal diagnosis: a directive approach to genetic counselling using decision analysis. *Yale Journal of Biological Medicine*, **50**, 275–289

Pauker, S.P. and Pauker, S.G. (1987) The amniocentesis decision: ten years of decision analytic experience. *Birth Defects: Original Article Series,* **23**, (2), 151–169, March of Dimes Birth Defects Foundation

Pauker, S.G., Pauker, S.P. and McNeil, B.J. (1981) The effect of private attitudes on public policy: prenatal screening for neural tube defects as a prototype. *Medical Decision Making*, **1**, 103–114

Raiffa, H. (1968) *Decision analysis: introductory lectures on choices under uncertainty.* Reading, MA: Addison-Wesley, p. 271

Tabor, A., Madsen, M., Obel, E.B., Philip, J., Bang, J. and Norgaard-Pedersen, B. (1986) Randomised controlled trial of genetic amniocentesis in 4606 low-risk women. *Lancet,* **i**, 1293–1298

Thornton, J.G., Bryce, F.C. and Bhabra, K. (1988) Withholding intensive care from premature babies. *Lancet,* **ii**, 332–333

Thornton, J.G., Howel, D. and Lilford, R.J. (1989) Prenatal diagnosis of Down's syndrome; a method for measuring the consistency of womens' decisions. *Medical Decision Making*, (in press)

Tyrrell, S., Howell, D., Bark, M., Allibone, E. and Lilford, R.J. (1988) Should maternal alpha-fetoprotein estimation be carried out in centers where ultrasound screening is routine. *American   Journal of Obstetrics and Gynecology*, **158**, 1092–1099

Tversky, A. and Kahnemann, D. (1974) Judgement under uncertainty: heuristics and biases. *Science*, **185**, 1124–1131

Weinstein, M.C. and Fineberg, H.V. (eds) (1980) *Clinical Decision Analysis.* Philadelphia: W.B. Saunders

Index